Clinical Guide to Depression in Children and Adolescents

Clinical Guide to Depression in Children and Adolescents

Edited by

Mohammad Shafii, M.D.

Professor of Psychiatry
Director, Child Psychiatry Training Program
Department of Psychiatry and Behavioral Sciences
University of Louisville School of Medicine

Sharon Lee Shafii, R.N., B.S.N.

Editor-in-Residence
Formerly Assistant Head Nurse, Adolescent Service
Neuropsychiatric Institute
University of Michigan Medical Center

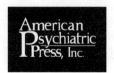
American Psychiatric Press, Inc.

Washington, DC
London, England

1992

Copyright © 1992 American Psychiatric Press, Inc.
ALL RIGHTS RESERVED
Manufactured in the United States of America on acid-free paper
95 94 93 92   4 3 2 1

American Psychiatric Press, Inc.
1400 K Street, N.W., Washington, DC 20005

Library of Congress Cataloging-in-Publication Data
Clinical guide to depression in children and adolescents / edited by
Mohammad Shafii and Sharon Lee Shafii.
    p. cm.
Includes bibliographical references and index.
ISBN 0-88048-356-3 (alk. paper)
    1. Depression in children. 2. Depression in adolescence. 3. Manic-depressive psychoses in children. 4. Manic-depressive psychoses in adolescence.   I.
Shafii, Mohammad. II. Shafii, Sharon Lee.
    [DNLM: 1. Bipolar Disorder—in adolescence. 2. Bipolar Disorder—in
infancy & childhood. 3. Depression—in adolescence. 4. Depression—in
infancy & childhood. 5. Depression therapy. WM 171 C6412]
    RJ506.D4C59 1992
    618.92'8527—dc20
    DNLM/DLC
    for Library of Congress   91-22112
                                                                                    CIP

British Library Cataloguing in Publication Data
A CIP record is available from the British Library.

Dedicated to

RAYMOND W. WAGGONER, SR., M.D.

Chairman Emeritus
Department of Psychiatry
University of Michigan Medical Center
and
Past President
American Psychiatric Association

An outstanding mentor and a good friend

On Joy and Sorrow

Your joy is your sorrow unmasked.
And the selfsame well from which your laughter rises was oftentimes filled
    with your tears.
And how else can it be?

The deeper that sorrow carves into your being, the more joy you can contain.
Is not the cup that holds your wine the very cup that was burned in the
    potter's oven?
And is not the lute that soothes your spirit, the very wood that was hollowed
    with knives?

When you are joyous, look deep into your heart and you shall find it is only
    that which has given you sorrow that is giving you joy.
When you are sorrowful look again in your heart, and you shall see that in
    truth you are weeping for that which has been your delight.

Some of you say, "Joy is greater than sorrow," and others say, "Nay, sorrow is
    the greater."
But I say unto you, they are inseparable.
Together they come, and when one sits alone with you at your board,
    remember that the other is asleep upon your bed.

Kahlil Gibran

Reprinted from *The Prophet* by Kahlil Gibran, by permission of Alfred A. Knopf Inc. Copyright 1923 by Kahlil Gibran and renewed 1951 by Administrators C.T.A. of Kahlil Gibran Estate and Mary G. Gibran.

CONTENTS

CONTRIBUTORS

Robert F. Baxter, M.D.
Associate Professor of Psychiatry and Behavioral Sciences
Director, Child Psychiatric Services
University of Louisville School of Medicine
Louisville, Kentucky

Gabrielle A. Carlson, M.D.
Professor of Psychiatry
Director of Child Psychiatry
Department of Psychiatry
State University of New York at Stony Brook
Stony Brook, New York

Javad H. Kashani, M.D.
Professor of Psychiatry, Psychology, Pediatrics, and Medicine
Director of Child and Adolescent Services
Director of Training in Child Psychiatry
Mid-Missouri Mental Health Center
Department of Psychiatry, Section of Child Psychiatry
University of Missouri
Columbia, Missouri

James F. Kennedy, Ph.D.
Associate Clinical Professor of Psychiatry
Child Psychiatric Services
University of Louisville School of Medicine
Louisville, Kentucky

Hartmut B. Mokros, Ph.D.
Director of Research
Department of Communication
Rutgers University
New Brunswick, New Jersey

Caroly S. Pataki, M.D.
Assistant Professor of Psychiatry (Child)
Medical Director, Inpatient Child Psychiatry
University Hospital
State University of New York at Stony Brook
Health Sciences Center
Stony Brook, New York

Cynthia R. Pfeffer, M.D.
Professor of Psychiatry
Cornell University Medical College
Chief, Child Psychiatry Inpatient Unit
New York Hospital—Westchester Division
White Plains, New York

Elva O. Poznanski, M.D.
Professor, Department of Psychiatry
Chief, Section of Child Psychiatry
Rush-Presbyterian-St. Luke's Medical Center
Chicago, Illinois

Katherine A. Raymer, M.D.
Assistant Professor of Psychiatry
Assistant Director of Adolescent Affective Treatment Service
Western Psychiatric Institute and Clinic
Pittsburgh, Pennsylvania

Neal D. Ryan, M.D.
Associate Professor of Psychiatry
University of Pittsburgh School of Medicine
Director, Child and Adolescent Depression Program
Western Psychiatric Institute and Clinic
Pittsburgh, Pennsylvania

Lynette S. Schmid, M.D.
Clinical Assistant Professor of Psychiatry
Mid-Missouri Mental Health Center
Department of Psychiatry
Section of Child Psychiatry
University of Missouri
Columbia, Missouri

G. Randolph Schrodt, Jr., M.D.
Associate Professor of Psychiatry
University of Louisville School of Medicine
Associate Clinical Director
Norton Psychiatric Clinic
Louisville, Kentucky

Mohammad Shafii, M.D.
Professor of Psychiatry
Director, Child Psychiatry Training Program
Department of Psychiatry and Behavioral Sciences
University of Louisville School of Medicine
Louisville, Kentucky

Sharon Lee Shafii, R.N., B.S.N.
Editor-in-Residence, formerly Assistant Head Nurse
Adolescent Service
Neuropsychiatric Institute
University of Michigan Medical Center
Ann Arbor, Michigan

William A. Sonis, M.D.
Assistant Professor
University of Pennsylvania
Outpatient Medical Director
Philadelphia Child Guidance Center
Philadelphia, Pennsylvania

Michael Strober, Ph.D.
Professor of Psychiatry and Biobehavioral Sciences
Director, Adolescent Mood Disorders Program
Neuropsychiatric Institute and Hospital
Los Angeles, California

Elizabeth B. Weller, M.D.
Professor of Psychiatry and Pediatrics
Director, Division of Child and Adolescent Psychiatry
Ohio State University Hospitals
Columbus, Ohio

Ronald A. Weller, M.D.
Professor of Psychiatry
Director of Training
Ohio State University Hospitals
Columbus, Ohio

Shahnour Yaylayan, M.D.
Assistant Professor of Psychiatry
Ohio State University Hospitals
Columbus, Ohio

INTRODUCTION

Depression is a disorder of mood, so mysteriously painful and elusive in the way it becomes known to the self—to the mediating intellect—as to verge close to being beyond description. It thus remains nearly incomprehensible to those who have not experienced it in its extreme mode . . .

William Styron (1990)

The prevalence of emotional disorders in children and adolescents is unknown. The Institute of Medicine, in *Research on Children and Adolescents With Mental, Behavioral and Developmental Disorders* (1989), estimates that "in this country, at least 12% (or about 7.5 million) of the 63 million children under age 18 suffer from one or more mental disorders . . ." (p. 13). According to the National Institute of Mental Health Epidemiological Catchment Area Studies (Myers et al. 1984), in the adult population the 6-month prevalence of emotional disorders in the United States is 19.6%. Many investigators and clinicians believe that the prevalence of emotional disorders in children and adolescents is similar to that in adults.

The prevalence of depressive disorders in children and adolescents is estimated to be between 1.9% and 4.7% (1–3 million). Frequently, depressive disorders in children and adolescents are associated with other psychiatric disorders (comorbidity), such as anxiety disorders, oppositional-defiant disorder, attention-deficit hyperactivity disorder, conduct disorders, and alcohol and drug abuse. Depressive disorders in this age group may also be related to physical and sexual abuse and/or family dysfunction (e.g., parental neglect, drug or alcohol abuse, depression, and other psychiatric disorders).

Data-based research in child and adolescent psychiatry lags behind that in adult psychiatry. In recent years, significant strides have been made to close this gap. One area of intensive investigation is the study of depressive disorders in children and adolescents. Phenomenological investigation and longitudinal, psychopharmacological, and neurobiological studies have brought these distressing and debilitating disorders to the forefront. Now we recognize that depressive disorders in children and adolescents are, for the most part, similar to those in adults. We are beginning to explore more specifically the developmental factors that affect the expression of depressive disorders in infancy, childhood, and adolescence. Also, we are more aware of the cyclic and chronic nature of depressive disorders in children and adolescents. Through the method of psychological autopsy, we are beginning to recognize a relationship between actual suicide and the presence of diagnosable psychiatric disorders, especially major depression with comorbidity.

Clinical Guide to Depression in Children and Adolescents summarizes, synthesizes, and brings together significant advances that have occurred in the recognition, diagnosis, management, and treatment of depressive disorders and bipolar disorders in infancy, childhood, and adolescence. Most of the contributing authors have had many years of clinical experience and research activities in this area.

This book is divided into three parts. Part I, "Clinical Manifestations of Depressive Disorders in Children and Adolescents," examines depression both as an adaptive behavior and as a psychopathological disorder. Epidemiology, etiology, and neurobiology of depression in children and adolescents are reviewed. The emerging field of the study of biological rhythms (chronobiology) opens new vistas in understanding seasonal mood disorders. The relationship between suicidal behaviors and depression in children and adolescents is examined.

In Part II, "Diagnostic Assessment and Treatment of Depressive Disorders in Children and Adolescents," standardized instruments and structured and semistructured interviews used in clinical research are described and discussed. Employment of these instruments by the clinician could facilitate a more systematic and thorough assessment, more accurate diagnosis, and an increased awareness of the severity and the possible presence of other psychiatric disorders. Using these instruments throughout the treatment process and in follow-up helps to measure changes in the patient's depressive profile. Present psychotherapeutic approaches such as dynamic psychotherapy, group therapy, and cognitive-behavioral therapy are described. No matter which psychotherapeutic approach the clinician employs, working with and treating the family is essential. Also, indications for and side effects of pharmacological agents are examined. A chapter on inpatient psychiatric treatment along with a brief description of the therapeutic milieu concludes Part II.

In Part III, "Bipolar Disorders in Children and Adolescents," the clinical manifestation, natural history, genetics, and treatment of bipolar disorders are examined. At the present time, our knowledge of bipolar disorders is limited. Some clinical investigators hold the view that bipolar disorders manifest during adolescence—not at younger ages. However, in clinical practice one sees cases of bipolar disorders in preschool-aged and school-aged children. Also, occasional case descriptions and anecdotal reports of younger children with bipolar disorders are found in the literature. Our knowledge of bipolar disorders in children and adolescents is in an early phase and resembles our knowledge of depressive disorders in this age group more than a decade ago.

Throughout this book the role of the family in the genesis, expression, and amelioration of depressive and bipolar disorders is emphasized. We believe that children are the thermometers of the family. Working with the family at the initial assessment, throughout the course of treatment, and in the follow-up period is indispensable whether this work is in the form of family therapy, conjoint marital therapy, individual therapy, and/or parental education and training.

We hope that the *Clinical Guide to Depression in Children and Adolescents* will be useful to child and adolescent psychiatrists, general psychiatrists, residents in general, child and adolescent psychiatry, developmental pediatricians, pediatric neurologists, family physicians, medical students, psychologists, psychiatric nurses, psychiatric social workers, art and activity therapists, and other health and mental health professionals.

The planning and organization of this book took place when we were on sabbatical from the University of Louisville School of Medicine in the winter of 1989 in Nice, France. Writing and editing were done jointly and reflect our clinical work and research over the past decade in Louisville on the psychological autopsy of suicide in children and adolescents and on the neurobiology of depressive disorders in children and adolescents, specifically the role of melatonin, a hormone of the pineal gland.

We are grateful to Carol Nadelson, M.D., Editor-in-Chief of American Psychiatric Press, Inc., for suggesting the idea of this book. We are thankful to Amy Willard, Program and Research Assistant, for the typing and retyping of this manuscript and for carefully checking the accuracy of references.

Mohammad and Sharon Shafii

REFERENCES

Institute of Medicine: Research on Children and Adolescents With Mental, Behavioral, and Developmental Disorders. Washington, DC, National Academy Press, 1989

Myers JK, Weissman MM, Tischler GL, et al: Six-months prevalence of psychiatric disorders in three communities. Arch Gen Psychiatry 41:959–967, 1984

Styron W: Darkness Visible: A Memoir of Madness. New York, Random House, 1990, p 7

PART I

CLINICAL MANIFESTATIONS OF DEPRESSIVE DISORDERS IN CHILDREN AND ADOLESCENTS

One may not reach dawn
save by the path of the night.

Kahlil Gibran

CHAPTER 1

Clinical Manifestations and Developmental Psychopathology of Depression

Mohammad Shafii, M.D.
Sharon Lee Shafii, R.N., B.S.N.

Depression can be a sign, symptom, syndrome, or disorder. As a sign or signal, depression in the form of sad affect or sad mood (dysphoria) is one of the most commonly experienced human emotions from infancy to aging. Depression as a symptom differs from depression as a sign or signal in that it is more intense and prolonged and interferes with the well-being or adaptation of the individual. When depression is referred to as a syndrome or disorder, it not only includes intense and prolonged sad mood, but also other symptoms such as anhedonia (loss of interest or enjoyment in everyday activities); increase or decrease of sleep; increase or decrease in appetite; decrease of energy or fatigue; psychomotor agitation or retardation; feelings of worthlessness; self-blame or excessive guilt; diminished ability to concentrate or think; and morbid thoughts, suicidal ideation, or suicide attempt.

DEPRESSION AS A SIGN OR SIGNAL

Depression as an affect is expressed behaviorally by a sad facial expression, decrease in body movement, slowing down of body functions, and a temporary, partial, or total withdrawal.

At a time of distress or danger, a living organism either fights or flees or,

Parts of the chapter "Depression in Infancy, Childhood, and Adolescence" from *Pathways of Human Development: Normal Growth and Emotional Disorders in Infancy, Childhood and Adolescence*, by Shafii, M., and Shafii, S.L. (New York: Thieme-Stratton, 1982, pp. 77–95) are integrated into this chapter.

We acknowledge the contribution of Andrea Minyard, a medical student, University of Louisville School of Medicine, for reviewing the literature for some parts of this chapter.

3

in some situations, withdraws. In mammals, primates, and particularly human beings, the fight-flight response is called anxiety or signal anxiety (Cannon and de la Paz 1911; Freud 1926; Kandel and Davies 1982; Selye 1946, 1950). When an organism experiences failure in a distressful situation, it generally withdraws. This withdrawal serves to *conserve* energy and facilitate survival. Engel et al. (1956) studied a 15-month-old female, Monica, who had a gastric fistula. Monica experienced withdrawal and depression whenever she felt acutely distressed, such as when someone she loved or was attached to left her. Engel et al. noticed that, along with withdrawal and depression, Monica's gastric secretions also decreased significantly. They postulated that Monica's depression and withdrawal had survival value and helped her conserve energy and resources. "Withdrawal-conservation" in human beings has an adaptive significance that is similar to withdrawal and hibernation in animals.

Before these studies, withdrawal and depression were perceived as severe psychopathological disturbances or as pathological defensive reactions to anxiety. Now it is understood that withdrawal and depression are primary affective responses that help the individual conserve emotional and physiological resources for further adaptation. When depression is a sign or signal, we refer to it as *signal depression* or *adaptive depression*.

SIGNAL DEPRESSION, OR ADAPTIVE DEPRESSION

Until recently, it was thought that children began to manifest depression as a primary affect between ages 1 and 2 years, following the development of object relationship and symbolic thought processes (Dorpat 1977). Studies by Tronick et al. (1978) have thrown a new light on the possible existence of depression as a primary affect soon after birth. They videotaped face-to-face interactions between mothers and their infants from ages 2 through 20 weeks. There were two types of experimental situations, each lasting 3 minutes. In the first, the mother had a natural face-to-face interaction with her baby. In the second, she sat face-to-face with her baby while ". . . remaining unresponsive and maintaining an expressionless face" (p. 2).

To emphasize the infants' sensitivity, responsiveness, and affective reaction in reciprocal communications with their mothers, we have used extensive, direct quotations from Tronick et al.'s (1978) fascinating observations. A 2-month-old baby sits quietly alone in an infant seat, ". . . face serious, cheeks droopy, mouth half open, corners down, but there is an expectant look in his eyes as if he were waiting" (p. 5). As soon as his mother comes into the room and says, "Hello," his face and hands reach out in her direction. He follows his mother with his head and eyes as she comes toward him.

His body builds up with tension, his face and eyes open up with a real greeting which ends with a smile. His mouth opens wide and his whole body orients toward her. He subsides, mouths his tongue twice, his smile dies, and he looks down briefly, while she continues to talk in an increasingly eliciting voice. (p. 5)

The mother begins to touch the infant and gently move his hips and legs.

He looks up again, smiles widely, narrows his eyes, brings one hand up to his mouth, grunting, vocalizing, and begins to cycle his legs and arms out toward her. With this increasing activity, she begins to grin more widely, to talk more loudly and with higher-pitched accents, accentuating his vocalizations with hers and his activity with her movement of his legs. (p. 5)

The mother continues to accentuate the interaction with the infant and, after 40 seconds,

he looks down again, gets sober . . . makes a pouting face. She looks down at his feet at this point, then comes back to look into his face and he returns to look up at her. She lets go of his legs, and they draw up into his body. He bursts out with a broad smile and a staccato-like vocalization for three repetitions. (pp. 5–6)

Whenever the baby's face "broadens and opens wide," and his arms and legs move toward the mother, she

. . . seems to get caught up in his bursts, and smiles broadly, her voice also getting brighter. After each burst, he subsides to a serious face, limbs quiet, and her quieting response follows his.
    At 70 seconds, he subsides completely, and looks down at his feet with a darkly serious face. She gets very still, her face becomes serious, her voice slows down and almost stops, the pitch becomes low. Her mouth is drawn down, reflecting his serious mouth. After 3 seconds, he begins to brighten again into a wide, tonguing smile. (p. 6)

The mother immediately responds coyly with a gentle smile and gentle voice. The baby responds with staccato-like vocalization and the cycling of his legs toward her. At 90 seconds,

his movements subside and his face becomes serious. She also is quite serious. . . . (p. 6)

This interaction continues with intermittent encouraging smiles, serious looks, and quiescence in harmony between mother and infant. The mother becomes quiet when the baby becomes quiet. Then the baby entices mother toward interaction. When the baby becomes very excited, the mother gently holds the baby's hips and legs to contain the peak of his excitement.
    This observation clearly documents the emotional and affective exchanges and reciprocal interactions between the infant and his mother.

When the interaction reaches a crescendo of excitement, the infant actively begins disengagement by looking serious or sober, or by looking away, thereby modulating and decreasing mother's input. When the infant wants more contact with his mother, he invites renewed involvement by a look, smile, gesture of hands, cycling of the legs, and change in the shape of his mouth or in the pitch of his voice. Mother's sensitivity and receptivity to her infant's affective communication reinforce his behavior and facilitate his sense of effectiveness and competency.

In the second experimental situation with the same infant, the mother remains expressionless for 3 minutes. The infant is sitting alone in an infant seat, looking down at his hands,

> . . . fingering the fingers of one hand with the other. As the mother enters, his hand movements stop. He looks up at her, makes eye-to-eye contact and smiles. Her masklike face does not change. He looks away quickly to one side and remains quiet, his facial expression serious. He remains this way for 20 seconds. Then he looks back at her face, his eyebrows and lids raised, his hands and arms startling slightly out toward her. He quickly looks down at his hands, stills for 8 seconds, and then checks her face once more. This look is cut short by a yawn, with his eyes and face turning upward. (p. 7)

He begins to pull at the fingers of the other hand while his whole body is motionless. After the yawn, which lasts 5 seconds, he looks at mother's face briefly. When mother does not respond, his arm movements become jerky,

> . . . his mouth curves downward, his eyes narrow and partially lid. He turns his face to the side, but he keeps his mother in peripheral vision. He fingers his hand again, his legs stretch toward her and rapidly jerk back again. He arches forward, slumps over, tucks his chin down on one shoulder, but he looks up at her face from under his lowered eyebrows. This position lasts for over a minute, with brief checking looks at the mother occurring almost every 10 seconds. He grimaces briefly and his facial expression becomes more serious, his eyebrows furrowing. Finally, he completely withdraws, his body curled over, his head down. He does not look again at his mother. He begins to finger his mouth, sucking on one finger and rocking his head, looking at his feet. He looks wary, helpless, and withdrawn. As the mother exits at the end of the 3 minutes, he looks halfway up in her direction, but his sober facial expression and his curled body position do not change. (pp. 7–8)

According to Tronick et al., this is a typical pattern of the infant's reaction to the mother's expressionless face. Initially, the infant responds to the mother and greets her. When she does not respond, the infant becomes sober and wary. He tries to engage her with brief smiles. When he does not receive any response, he looks away. He continues to persist. When consistent persistence for contact meets failure, he

> ... eventually withdraws, orients his face and body away from his mother with hopeless expression, and stays turned away from her. None of the infants cried, however. (p. 8)

The mothers felt that it was extremely taxing and difficult to remain emotionally unresponsive to their babies for 3 minutes. When they returned after this experiment, it took at least 30 seconds for the babies to warm up to their mothers again. Initially, the baby showed "wary monitoring" of the mother. On occasion, the baby "... would arch away from the mother as if he had not forgiven her the previous insult" (p. 10).

Infants have an innate ability to respond discriminately to other human beings even in the first day of life. The studies conducted by Tronick et al. demonstrated the infant's rich affective and emotional responses to other human beings. They convincingly demonstrated that failure in human contact, even in a 3-minute time period, creates sadness, soberness, withdrawal, helplessness, and hopelessness in the infant. We propose that these signs in toto could be called a *signal depression* or *adaptive depression*.

Signal depression is a mild to moderate transient form of depression that usually lasts a short period of time—a few minutes to a few hours. It is experienced on a sensory-motor, proprioceptive, and visceral level. This experience is not retrievable through memories, recall, or free associations. Signal depression is related to a disturbance in the biological rhythm of engagement and disengagement in human contact. Disengagement, withdrawal, and signal depression modulate and "tone down" mood and affective responses, facilitate the conservation of energy and resources, and stimulate more effective ways of adaptation. Signal depression activates attachment behavior in the mothering person, modulates affective responses, and stimulates initiation of new contacts.

Melanie Klein's (1957) observation of the "depressive position" in normal infants between the ages of 3 and 6 months and Margaret Mahler's (1972) description of "mini anaclitic" depression in children in the subphase of rapprochement (ages 16–25 months) reveal behavioral manifestations of signal depression.

A certain amount of signal-depressive experiences are inevitable and promote further growth and development. Temporary, but adaptive depression during adolescence, midlife crisis, retirement, and aging, and the experience of loss and grief, are manifestations of cumulative signal depressions. Disengagement and withdrawal for the sake of new engagement, commitment, and integration are essential features of human development from birth to death.

DEPRESSION AS A DISORDER

Historical Perspective

In the past, the existence of depression as an emotional disorder in infancy and childhood was a matter of controversy. Some psychoanalysts thought that infants and children did not experience "depressive neurosis" because they had not, as yet, internalized the superego and therefore were unable to experience guilt (Rie 1966; Rochlin 1959). In classical psychoanalytic theory, internalization of the superego and the experience of guilt were prerequisites for depressive disorders (Abraham 1911, 1916; Freud 1917, 1923, 1938).

Careful observation of infants during the first year of life by Spitz (1945, 1946, 1965) and Spitz and Wolf (1946) documents the presence of severe depression following maternal deprivation. Bowlby (1946, 1951, 1960) related the loss of maternal attachment in childhood and the accompanying pathological grief, mourning, and depression to the occurrence of juvenile delinquency. Harlow (1958, 1959, 1960) studied the effect of maternal deprivation on infant monkeys. He found that maternal deprivation and disturbance in attachment behavior led to the development of severe psychopathology, including profound depression, delay of development, and the possibility of psychosis.

Anthony and Scott (1960) and Anthony (1970, 1978) documented the existence of depression in children and adolescents. Sandler and Joffe (1965) related the existence of depression and depressive affect in children to the loss of the feeling of well-being, rather than to the loss of self-esteem or guilt.

During the last two decades, interest in the study of depression in children and adolescents has flourished. Glaser (1967) described masked depression in childhood and adolescence. Annel (1972), Brumback and Weinberg (1977), Cantwell and Carlson (1979), Cytryn (1972), Cytryn and McKnew (1974, 1979), Dorpat (1977), Geller (1983a, 1983b), Kashani and Simonds (1979), Kashani et al. (1983, 1986, 1987), Kazdin (1989), Kazdin et al. (1986), Kovacs (1980/1981), Kovacs and Beck (1977), Malmquist (1971), Nurcombe et al. (1989), Phillips (1979), Poznanski (1980, 1982), Poznanski and Zrull (1970), Puig-Antich and Chambers (unpublished manuscript, 1978), Puig-Antich et al. (1984a, 1984b, 1984c, 1984d, 1985), Ryan et al. (1987), Shafii and Shafii (1982a, 1982b), Shafii et al. (1979, 1984, 1985, 1988, 1990), Weinberg et al. (1973), Weller et al. (1984, 1986), and Welner (1979) have contributed significantly to the study, documentation, classification, and development of behavioral scales and psychoneuroendocrinological measurements for depression in children and adolescents.

The above studies led to the realization that, for depressive disorders, adult criteria with some minor variations also apply to children and adolescents (American Psychiatric Association 1980; American Psychiatric Associ-

ation 1987). Using adult criteria in clinical practice and research has significantly furthered data-based research in mood disorders in children and adolescents. With these studies has also come the understanding that, along
with similarities to adult depression, one needs to consider developmental
differences (Kazdin 1989).

TYPES OF DEPRESSIVE DISORDERS

Mood disorders (affective disorders) are divided into depressive disorders
and bipolar disorders. Depressive disorders are further divided into major
depression (unipolar disorder), dysthymia (dysthymic disorder or depressive neurosis), and depressive disorder not otherwise specified (NOS). In
major depression the patient experiences single or recurrent episodes of depression associated with other symptoms lasting at least 2 weeks but without mood elevation, elation, or mania. Thus, this disorder is sometimes referred to as unipolar disorder. In dysthymia the patient experiences chronic
depressed mood in association with other symptoms. The severity of symptoms in dysthymia is less than in major depressive episodes. The duration of
dysthymia is usually 2 years for adults and 1 year for children and adolescents. Also, children and adolescents may have irritable rather than depressed mood. In depressive disorder NOS the patient experiences depressive features that do not fulfill the criteria for major depressive disorder
(MDD) or dysthymia.

Bipolar disorders are divided into bipolar disorder (classic manic depression disorder, bipolar I), cyclothymia (bipolar II), and bipolar disorder
NOS. In bipolar disorder the patient experiences manic episodes in the form
of predominant elevation of mood, expansiveness, irritability, hyperactivity,
pressure of speech, flight of ideas, and inflated self-esteem. Later, the patient
may experience a period or periods of depression. Because of mood fluctuation between the two opposite poles of elation and depression, this disorder
is called bipolar disorder. The episodes are severe enough to impair the
patient's relationships with others, work performance, and social activities.
In cyclothymia the patient experiences chronic mood disturbances involving
episodes of hypomania and periods of depressed mood. The severity and
duration of cyclothymia are less than the severity and duration of bipolar
disorder, usually 2 years for adults and 1 year for children and adolescents.
The patient is not free for more than 2 months from hypomanic or depressive
symptoms. In bipolar disorder NOS the patient experiences manic or hypomanic features that do not fulfill the diagnostic criteria for bipolar disorder
or cyclothymia (American Psychiatric Association 1987).

In the next section we will discuss the diagnostic criteria of major depression and dysthymia, followed by specific developmental consideration
of depressive disorders from birth to age 18 years. Seasonal mood disorders

in children and adolescents are discussed in Chapter 4. The description, follow-up, and treatment of bipolar disorders in children and adolescents are
discussed in Chapters 12 and 13.

DIAGNOSTIC CRITERIA OF MAJOR DEPRESSIVE EPISODE

Cytryn et al. (1980) have made a "point by point comparison between the
diagnostic criteria" of their own work, Weinberg's criteria, Kovacs's
Children's Depression Inventory (CDI) (1980/1981), and DSM-III criteria for
depression. They found that ". . . childhood and adult diagnostic criteria for
affective disorders are very similar, and DSM-III is a valid instrument for
diagnosing childhood affective disorder" (p. 22).

The following clinical features or diagnostic criteria of major depressive
episodes apply to infants, children, adolescents, and adults (American Psychiatric Association 1987).

Essential Features

The patient must have one or both of the following symptoms for at least 2
weeks:

1. Depressed or dysphoric mood for most of the day almost every day as
   reported by the patient or as observed by others. In children and
   adolescents irritable mood may replace depressed mood.
2. Significantly decreased interest or pleasure (anhedonia) in all or nearly
   all activities for most of the day almost every day as reported by the
   patient or as observed as apathy by others.

Associated Symptoms

The patient must have a total of at least five symptoms occurring almost
every day for at least 2 weeks. Of these five symptoms, one or two must be
essential features of depression, with the remaining three or four being associated symptoms:

1. Increase or decrease in appetite or increase or decrease of more than 5%
   of the body weight in 1 month when not dieting. In children, a lack of
   expected increase in weight.
2. Increase or decrease of sleep.
3. Psychomotor retardation or agitation as observed by others.
4. Fatigue or loss of energy.
5. Feelings of worthlessness or excessive or inappropriate guilt.
6. Diminished concentration or indecisiveness.
7. Morbid ideations, recurrent thoughts of death and dying, recurrent

suicidal ideation either with or without a specific plan to commit suicide or a suicide attempt.

The symptoms should not be related to underlying organic factors or other psychiatric disorders or to uncomplicated bereavement. The symptoms must be severe enough to affect the patient's functioning.

Types of Major Depressive Disorder

MDDs are described as single episode or recurrent; mild, moderate, or severe either with or without psychotic features; in partial or full remission; chronic; or unspecified.

A subtype of recurrent MDD is melancholic type. The patient must meet five of the following diagnostic criteria:

1. Anhedonia.
2. No reaction to pleasurable stimuli.
3. Depression that is worse in the morning.
4. Early morning awakening.
5. Psychomotor retardation or agitation.
6. Anorexia or weight loss.
7. No previous personality disorder.
8. Previous major depressive episode (one or more) with almost or complete recovery.
9. History of good response to antidepressant therapy such as electroconvulsive therapy, tricyclics, monoamine oxidase inhibitors, and lithium.

DIAGNOSTIC CRITERIA OF DYSTHYMIA

Dysthymia is a form of depressive disorder less severe than major depression. Frequently, major depression can be superimposed on dysthymia.

Essential Features

The patient must have depressed mood for most of the day most of the time, as reported by the patient or observed by others for at least 2 years. In children and adolescents the duration must be at least 1 year, and irritable mood may replace depressed mood. Patients are not without symptoms of depressed mood for more than 2 months at a time.

Associated Symptoms

In dysthymia, the patient must have at least two of the following associated symptoms, in addition to depressed mood:

1. Increase or decrease in appetite.
2. Increase or decrease in sleep.
3. Low energy or fatigue.
4. Low self-esteem.
5. Difficulty in concentration or decision making.
6. Feelings of hopelessness.

Types of Dysthymia

Dysthymia can be either a primary type or a secondary type. The primary type is not related to a preexisting psychiatric non-mood disorder or a physical disorder, whereas the secondary type is related to a preexisting psychiatric non-mood disorder or a physical disorder. Dysthymia is also divided into early onset (beginning before age 21 years) or late onset (beginning at age 21 years or older).

DEVELOPMENTAL PSYCHOPATHOLOGY

Applying adult criteria to the diagnosis of depressive disorder in infancy, childhood, and adolescence has been a major step in helping the clinician to make an appropriate diagnosis and to develop an appropriate treatment plan. Some of the developmental issues concerning infants, children, and adolescents have been taken into consideration, such as irritable mood replacing depressed mood, 1-year instead of 2-year duration for dysthymia, and lack of expected weight gain instead of weight loss. However, still more emphasis is needed on developmental perspectives regarding the onset, symptomatic expression, and evolution of specific disorders.

Sroufe and Rutter (1984) are pioneers in the field of developmental psychopathology. According to them, developmental psychopathology explores the "ontological process whereby early patterns of individual adaptation evolve into latter patterns of adaptation" (p. 27). The major perspective of developmental psychopathology is that not only do normal patterns of behavior go through changes, but also psychopathological symptoms evolve and change throughout development. Trad (1986) wrote: "Central to the developmental perspective is the proposition that both normal and disordered individuals undergo a common course of development in which functioning at one level has predictable implications for subsequent functioning" (p. 3). Developmental psychopathology does not follow a linear development but rather favors "a model that allows for behavioral transformations as well as for regressions" (Trad 1986, p. 3).

Phenomenologically oriented classifications such as DSM-III and DSM-III-R do not take behavioral transformation and regressions into consideration in describing depressive disorders in infancy, childhood, and adolescence. This shortcoming will need to be addressed sooner or later. More direct clinical observations and data-based research integrating developmental perspectives with normative and psychological behavioral observations through the first year of life, ages 2–3 years, ages 4–5 years, ages 6–12 years, and ages 13–18 years will help to make evaluation and diagnosis more accurate and treatment intervention more effective.

In addition to the general clinical features of depression, depression in children expresses itself by regression. The child loses some acquired age-specific developmental skills and functions on an earlier level. The clinician needs to be familiar with the developmental tasks of each stage, so that absence, delay, or regression of any behavior will be readily apparent and serve as a signal of possible disturbance.

DEPRESSIVE DISORDERS IN THE FIRST YEAR OF LIFE

Depressive disorders in the first year of life are closely related to the disorders of attachment and mothering, child neglect, maternal deprivation, parental psychopathology, and placement of infants in institutions. Anaclitic depression, hospitalism, failure to thrive, and major depression in infancy will be discussed.

Anaclitic Depression—Partial Emotional Deprivation

Anaclitic depression is a term used by Spitz (1946) to describe partial emotional deprivation in infants. Spitz and Wolf (1946) observed 123 infants, the total population of an institution. Each infant was observed for 12–18 months or longer. The infant population was almost evenly distributed between males and females.

The infants were in a "nursery" of a penal institution for delinquent girls who were pregnant at the time of incarceration. The infants' mothers were mostly young adolescents with a multitude of problems, such as delinquency, mental retardation, or immaturity.

The infants were cared for by their mothers with some supervision from a small nursing staff. Spitz (1965) noted that during the first 6 months the infants had a good relationship with their mothers and showed appropriate developmental progress.

> However, in the second half of the first year, some [$n = 19$] of them developed a weepy behavior that was in marked contrast to their previous happy outgoing behavior. After a time, this weepiness gave way to withdrawal. They would lie prone in their cots, face averted, refusing to take part in the life of their surroundings. (Spitz 1965, pp. 268–269)

Most of these troubled infants ignored adults. A few watched adults with "a searching expression." If the observers were insistent on interaction, ". . . weeping would ensue, and in some cases screaming" (p. 269).

The troubled infants demonstrated the following symptoms, beginning at approximately 6 months of age:

1. Weepy and withdrawal behavior, lasting 2–3 months.
2. Loss of weight instead of expected weight gain.
3. Insomnia in some cases.
4. Increased susceptibility to recurrent colds and infections.
5. Retardation in the rate of psychological and intellectual growth, followed by actual decline.
6. Frozen rigidity of expression replaced weepy behavior after 3 months. "Now these children would lie or sit with wide-open expressionless eyes, frozen immobile face, and a faraway look, as if in a daze, apparently not seeing what went on around them" (p. 269).
7. Human contact became ". . . increasingly difficult and finally impossible" (p. 269).

The infants' symptoms and facial expressions strongly reminded the investigators of the symptoms and facial expressions of depressed adults. Spitz discovered that all of these infants had

> . . . one experience in common: at some point between the sixth and eighth month of life all of them were deprived of the mother for a practically unbroken period of three months. This separation took place for unavoidable external administrative reasons. (p. 271)

Spitz noticed that "no child developed this syndrome whose mother had not been removed" (p. 271). Spitz referred to this syndrome as *anaclitic depression, anaclitic* meaning "leaning up against." In the first year, the infant "leans up against" the mother for physical and emotional growth.

Concerning intellectual development, these maternally deprived infants were brighter (Developmental Quotient mean, 130) than the control group (Developmental Quotient mean, 116–120). After separation from mother, the infant's intellectual development declined significantly. If the separation continued for more than 1 year, the infant's intelligence deteriorated to the moderate-to-severe retardation range (Developmental Quotient mean, 40–50), as compared with the control group (Developmental Quotient mean, 110).

Spitz observed that if the infant's deprivation from mother lasted not more than 3–5 months, most infants recovered, although not completely. However, if the deprivation exceeded 5 months ". . . the whole symptomatology changes radically and appears to merge into the prognostically poor syndrome of what I have described as 'Hospitalism' . . ." (p. 272).

Anaclitic depression also could be caused by disruption in the relationship between the infant and the primary caregivers rather than the mother. Emde et al. (1965) reported on a case of a 9-month-old infant named George. George lived all of his life in a residential nursery. After he was transferred to another section of the nursery that had fewer caregivers, he began to manifest symptoms of anaclitic depression. When this disorder was diagnosed in George, the nursery staff increased their care and attention to him. George recovered 7 ½ months after the onset of anaclitic depression.

Harmon et al. (1982) reported on George's follow-up. During George's preschool years, he experienced three episodes of major depression, each resulting from separation from his primary caregiver. Each time after separation, he became agitated, followed by depression and withdrawal. Separations were also associated with a flare-up of severe atopic dermatitis.

Hospitalism—Total Emotional Deprivation

According to Spitz (1965), if emotional deprivation continues for more than 5 months, the infant will show "... the symptoms of increasingly serious deterioration, which appears to be, in part at least, irreversible" (p. 277).

In another study, Spitz observed 91 infants in a foundling home. These infants were breast-fed for the first 3 months by their mothers or by someone else. They grew normally. At age 3 months, the infants were separated from their mothers. The medical care, food, and hygiene provided for these infants were as good as or superior to those provided by any other institution, but one nurse had to care for 8–12 infants.

> After separation from their mothers, these children went through the stages of progressive deterioration.... The symptoms of anaclitic depression followed one another in rapid succession and soon, after the relatively brief period of three months, a new clinical picture appeared. (Spitz 1965, p. 278)

In addition to all of the signs and symptoms of anaclitic depression, the observers now saw the following symptoms:

1. Significant motor retardation.
2. Complete passivity—the infants would lie supine on their cots and would not turn around or assume a prone position.
3. Vacuous facial expression.
4. Defect in eye coordination.
5. Spasticity in body movement even after extensive rehabilitation.
6. Bizarre finger movements similar to decerebrate or athetoid movements.
7. Progressive decline in developmental quotient—by the end of the second year, the average developmental quotient was in the moderately to severely retarded range.
8. Extremely high mortality rate—29.6% died in the first year.

The authors followed some of these children up to age 4 years. Most of them, even by this age, could not sit, stand, walk, or talk.

Anaclitic depression and hospitalism are manifestations of infantile depression and maternal deprivation in its most severe form. A number of studies have documented that disorders in mothering, such as maternal depression, parental immaturity, family disharmony, drug and alcohol abuse, child abuse, and emotional neglect can also contribute to the development of depression in infancy, delayed development, and growth failure. Failure to thrive in infancy is one of the most frequent results of attachment disorders.

Failure to Thrive

Failure to thrive is a clinical syndrome common in pediatric practice. Because of the child's age, it usually does not come to the attention of child psychiatrists. Failure to thrive may be considered the severe form of reactive attachment disorder of infancy or early childhood.

Incidence

The actual incidence is unknown, but this is "... one of the most common reasons for admission of infants to the hospital" (Reinhart 1979, p. 594). Failure to thrive frequently occurs in multiple-problem families, families prone to child abuse and neglect, and lower socioeconomic families. However, clinicians also need to be aware of the possibility of failure to thrive in middle- or upper-class families.

Etiology

Approximately 50% of the infants suffering from failure to thrive do not show any organic or physical cause of growth failure. The other half may suffer from growth failure because of kidney, heart, gastrointestinal, metabolic, or central nervous system abnormalities, malnutrition, or chronic infection.

Clinical Features

Failure to thrive, which is also referred to as reactive attachment of infancy (DSM-III-R, pp. 91–93), has the following features.

Onset before age 5 years. But even in the first month of life, diagnosis can be made.

Evidence of lack of care. Gross emotional neglect, institutionalization, or disorders in the development of attachment behavior and human bonding are evident.

Delay in development. The infant is behind in many areas of development, such as affective response, cognitive development, and physical development.

Failure to thrive should be considered one of the major diagnostic possibilities if the infant has not developed or has significant delay in the following psychosocial behaviors:

1. Visual tracking of eyes and human face by age 2 months.
2. Social smile at human face by age 2 months.
3. Visual reciprocity by age 2 months.
4. Alerting and turning to the caretaker's verbal communication by age 4 months.
5. Spontaneous reaching to mother by age 4 months.
6. Vocal reciprocity by age 5 months.
7. Anticipatory response when the infant is approached to be picked up by age 5 months.
8. Involvement and participation in playful games with mother or caregiver by age 5 months.

Weight.   Most of these infants have gained very little weight or have lost weight. Usually, the weight is below the third percentile at the time of evaluation. The infant gains weight rapidly after hospital admission or environmental changes in maternal care.

Height.   Height is usually affected, but not as severely as weight. If the child suffers from failure to thrive for a long period of time, a significant decrease in height will result.

Head size.   Head size is normal.

Absence of physical disorder, mental retardation, or infantile autism. The mother or primary caregiver of a great majority of infants suffering from failure to thrive is ". . . depressed, angry, helpless, and desperate and with poor self-esteem" (Reinhart 1979, p. 596). One of the most striking clinical features of children suffering from failure to thrive, besides weight loss, is apathy. These infants appear joyless and lifeless. Evidence of sadness or depression, instead of overwhelming apathy, indicates that the infant is still experiencing and communicating internal feeling. This is a favorable sign.

Additional signs.   Some of the following may also be present:

1. Weak cry.
2. Hypersomnia (excessive sleep).
3. Apathy (lack of interest in the environment).
4. Hypotonia of the muscles due to lack of stimulation and movement.
5. Hypomotility.
6. Weak rooting and grasping reflexes when feeding.

Sensory-Motor Depression

In infancy, anaclitic depression, hospitalism, and failure to thrive represent severe and prolonged forms of depression and deprivation with dire consequences. However, other clinical symptomatologies have been observed in infants that are not consistent with the above syndromes but that do have significant features of depression. For example, Robertson (1965) reported on the presence of depression in a 2-month-old infant who improved significantly when the mother became more involved. Wisdom (1977) reported on an acute form of depression in a 6-month-old boy from an intact family. This depression lasted 3–4 days after the loss of a "nanny." Fraiberg and Freedman (1964) and Fraiberg (1968, 1977) found that parental depression and withdrawal contributed to sadness, withdrawal, autoerotic, autistic-like behavior, and developmental retardation in blind infants.

Brazelton et al. (1971) described an infant girl who manifested soberness, sadness, withdrawal, and unresponsiveness beginning 10 days following birth. The research team had observed that, at birth and during the ensuing week, this infant ". . . was an alert, wide-eyed newborn who looked vigorous and mature. She was entirely normal in all neurological and behavioral responses . . ." (p. 303).

The research team, on a home visit 3 days later, reported that the mother appeared "quiet and unresponsive." The baby ". . . was curled in fetal position . . . and moved very little as we handled her" (p. 304). She was, to some extent, responsive to auditory and visual stimuli. By age 3 weeks, the infant was subdued, in a semialert state, and was preoccupied most of the time with sucking her fist. Observations at 10 weeks and 3, 4, 7, and 8 months revealed that the infant continued to deteriorate cognitively and emotionally, was significantly behind in developmental milestones, and had very little facial animation. However, there was no report of weight loss or failure to gain weight—a prerequisite of failure to thrive.

At 8 months the infant was seen by a neurologist. The neurologist told the mother that her infant was retarded and that her brain was ". . . not normal and that her prognosis for ultimate development was probably poor" (p. 306).

When the research team made a home visit 2 weeks later, they noticed a profound change in the mother's attitude. She had mobilized her resources to overcome her own depression and apathy and had begun active involvement with her baby by an increase in body contact, talking, and playing. The observers noticed that the infant was already more active, rolled around in the playpen, tried to creep, and sat without support. The infant continued to improve dramatically. By age 12 months, her motor coordination was age-appropriate, by 18 months she walked alone, and by 21 months she played with dolls. At age 2 years, this child was warm, expressive, affectionate, and functioning close to chronological age.

This infant, who at one time was diagnosed "brain-damaged and retarded" by a neurologist and "possibly autistic" by the research team, dramatically improved after her mother's sensory-motor and affective contact increased. This case illustrates a severe form of depression that does not follow the criteria for failure to thrive, anaclitic depression, or hospitalism. Disturbance in human contact and mothering contributed to the development of withdrawal behavior, soberness, apathy, and significant delay in sensory-motor and affective development.

Smart and Taylor (1973) reported on a case of a 9-week-old baby. The mother and the infant had formed a close and happy relationship. The mother's older child was hospitalized. The mother continued to function as the baby's main caregiver, feeding him quickly and putting him back to bed. The baby was not unattended but received minimal care from his mother compared with the first 9 weeks of life. Soon after, the baby became very pale and listless. After that, he became lethargic. His fontanel was depressed and skin was inelastic. After realizing that the infant might be suffering from depression due to minimal contact with her, the mother began spending more time with the infant and actively caring for him. In a 1-week period, the infant recovered.

Based on case reports in the literature and clinical observation, we noticed that in infants there is a cluster of behaviors related to depression that does not follow the classic descriptions of anaclitic depression and hospitalism or the criteria for failure to thrive, major depression (at least 2 weeks' duration), or dysthymia (at least 1 year's duration). Because of the infant's cognitive stage, we have chosen the term *sensory-motor depression* to describe this mood disorder in infancy. This term emphasizes the two major components of this disturbance—cognitive and affective.

The use of the term *sensory-motor* refers to the sensory-motor stage of intelligence—the first stage of human cognition—from birth to age 18 months (Piaget 1962). According to Piaget, human cognition based on inborn patterns of response (schema) originate from environmental and bodily stimuli and the motoric responses to these stimuli. Decrease, disturbance, or failure in human contact and stimulation have immediate effect on the infant's cognitive and affective development.

The use of the term *depression* describes the affective and emotional component of the infant's response of soberness, sadness, and withdrawal. Clinical manifestations of sensory-motor depression using the developmental psychopathological perspectives of developmental continuity and discontinuity, developmental arrest, regression, and transformation follow.

Onset

Sensory-motor depression can occur immediately after birth, but usually becomes noticeable in the second to third week of life or later. The infant cannot verbally express feelings of sadness and dysphoria, but the informed and sensitive clinician can detect the infant's emotional state through observation of facial expression and behavior.

Duration

In the acute form, sensory-motor depression is of short duration, lasting a few hours to a few days. If the mothering person does not alleviate the depression through human contact, it can become cyclical and eventually chronic.

Clinical Features

Facial expression. The infant has a persistently sober, sad, and joyless facial expression. This sadness and lack of joy are contagious. Sensitive parents, observers, and clinicians, when seeing the infant's face, often feel profound sadness within. When the clinician experiences this empathic sadness, it has diagnostic significance and often helps in differentiating depression from other forms of withdrawal behavior, such as in cases of physical illness, childhood autism, or severe mental retardation.

The infant's sad face reactivates maternal and caregiving behavior in the observer. The observer may spontaneously feel like picking up and hugging the infant to give comfort.

Crying. Initially, the crying of the depressed infant has the quality of a "pain" cry, but it gradually loses forcefulness and becomes a cranky, irritable cry or whimper. When an adult approaches, the infant gazes at his or her eyes with a long, wary, and deeply sad look and then bursts into a pain cry. As the infant's depression becomes more prolonged, the pain cry may disappear, and only a cranky, irritable cry or whimper remains. After a while, the infant may stop crying completely. Parents might feel that the infant is doing much better and is becoming a "good baby." Significant decrease in crying or absence of crying in a depressed infant is an ominous sign.

Eye contact. The eye contact of normal infants has a bright-eyed quality, which usually creates a feeling of joy in the observer. The depressed infant, especially in the early phases of depression, has prolonged eye contact, but without "brightness." The infant's eyes emanate wariness and sadness, as though communicating internal misery.

As depression progresses, the infant continues to have eye contact, but it is usually brief. However, in profound depression, the infant might gaze at the observer in an empty and apathetic manner or avoid eye contact. Facial expression and eye contact are the two major clues that alert the clinician to the possibility of sensory-motor depression and disorders in mothering.

Language. Cooing and babbling, usually seen between ages 1 and 2 months, do not occur in depressed infants. The infant will continue to be fussy. The infant, it appears, has not been able to learn new schemata for expression of internal states, such as cooing, babbling, and vocally responding to maternal stimulation. In the older infant, imitative behavior and acquired language skills decline and the infant regresses to more fussiness and crying behavior.

Smile. When the infant becomes depressed, one of the first behaviors to disappear is the social smile, which usually occurs at age 2 months, and the recognition smile, which usually appears at age 4 months. The infant may have an anemic smile or grimace, but it connotes internal sadness rather than joy and pleasure.

Motor behavior. The depressed infant has hypomotility and motor retardation, particularly in the first 6 months of life. In the second 6 months of life, with the emergence of separation and stranger anxiety, the acutely depressed infant exhibits restlessness, agitation, and fidgetiness, in addition to hypomotility.

The motor skills acquired last will be the first to disappear. Also, there will be a delay in the development of new skills such as sitting, crawling, standing, and walking. The more prolonged the depression, the more profound the motor retardation.

Eating behavior. The depressed infant does not suck at the breast or bottle vigorously. The infant does not appear to experience pleasure and relief following eating and becomes a fussy eater. Vomiting, spitting up food, rumination, and occasionally overeating may develop if the depression continues. Lack of expected weight gain or weight loss signals a failure to thrive.

Sleep. Sleep becomes dysrhythmic. Depressed infants sleep significantly more (hypersomnia) than normal infants. This sleep is restless, with frequent whimpering. Older infants may wake up agitated and crying or regress to dysrhythmic sleep.

Lack of assertiveness and curiosity. Depressed infants lose their assertiveness and their curiosity for new experiences. They become withdrawn and resigned. This resignation, however, is different from passivity, because there is an underlying tone of sadness, depression, and apathy.

Apathy. As the depression progresses, a sober, sad facial expression is replaced with an unresponsive and vacuous expression. Apathy signals the child's profound feeling of helplessness and hopelessness. The presence of apathy is an ominous sign of anaclitic depression or failure to thrive.

Mother-child interaction. If the depression occurs in the first 6 months of life, the development of the mother-child interaction may suffer profoundly. There will be a significant fracture in the attachment behavior between the infant and mother: for instance, lack of or delay in both the recognition smile at age 4 months and stranger-separation anxiety at age 8–10 months.

The older infant (age 10–12 months) may regress and show intensified and overwhelming stranger-separation anxiety and become clingy to the mother. If depression continues, the older infant will regress further and become apathetic and unresponsive to either mother's presence or absence.

Cognitive development. Depending on when the infant becomes depressed, significant delay or regression in cognitive development such as reciprocity by age 2 months, imitative behavior by age 4 months, and object permanency by age 10–18 months occurs. Prolonged infantile depression has more profound impact on cognitive development.

Health. The depressed infant suffers from a variety of physical illnesses, such as frequent respiratory infections, vomiting, diarrhea, and weight loss. Psychophysiological disorders, such as infantile eczema, dermatitis, asthma, and a variety of food or milk allergies, are more prevalent. If the depression continues and becomes prolonged, failure to thrive with significant weight loss and, in severe cases, hospitalism will follow.

DEPRESSION: AGES 1–3 YEARS

As the depression continues and becomes more severe, the symptoms of failure to thrive may emerge. In addition to the clinical features of sensory-motor depression discussed earlier, at this age depression interferes with newly acquired developmental skills. Following the developmental psychopathology perspective, regression, developmental arrest, behavior continuity-discontinuity, and transformation of behavior occur in depressed children. Some of the age-specific clinical features of depression in children ages 1–3 years follow.

Age-Specific Clinical Features

Dysphoric mood. Dysphoric or depressed mood in infants and children ages 1–3 years may manifest as sad or expressionless face, gaze aversion, staring, and irritability (Carlson and Kashani 1988).

Motor behavior. Delay or regression occurs in standing, walking, and running.

Eating behavior. The child stops feeding himself or herself and becomes a fussy eater with a poor appetite. Indiscriminate mouthing, pica (eating everything), and frequent coprophagy (eating feces) occur and are closely associated with depression or maternal deprivation or neglect.

Sleep. The child experiences disturbances in sleep, increase in the amount of sleep, frequent wakefulness, increase of nightmares and night terrors, and occasional insomnia.

Cognitive development. There is delay in the development of symbolic thought representation.

Language. Delay or regression in language development is profound. The child is not motivated to use language and might lose some already acquired language skills temporarily until the depression is over.

Autoerotic behavior. Self-stimulating behaviors, such as masturbation, rocking, head-banging, scratching oneself, and self-biting, become predominant (Shafii and Shafii 1982a, p. 87).

Transitional object. In the early phase of depression, the child's clinging to a transitional object may greatly increase, whereas in severe depression the child may lose interest in the favorite object—a serious sign.

Negativism and oppositional behavior. Initially the child's negativistic and oppositional behavior intensifies. Later a feeling of distrust or even paranoid behavior is manifested, but this behavior decreases as the depression becomes more severe.

Toilet training. Delay or loss of bowel or bladder control occurs.

Play behavior. Interest in playing with adults or parallel play with peers decreases, and there is a loss of interest in manipulating objects and making discoveries.

Developmental and psychodynamic considerations. Depression in the subphase of rapprochement (Mahler 1972), ages 15–25 months, significantly interferes with the development of object constancy (internalization of the maternal imago, seeing good and bad qualities in the same person) and with the psychological birth of the self, which usually occurs between the ages of 25 and 36 months. In the early stages of depression, the child may become much more clinging and manifest intensified forms of separation and stranger anxiety, similar to those manifested by an infant between the ages of 8 and 10 months. These behaviors are frequently associated with intense ambivalence toward parents, such as crying outbursts, hitting, kicking, and biting, along with constant clinging and dread of separation.

The depressed child between ages 2 and 3 years may verbalize overwhelming fear of being killed or of being "eaten up" by humans or animals (intensified oral-incorporative fantasies). Nightmares often have these themes.

Depression during early childhood is closely related to the loss of the love object because the child has not internalized the maternal imago, which is referred to as object constancy. The child mourns and grieves over this loss in a pathological way. The child's grief and mourning resemble the chronic unresolved mourning of adults, which usually manifests itself in the form of clinical depression (Abraham 1927; Bowlby 1960; Freud 1917).

According to Bowlby (1960), grief and mourning in both children and adults include protest, despair, and detachment. Protest is expressed through anger, hostility, and crying. Despair is affective sadness and temporary regression and depression. Detachment is the withdrawal of the affect and love invested in the lost love object. These processes occur concomitantly and help the individual work through and come to terms with the loss. According to Bowlby, children, particularly those under age 6 years, are not able to work through a loss effectively. The mourning process in children becomes lifelong and chronic, similar to unresolved and pathological mourning in adulthood.

According to psychodynamic theory, depression in children and adults is often related to loss of the love object, loss of self-esteem, or loss of the feeling of well-being. Unresolved and untreated depression in childhood, along with lack of at least partial replacement of the love object, may lead to the development of lack of empathy, resulting in cruelty to animals and other children. Later, in adolescence and adulthood, sadistic, destructive, and occasionally homicidal behavior may be the outcome.

According to Lorenz (1966), human beings do not have innate inhibition against intraspecies destructive behavior. Only the establishment of attachment to another human being, usually the mothering person, can contain destructive tendencies. Through the establishment of the human bond, the child learns to love other human beings and to respect life (Fraiberg 1967).

Depression in the first 3 years of life may contribute to the development of a multitude of psychopathologies in later childhood, adolescence, and adulthood, such as major depression, narcissistic personality disorder, borderline psychosis, delinquency, alcohol and drug abuse, psychophysiological disorders, and psychosis.

MAJOR DEPRESSION: AGES 3–5 YEARS—PRESCHOOLERS

Major depression in children between the ages of 3 and 5 years has the greatest impact initially on developmental tasks and newly acquired skills. In a study of preschoolers ages 2–6 years, Kashani et al. (1986), using DSM-III criteria, found that 60% of depressed preschoolers versus 22% of nondepressed preschoolers had the following symptoms: sad appearance, appetite or weight changes, sleep disturbances, fatigue, hypoactivity, expressed worthlessness, and suicidal ideations. Also, depressed preschoolers were found to be more angry, less cooperative, and more apathetic. Other common symptoms were frequent crying, irritability, sulkiness, social withdrawal, refusal to go to nursery, and somatic complaints. Tables 1–1 and 1–2 show the frequency of depressive symptoms in both nonpatients and patients with MDD.

Age-Specific Clinical Features

Dysphoric mood. Dysphoric and depressed mood in children ages 3–5 years may be manifested by sad expression, somberness, or labile mood and irritability (Carlson and Kashani 1988). Overwhelming sadness, helplessness, lack of joy, and preoccupation with punishment fill the child's world. Themes of failure, hurt, destruction, and death permeate fantasy play and the world of make-believe. In the early phase of depression, omnipotent and magical fantasies may temporarily alleviate the pain of despair. As depression continues, omnipotent fantasies disappear, and themes of overwhelming failure prevail in play and fantasy.

In prolonged and severe forms of depression, the forest of fantasies becomes an empty desert of loneliness and detachment. Usually, it is so painful for these children to share their morbid fantasies with others that they keep them within; however, some may act out with aggressive and destructive behavior. When the child begins to share fantasies with a caring listener, the child is already on the road to recovery (see Chapter 7).

Motor behavior. There may be loss of interest in newly acquired skills such as running, climbing, buttoning clothes, putting on shoes, and riding a bicycle. One of the first activities to decline is involvement in group games and play with peers.

Sphincter control. The child between the ages of 5 and 6 years, who had been dry at night for some time, may become enuretic or encopretic.

Cognitive development. A decline in cognitive functions, such as interest in reading, writing, or drawing, occurs. The cognitive ability for drawing images without relying on immediate sensory input (deferred imitation) may decrease or disappear. Language ability declines. The more depressed the child becomes, the more the child will lose cognitive schemata of the preoperational stage of intelligence and rely on sensory-motor intelligence. Due to the decline in cognitive ability, the child may feel "dumb" or "stupid."

Play behavior. Play with peers decreases significantly; daydreaming and isolation increase. When parents ask the child why he or she is not playing with others, the child might burst into tears and say, "Nobody likes me," "Everybody hates me," or "Everyone says I'm stupid."

Eating behavior. There is overemphasis on food fads and loss of pleasure in eating. The fantasies of prowess from eating certain foods are replaced by apprehension about the dangers of food. Extreme weight loss may result in anorexia. Occasionally the child may gorge.

Sleep. Sleep is disturbed with frequent nightmares, night terrors, difficulties going to sleep, or awakening during the night. Nightmares may have overwhelming themes of death, destruction, threats, and danger without any hope of rescue. On occasion, dreams of denial prevail; for instance, the

Table 1–1. Frequency of depressive symptoms in nonpatient children and adolescents

Symptom	Preschoolers (%) Kashani et al. 1987 (N = 18)	School-age children (%) Kashani and Simonds 1979 (N = 103)	Adolescents (%) Teri 1982 (N = 568)	Adolescents (%) Schoenbach et al. 1982 (N = 384)	Adolescents (%) Kaplan et al. 1984 (N = 385)	Adolescents (%) Garrison et al. 1989[a] (N = 677)
Depressed mood	0		5.4	19	2.9	56
Irritability	33		14.3		8.9	59
Anhedonia	0		5			
Weight gain	0			27		
Weight loss	0		13.5	14	6.8	41
Insomnia	22		7.1	21	6.2	47
Hypersomnia				24		
Psychomotor retardation	11	3.5				
Psychomotor agitation	67	3.5				
Fatigue	0		7.2	19	2.3	61
Low self-esteem	44	11		39	2.3	65
Guilt	0		3.7		2.1	
Low concentration	55		7.2	30	7.5	78
Suicidal ideation	0		5.4		1.5	
Somatic complaints	0	9				

[a]Garrison et al. (1989) included those who felt the symptoms "some" of the time as well as "most" and "a lot" of the time. The others included only those replying "most" and "a lot" of the time.

Table 1–2. Frequency of depressive symptoms in children and adolescents with major depressive disorder

Symptom	Preschoolers (%) Kashani et al. 1987 (N = 9)	School-age children (%) Kashani and Simonds 1979 (N = 103)	Eastgate and Gilmour 1984 (N = 19)	Ryan et al. 1987 (N = 95)	Mitchell et al. 1989 (N = 45)	Adolescents (%) Carlson 1981 (N = 28)	Ryan et al. 1987 (N = 92)	Mitchell et al. 1989 (N = 50)
Depressed mood	100		100	91	95	93	88	92
Irritability	78							
Anhedonia	22			67	89	46	74	92
Weight gain	100		31	6	9	61	12	14
Weight loss	100		31	6	18		20	32
Insomnia	100		68	60	82	61	63	64
Hypersomnia				10	24		25	60
Psychomotor retardation	78	44		29	56	21	36	48
Psychomotor agitation	33	44		60	51	18	41	70
Fatigue	89		89	66	62	61	71	92
Low self-esteem	89	12	84	63	93	64	57	94
Guilt	55			33	44		33	56
Low concentration	44			75	80	82	79	82
Suicidal ideation	67			51	67	61	49	68
Somatic complaints	100	72	63	58	77	50	49	78

child dreams that he or she is happy and that he or she does not have any worries or concerns.

Nursery school. The joy of going to nursery school or kindergarten decreases or disappears. The child may cling to mother, express fear of leaving her, and manifest signs of school phobia (separation anxiety disorder).

Psychophysiological symptoms. Frequent complaints of headaches, stomachaches, or upset stomach are common. Weight loss, anorexia, asthma, dermatitis, and allergies may occur.

Suicidal and self-destructive behavior. Until recently, it was thought that depressed preschool or latency-age children did not manifest suicidal behavior. However, we have seen a number of children between the ages of 3 and 5 years who have openly verbalized suicidal ideas and death wishes and, at times, have even attempted suicide. These children have tried to hang themselves, have run deliberately in front of a car, or have jumped out of a window.

Some children do not openly verbalize suicidal ideas, but they demonstrate self-destructive behavior, in the form of severe head-banging, biting, scratching themselves severely enough to bleed, swallowing sharp objects, or becoming accident prone.

Physical abuse and neglect. Some depressed preschool children have been physically abused or neglected or have witnessed frequent physical violence at home. Kashani et al. (1986) also found that there were significantly more stressful life events (separation or divorce of parents) for depressed preschoolers than for nondepressed preschoolers. Kashani et al. (1987) also found that 100% of the depressed preschoolers versus 33% of the control preschoolers lived in broken homes and that 100% versus 22% had been abused or severely neglected. This study suggests a strong relationship in preschoolers between physical abuse and neglect and depressive symptoms.

Psychodynamic considerations. According to psychodynamic theory, during the phallic-oedipal phase, ages 3–6 years, emerging castration anxiety may become fused with depressive affect. In the early phase of depression, the irrational dread of bodily injury and autoerotic behavior significantly intensify. As the depression increases in intensity and duration, the child regresses further, giving up phallic-oedipal strivings of triangular relationships and retreating to the earlier dyadic relationship. Anal and oral behavior become more predominant.

MAJOR DEPRESSION: AGES 6–12 YEARS— SCHOOL-AGE CHILD

Most studies of childhood depression are reports on school-age (latency) children or adolescents. This is probably because mental health clinicians have more contact with these age groups. The child of this age is more verbal and can share depressive feelings with others. Frequently, teachers are the first to notice the child's persistent sadness, poor performance, withdrawal, and daydreaming. Parents are often unable to recognize their child's depression or tend to minimize or deny it.

Clinical Features

Symptoms of depression in children between the ages of 6 and 12 years are somewhat similar to those in adults. According to Poznanski (1982), depressed mood is the most important symptom in the clinical diagnosis of depression in school-age children: "The distinction between an unhappy child and a depressed child can be made in part by determining the duration of the child's downcast mood" (p. 309). The inability to have fun (anhedonia) is also a common symptom. When a child describes being bored 50–90% of the time, he or she may be depressed. When depressed, children will also tend to have a low opinion of themselves, describing themselves as "stupid" or "not popular," although, according to Poznanski (1982), it is difficult to obtain consistent and reliable information from children concerning self-esteem. Poor school performance, another major symptom, might be related to a lack of concentration. Eating and sleep disturbances, hypoactivity, retardation of speech and language, excessive fatigue, morbid ideation, suicidal ideation with and without a plan, and suicide attempts are common symptoms of depression.

Kashani et al. (1983) also noted the presence of headache, fighting, general disobedience, worrying, and irritability. Altmann and Gotlib (1988) found that depressed school-age children spent more time alone than nondepressed children, were more socially withdrawn, and showed more negative and aggressive behavior when interacting with peers. Surprisingly, they also found that these depressed school-age children initiated a greater number of interactions with others than their nondepressed peers. Also, depressed children were approached by others more frequently. According to Kashani et al. (1983) and Lefkowitz et al. (1985), there was no significant association between either sex or socioeconomic status and depression in this age group. Mother's rejection correlated significantly with the child's depressive syndrome (Lefkowitz et al. 1985; Poznanski and Zrull 1970). (See Tables 1–1 and 1–2.)

Age-specific clinical features are as follows.

Dysphoric mood. Dysphoric mood and depressive affect express themselves in morbid fantasies. Depressive themes such as "thwarting, blame or criticism, loss and abandonment, personal injury, death, and suicide" predominate in the child's play, dreams, and daydreams (Cytryn and McKnew 1979, p. 330).

These depressive themes play a significant role in the development and sustenance of depression. In some children, they are the only evidence of depression, as outward appearance and behavior may not be affected.

Cognitive development and school performance. Disturbances in academic performance and peer relationships in school are some of the earliest signs of depression in the school-age child. Loss of interest, lack of motivation, and decline in cognitive functioning all directly affect school performance. The most newly acquired or the weakest academic area is the most vulnerable. For instance, reading disturbances in an average or below-average child, or overwhelming apprehension and fear of failure in a bright child, might be early signs of depression. Obsessive preoccupation with schoolwork, undue concern about performance, and lack of pleasure in achievement may also be early signs of depression.

Decline of school performance in a bright child who had previously been performing well should be taken seriously. Also, a change in behavior, such as clowning in a formerly quiet child or withdrawal in a previously outgoing child, may also be a sign of depression.

Motor behavior. In most children who are depressed, hypomotility, fidgetiness, agitation, clumsiness, and accident-proneness are common. Some children, because of their temperament, exhibit hyperactive behavior or aggressive and disruptive behavior in school. Symptoms of hyperactivity, along with a decline in cognitive function, are often misdiagnosed as attention-deficit disorder. Careful attention to the presence of dysphoric mood, depressive affect, and low self-esteem will help in the accurate diagnosis of depression.

Guilt. With the further development of the superego and the cognitive development of morality, the depressed child becomes extremely self-critical. The child feels guilty about everything he or she says, does, or thinks about. The child may apologize over and over without relief or become oversolicitous, ingratiating, and "too kind" to others (the defense of reaction formation). Because of low self-esteem and overwhelming guilt, depressed children seek constant reassurance and praise. But, at the same time, undue reassurance and praise reinforce their guilt feelings and become ineffective. Judicious support and praise, properly timed, can be effective.

Expression of hostility and aggression. Because of overt inhibition, overcontrol, and hypomotility, aggressive impulses and hostile feelings are repressed. The depressed child unconsciously turns these aggressive and destructive feelings against the self. Overwhelming feelings of guilt, self-depreciation, and self-destructive behavior are manifestations of this pathological process.

The more the child is able to directly express aggressive and hostile feelings, either verbally or through play, the better will be the hope for recovery. Encouragement of physical activity and body motility channels repressed aggressive tendencies in a sublimated and effective manner. (See Chapters 7, 8, and 9.)

Suicidal behavior. In recent years, there has been an increase in the prevalence of suicidal behavior in younger children. Out of 340 children and adolescents referred for suicidal behavior to the Child Psychiatric Services, University of Louisville School of Medicine, 43% were age 12 years and younger (Shafii et al. 1979).

Active suicidal ideation and suicidal attempts have become prevalent. During recent years in the Louisville, Kentucky, area, the youngest child who committed suicide was 10 years of age. Nationally, there are more than 140 suicides in this age group annually. It is a tragedy that many clinicians still believe that suicidal behavior in the form of suicide attempts or actual suicide is rare in this age group. In children and adolescents, suicidal ideation, messages, behavior, and attempts must be taken seriously.

Psychodynamic considerations. The depressed school-age child loses interest in friendships and associations. According to psychodynamic theory, the child regresses to the early phallic-oedipal stage, with increased evidence of castration anxiety. If the depression continues, there is further regression to anal or oral behaviors.

Industry and enthusiasm for the development of skills give way to feelings of inferiority and self-doubt. Ambivalence (love and hate feelings) may predominate in the child's relationship with the parents. Because of the child's ability to experience guilt more intensely, ambivalence constantly torments the child and interferes with functioning.

DEPRESSION IN ADOLESCENCE: AGES 12–18 YEARS

Clinical Features

Developmentally, normal adolescents have a proclivity toward depression. It is important to clearly and carefully differentiate the normal depressive mood swings of adolescence from pathological depression. This differentiation taxes the ability of even experienced clinicians.

According to Carlson (1981), the symptoms of adolescent depression are difficult to distinguish from "adolescent turmoil." Thus, adolescent depression has been underdiagnosed. Frequently, psychiatrically ill adolescents become psychiatrically ill adults.

Carlson (1981) divides adolescent depression into primary and secondary types. Primary means that there was no preexisting psychiatric disorder before the current illness, and secondary means that the current illness is associated with a previous psychiatric disorder. According to Carlson, adolescents with secondary depressive disorder are more disturbed, are significantly more aggressive, have excessive somatic complaints, and more commonly manifest irritability, hopelessness, suicidal ideation, sleep problems, decreased school performance, low self-esteem, and disobedience.

Kaplan et al. (1984) gave the Beck Depression Inventory (BDI) (Beck 1967) to 385 junior and senior high school students. They found that age has a significant influence on depressive symptomatology. Eleven- to 13-year-olds had fewer depressive symptoms than 14- to 16-year-olds or 17- to 18-year-olds, except for two symptoms—regarding the self unattractive and losing weight on purpose. They also found that females did not have more symptoms. However, more females than males felt unattractive and fatigued, lost weight, and tried to lose weight on purpose. On the other hand, Teri (1982), who administered the BDI to 568 students in grades 9–12, found that there were more females than males in a group that had a high depression score.

Kandel and Davies (1982) administered a 90-item symptom checklist to 8,206 adolescents ages 14–18 years in public schools and made diagnoses according to DSM-III criteria. These investigators reported that "there were no meaningful differences on any of the . . . factors: age, race, religion, or social class status . . ." (p. 1207). However, they did find that adolescents from families with incomes below $3,000 were more depressed than any other group. They also found that those adolescents who were more peer-oriented (versus parent-oriented) and who had more delinquent tendencies were more depressed.

Schoenbach et al. (1982) surveyed 384 young adolescents to assess depressive symptoms. Compared with normal adolescents, depressed adolescents had more restless sleep, could not get going, had trouble concentrating, did not enjoy life, had crying spells, felt sad, and had hyposomnia. (See Tables 1–1 and 1–2.)

The major age-specific clinical features are as follows.

Dysphoric mood and depressive affect. The normal mood swings of adolescence are significantly intensified, and sadness and dysphoric mood are more commonly experienced. Volatile moods prevail, and the proclivity toward rage reactions increases. Adolescents are vulnerable to depressive disorders. The symptoms of depression in adolescence are similar to those in adulthood.

Puberty. The emergence of puberty may be delayed in a chronically depressed early adolescent, particularly if the depression is associated with weight loss and anorexia. The depressed adolescent may have great difficulty accepting or understanding the signs of puberty. Self-consciousness and self-doubt are intensified. A flood of hormonal secretions, along with a stressful environment, may plunge the adolescent into the depths of depression and possibly suicidal behavior.

Wet dreams and incestuous dreams add an extra burden to the already guilt-ridden depressed adolescent. The menstrual period of depressed adolescent females may be delayed, irregular, or associated with exaggerated pain and discomfort. Dysphoric moods are intensified during the premenstrual period. Depressed adolescent females may feel "blue," "down in the dumps," cry without provocation, become sulky and pouty, isolate themselves in their rooms, and sleep much longer.

Cognitive development. Temporary disorganization of cognitive functioning in pubescence becomes significantly exaggerated in depressed adolescents. In younger adolescents, the development of abstract thinking, which usually occurs around 12 years of age, is delayed. In older adolescents, this newly acquired ability decreases or disappears.

School performance is frequently affected. If an adolescent is doing well in school and suddenly his or her performance declines, depression should be considered as one of the possible factors. Skipping school, procrastination in finishing assignments, irritable behavior in the classroom, and lack of concern about achievement and future vocation can also be early signs of depression in adolescents.

In depressed adolescents, concrete thinking, withdrawal, isolation, and low energy level may give the impression of a schizoid personality or of an early form of schizophrenia. This misperception is one of the most common errors made in diagnosing depression in adolescents.

Self-esteem. Low self-esteem is one of the significant contributors to depression throughout life. In adolescents, depression intensifies low self-esteem. Depressed adolescents feel internally that they have failed themselves and others. Hopelessness and helplessness lower the self-esteem further, and a vicious cycle ensues. At times, the depressed adolescent tries to defend against low self-esteem by denial, by omnipotent fantasies, or by escaping from reality through the use of drugs and alcohol.

Antisocial behavior. Skipping school, stealing, fighting, and frequent driving tickets or accidents, particularly in an adolescent with a former history of good behavior, may be indicators of depression.

Alcohol and drug abuse. A large number of depressed adolescents abuse alcohol/drugs. Use of marijuana, "uppers" (amphetamines, mood-elevating drugs), "downers" (barbiturates, tranquilizers, sleep-inducing agents), and particularly alcohol is common. Some of these adolescents use cocaine, heroin, or other narcotic derivatives or hallucinogens.

Studies by Johnston (1981) at the University of Michigan of 17,000 high school seniors in the United States found that, although the daily use of marijuana had decreased by 12%, still nearly 10% smoked marijuana daily. Alarmingly, 65% reported that they have used some type of illicit drug during their lifetime. There is evidence of decline in the use of hallucinogens, uppers, downers, and cocaine. However, the use of alcohol has increased.

Further epidemiological studies are needed to determine what percentage of adolescents who regularly use alcohol and drugs are depressed.

Sexual behavior. Generally, depressed adolescents do not show interest in dating or heterosexual interactions. However, some depressed adolescents become involved in sexual acting out or even promiscuity as a defense against depression. Promiscuity in depressed adolescents frequently has a self-deprecating quality. Many adolescents do not take precautions to prevent pregnancy or venereal disease. Some wish to become pregnant to compensate for object loss or low self-esteem. Depressed adolescents might marry early to escape family conflicts. Often, these marriages do not work out and reinforce depression.

Health. Depressed adolescents appear pale and tired and lack the vigor and joy of youth. Frequently, these adolescents have a multitude of physical complaints, such as headaches, stomachaches, lack of appetite, and weight loss without any organic cause. Because the depressed adolescent does not usually verbalize feelings, physical symptoms may often be the only route of coming in contact with a clinician. The clinician's sensitivity in picking up clues of dysphoric mood or depression may prevent an adolescent's suicide.

Weight. A decrease in the velocity of weight gain or a loss of weight could indicate depression. At the same time, low self-esteem and lack of self-care may contribute to overeating and obesity.

Suicidal behavior. Some adolescents, because of dysphoric mood and mercurial self-esteem, occasionally have thoughts of committing suicide. Usually, these suicidal thoughts are fleeting, not well organized, and without a definite plan. Depressed adolescents are highly vulnerable to suicide. In a recent survey of 5,500 freshman and senior high school students in Kentucky, 30% reported that they had seriously thought about attempting suicide in the past 12 months, 19% had a specific plan for committing suicide, and 11% had attempted suicide (Jennings 1990). In the Louisville area, we found a significant increase in actual suicide in adolescents during a 5-year period. In early adolescence, there was more than an 80% increase in the suicide rate, and in late adolescence there was more than a 100% increase (Shafii et al. 1985).

Suicide is the third leading major cause of death in adolescents, following accidents and cancer. Most adolescents commit suicide through violent means. In the Louisville study of 60 child and adolescent suicides, 57% used firearms. Many of these adolescents showed signs of depression and an increase in drug and alcohol use. Almost all of them had verbalized suicidal ideas prior to committing suicide. Some had attempted suicide earlier. Unfortunately, 82% of this group had never received psychiatric help.

It is of the utmost importance for the clinician to take the symptoms of depression, suicidal ideas, "gestures," or attempts in children and adolescents seriously. The management of a suicidal adolescent is in some ways similar to the management of an abused child. The clinician should mobilize all resources to help the family and the adolescent. Consultation with a child psychiatrist or a psychiatrist who is qualified to work with adolescents is essential. Postponing, delaying, or waiting to "see what happens" may cost a young person's life. (See Chapters 5, 7, and 11.)

COMORBIDITY

With the use of structured and semistructured interviews (see Chapter 6) and DSM criteria, the research clinician frequently finds that a particular patient fulfills the diagnostic criteria for more than one psychiatric disorder. This situation is referred to as comorbidity. Usually it is difficult to determine which disorder came first. Kovacs et al. (1984a, 1984b) observed that 79% of school-age children with MDD had concurrent illnesses: dysthymia-double depression (38%), anxiety disorder (33%), and conduct disorder (7%). They also noticed that 93% of patients with dysthymic disorder had other coexisting disorders such as MDD (57%), anxiety disorder (36%), attention-deficit disorder (14%), and conduct disorder (11%).

Ryan et al. (1987) found that 16% of preadolescent patients and 11% of adolescents with MDD also had conduct disorders. These investigators also noticed that 45% of children and 27% of adolescents with MDD had phobias with avoidance.

Kashani et al. (1987) found that of the 4.7% of adolescents in the general population who had the diagnosis of MDD (see Chapter 2), 100% also had a diagnosis of dysthymia. These adolescents also had an additional diagnosis, such as anxiety disorder (75%), oppositional disorder (50%), conduct disorder (33%), alcohol abuse (25%), and drug abuse (25%).

In psychological autopsies of completed suicide in children and adolescents, Shafii et al. (1984, 1985, 1988) found that 95% of the suicide victims had a diagnosable psychiatric disorder, compared to 48% of the control group. Of the suicide victims, 81% had a comorbid diagnosis—76% had MDD and/or dysthymia associated with conduct disorder and/or alcohol and drug abuse, compared to 29% of the controls. In an unpublished study of 350 children and adolescents who were hospitalized in a psychiatric inpatient service, we found that twice as many children and adolescents had MDD and dysthymia with a comorbid diagnosis of other psychiatric disorders (particularly conduct, oppositional, and attention-deficit hyperactivity disorders or alcohol and drug abuse) than had only the diagnosis of MDD and/or dysthymia.

Most of these studies also show that the intensity, severity, duration, chronicity, relapse, and suicide risk are significantly greater in depressed children and adolescents with a comorbid diagnosis than they are in children and adolescents without comorbidity.

CLINICAL COURSE AND FOLLOW-UP

Poznanski and Zrull (1970) reported on the clinical manifestation of depressive disorders in children and adolescents. In addition to having depressive symptoms, these children were prone to violent temper tantrums, fighting, biting, and destructive behavior. In a reevaluation follow-up study 6 ½ years later, Poznanski found that 50% of these patients were overtly depressed, although none of them showed aggressive or violent behavior (Poznanski et al. 1976; Poznanski 1980, 1982). Many of the subjects did not perform well academically. As the group reached adulthood, the depressive disorders resembled those of adults, supporting the idea that depression in children and adolescents may persist and express itself similarly to adult forms of depression.

Kovacs et al.'s follow-up study (1984a, 1984b) also showed that children with MDD were unlikely to recover within the first 3 months of their episode. They found that if a child does not go into remission by 1½ years from the onset of MDD (when the maximal recovery rate is 92%), recovery is not likely during the following year. Dysthymic disorder had the longest recovery time: 6 years to reach the maximal recovery rate of 89%. Adjustment disorder with depressed mood showed a more favorable recovery rate, with 90% recovering by 9 months after the original diagnosis.

Eastgate et al. (1984) followed 19 depressed children and adolescents, ages 5–14 years. Seven to 8 years later, they found only 1 patient enrolled in a university, and 6 of the 19 had had four or more different jobs since leaving school. The researchers also noticed that the patients frequently reported being sad/depressed, irritable, and tired; they had trouble concentrating; and they were preoccupied with death and suicide. Carlson (1981) observed that "youngsters with good premorbid adjustment and supportive families have better outcomes than the converse" (p. 417).

Harrington et al. (1990) in London reported on an 18-year follow-up of 52 matched pairs of children and adolescents with depressive syndrome compared with nondepressed psychiatric controls. They found cumulative probability of adult depression in the depressed group to be 0.6 compared to 0.27 in the control group. The depressed group had a high risk of hospitalization and use of psychotropic medication. Also, 37% of the depressed group versus 12% of the control group had made at least one suicide attempt during adulthood. In both groups the researchers noticed that although mood disorders were the most common, nonmood psychiatric disorders were also quite prevalent—85% in the depressed group versus 75% in the controls. The authors concluded that there was significant continuity between depression in childhood and depression in adulthood. At the same time, they observed that depressed children were not more likely than controls to have other psychiatric disorders.

From all of these studies, it is clear that MDD and dysthymia in children and adolescents are not acute disorders with a short duration. MDDs and dysthymia may manifest acutely but soon become chronic with or without cyclic episodes.

Depressive disorders in children and adolescents can be a common pathway for expression of other psychiatric disorders such as conduct disorder, alcohol and drug abuse, bipolar disorder (see Chapters 12 and 13), or suicide. Depressive disorders could be conceptualized as similar to a metabolic disorder such as diabetes mellitus in that genetic and environmental factors contribute significantly to the clinical manifestation of the disorder. Effective management and treatment can significantly alleviate the symptoms of the disorder, but the underlying neurobiological, genetic, developmental, and environmental factors continue to exist.

REFERENCES

Abraham K: Notes on the psychoanalytic investigation and treatment of manic-depressive insanity and allied conditions (1911), in Selected Papers on Psychoanalysis. Translated by Bryan D, Strachey A. New York, Basic Books, 1968, pp 137–156

Abraham K: The first pregenital stage of the libido (1916), in Selected Papers on Psychoanalysis. Translated by Bryan D, Strachey A. New York, Basic Books, 1968, pp 248–279

Abraham K: A short study of the development of the libido, viewed in the light of mental disorders (1924), in Selected Papers on Psychoanalysis. Translated by Bryan D, Strachey A. New York, Basic Books, 1968, pp 418–501

Altmann EO, Gotlib IH: The social behavior of depressed children: an observational study. J Abnorm Child Psychol 16(1):29–44, 1988

American Psychiatric Association: Diagnostic and Statistical Manual of Mental Disorders, 3rd Edition. Washington, DC, American Psychiatric Association, 1980

American Psychiatric Association: Diagnostic and Statistical Manual of Mental Disorders, 3rd Edition, Revised. Washington, DC, American Psychiatric Association, 1987

Annel AL: Depressive States in Children and Adolescents. New York, Halstead Press, 1972

Anthony E: Two contrasting types of adolescent depression and their treatment. J Am Psychoanal Assoc 18:841–859, 1970

Anthony EJ: Affective disorders in children and adolescents with special emphasis on depression, in Depression: Biology, Psychodynamics and Treatment. Edited by Cole J, Schatzberg A, Frazier S. New York, Plenum, 1978, pp 173–184

Anthony EJ, Scott P: Manic-depressive psychosis in childhood. J Child Psychol Psychiatry 1:53–72, 1960

Beck AT: Depression: Clinical, Experimental, and Theoretical Aspects. New York, Harper & Row, 1967

Bowlby J: Forty-Four Juvenile Thieves. London, Bailliere, Tindall & Cox, 1946

Bowlby J: Maternal Care and Mental Health. Geneva, World Health Organization Monograph, 1951

Bowlby J: Grief and mourning in infancy and early childhood. Psychoanal Study Child 15:9–52, 1960

Brazelton TB, Young GC, Bullowa M: Inception and resolution of early developmental pathology, in Infant Psychiatry, A New Synthesis. Edited by Rexford EN, Sander W, Shapiro T. New Haven, CT, Yale University Press, 1971, pp 301–310

Brumback RA, Weinberg WA: Childhood depression: an exploration of a behavior disorder of children. Percept Mot Skills 44:911–916, 1977

Cannon WB, de la Paz D: Emotional stimulation of adrenal secretion. Am J Physiol 28:64, 1911

Cantwell D, Carlson G: Problems and prospects in the study of childhood depression. J Nerv Ment Dis 167:522–529, 1979

Carlson GA: The phenomenology of adolescent depression. Adolesc Psychiatry 9:411–421, 1981

Carlson GA, Kashani JH: Phenomenology of major depression from childhood through adulthood: analysis of three studies. Am J Psychiatry 145:1222–1225, 1988

Cytryn L: Proposed classification of childhood depression. Am J Psychiatry 129:149–155, 1972

Cytryn L, McKnew D: Factors influencing the changing clinical expression of the depressive process in children. Am J Psychiatry 131:879–881, 1974

Cytryn L, McKnew DH: Affective disorders, in Basic Handbook of Child Psychiatry, Vol 2. New York, Basic Books, 1979, pp 321–341

Cytryn L, McKnew D, Bunney W Jr: Diagnosis of depression in children: a reassessment. Am J Psychiatry 137:22–25, 1980

Dorpat TL: Depressive affect. Psychoanal Study Child 32:3–27, 1977

Eastgate J, Gilmour L: Long-term outcome of depressed children: a follow-up study. Dev Med Child Neurol 26:68–72, 1984

Emde RN, Polak PR, Spitz R: Anaclitic depression in an infant raised in an institution. J Am Acad Child Psychiatry 4:545–553, 1965

Engel GL, Reichsman F, Segal HL: A study of an infant with a gastric fistula. Psychosom Med 18:374–398, 1956

Fraiberg S: The origins of human bonds, in Commentary (journal). New York, American Jewish Committee, 1967, pp 1–12

Fraiberg S: Parallel and divergent patterns in blind and sighted infants. Psychoanal Study Child 23:264–300, 1968

Fraiberg S: Every Child's Birthright: In Defense of Mothering. New York, Basic Books, 1977

Fraiberg S, Freedman DA: Studies in ego development of the congenitally blind child. Psychoanal Study Child 19:113–169, 1964

Freud S: Mourning and melancholia (1917), in The Standard Edition of the Complete Psychological Works of Sigmund Freud, Vol 14. Translated and edited by Strachey J. London, Hogarth Press, 1968, pp 239–258

Freud S: The ego and the id (1923), in The Standard Edition of the Complete Psychological Works of Sigmund Freud, Vol 19. Translated and edited by Strachey J. London, Hogarth Press, 1968, pp 3–66

Freud S: Inhibitions, symptoms and anxiety (1926), in The Standard Edition of the Complete Psychological Works of Sigmund Freud, Vol 20. Translated and edited by Strachey J. London, Hogarth Press, 1968, pp 1–307

Freud S: Splitting of the ego in the process of defense (1938), in The Standard Edition of the Complete Psychological Works of Sigmund Freud, Vol 23. Translated and edited by Strachey J. London, Hogarth Press, 1968, pp 271–278

Garrison CZ, Schluchter MK, Schoenbach VJ, et al: Epidemiology of depressive symptoms in young adolescents. J Am Acad Child Adolesc Psychiatry 28(3):343–351, 1989

Geller B, Perel JM, Knitter EF, et al: Nortriptyline in major depressive disorder in children: response, steady-state plasma levels, predictive kinetics, and pharmacokinetics. Psychopharmacol Bull 19:62–65, 1983a

Geller B, Rogol AD, Knitter EF, et al: Preliminary data on the dexamethasone suppression test in children with major depressive disorder. Am J Psychiatry 140:620–622, 1983b

Glaser K: Masked depression in children and adolescents. Am J Psychother 21:565–574, 1967

Harrington R, Fudge H, Rutter M, et al: Adult outcomes of childhood and adolescent depression, I: psychiatric status. Arch Gen Psychiatry 47:465–473, 1990

Harlow HF: The nature of love. Am Psychol 13:673–685, 1958

Harlow HF: Love in infant monkeys. Sci Am 200:68–74, 1959

Harlow HF: Primary affectional patterns in primates. Am J Orthopsychiatry 30:676–684, 1960

Harmon RJ, Wagonfeld S, Emde RN: Anaclitic depression—a follow-up from infancy to puberty. Psychoanal Study Child 37:67–94, 1982

Jennings M: Students' replies on sex, suicide, alcohol alarm education chief. Courier-Journal (Louisville, KY), Nov 13, 1990, pp 1, 10

Johnston L: in International Herald Tribune 30(484):3 (Feb 20, 1981)

Kandel DB, Davies M: Epidemiology of depressive mood in adolescents. Arch Gen Psychiatry 39:1205–1212, 1982

Kaplan S, Hong G, Weinhold C: Epidemiology of depressive symptomatology in adolescents. J Am Acad Child Psychiatry 23(1):91–98, 1984

Kashani J, Simonds JF: The incidence of depression in children. Am J Psychiatry 136:1203–1205, 1979

Kashani JH, McGee RO, Clarkson S, et al: Depression in a sample of 9-year-old children: prevalence and associated characteristics. Gen Psychiatry 40(11): 1217–1223, 1983

Kashani JH, Holcomb WR, Orvaschel H: Depression and depressive symptoms in preschool children from the general population. Am J Psychiatry 143: 1138–1143, 1986

Kashani JH, Carlson GA, Beck NC, et al: Depression, depressive symptoms, and depressed mood among a community sample of adolescents. Am J Psychiatry 144:931–934, 1987

Kazdin AE: Evaluation of the pleasure scale in the assessment of anhedonia in children. J Am Acad Child Adolesc Psychiatry 28(3):364–372, 1989

Kazdin AE, Rodgers A, Colbus D: The Hopelessness Scale for Children: psychometric characteristics and concurrent validity. J Consult Clin Psychol 54(2):241–245, 1986

Klein M: The psycho-analytic play technique: its history and significance, in New Directions in Psychoanalysis. Edited by Klein M, Heinmann P, Money-Kyrle RE. New York, Basic Books, 1957, pp 3–22

Kovacs M: Rating scales to assess depression in school-aged children. Acta Paedopsychiatr 46(5–6):305–315, 1980/1981

Kovacs M, Beck A: An empirical-clinical approach toward a definition of childhood depression, in Depression in Childhood. Edited by Schulterbrandt JG, Raskin A. New York, Raven, 1977, pp 4, 8–9

Kovacs M, Feinberg TL, Crouse-Novak MA, et al: Depressive disorders in childhood, I. Arch Gen Psychiatry 41:229–237, 1984a

Kovacs M, Feinberg TL, Crouse-Novak MA, et al: Depressive disorders in childhood, II. Arch Gen Psychiatry 41:643–649, 1984b

Lefkowitz MM, Tesiny EP: Depression in children: prevalence and correlates. J Consult Clin Psychol 53(5):647–656, 1985

Lorenz K: On Aggression. New York, Harcourt, Brace & World, 1966, p 159

Mahler M: On the first three subphases of the separation-individuation process. Int J Psychoanal 53:333–338, 1972

Malmquist C: Depressions in childhood and adolescence (Part One). N Engl J Med 284:887–893, 1971

Mitchell J, McCauley E, Burke P, et al: Psychopathology in parents of depressed children and adolescents. J Am Acad Child Adolesc Psychiatry 28(3):352–357, 1989

Nurcombe B, Seifer R, Sciole A, et al: Is major depressive disorder in adolescence a distinct diagnostic entity? J Am Acad Child Adolesc Psychiatry 28(3):333–342, 1989

Phillips I: Childhood depression: interpersonal interactions and depressive phenomena. Am J Psychiatry 136:511–515, 1979

Piaget J: The stages of the intellectual development of the child. Bull Menninger Clin 26:120–128, 1962

Poznanski E: Childhood depression: the outcome. Acta Paedopsychiatr 46:297–304, 1980

Poznanski EO: The clinical phenomenology of childhood depression. Am J Orthopsychiatry 52(2):308–313, 1982

Poznanski E, Zrull J: Childhood depression, clinical characteristics of overtly depressed children. Arch Gen Psychiatry 23:8–15, 1970

Poznanski EO, Krahenbuhl V, Zrull JP: Childhood depression. J Am Acad Child Psychiatry 15(3):491–501, 1976

Puig-Antich J, Novacenko H, Davies M, et al: Growth hormone secretion in prepubertal children with major depression, I: final report on response. Arch Gen Psychiatry 41:455–460, 1984a

Puig-Antich J, Goetz R, Davies M, et al: Growth hormone secretion in prepubertal children with major depression, II: sleep-related plasma. Arch Gen Psychiatry 41:463–466, 1984b

Puig-Antich J, Novacenko H, Davies M, et al: Growth hormone secretion in prepubertal children with major depression, III: response to insulin-induced hypoglycemia after recovery from a depressive episode and in a drug-free state. Arch Gen Psychiatry 41:471–475, 1984c

Puig-Antich J, Goetz R, Davies M, et al: Growth hormone secretion in prepubertal children with major depression, IV: sleep-related plasma. Arch Gen Psychiatry 41:479–493, 1984d

Puig-Antich J, Lukens E, Davies M, et al: Psychosocial functioning in prepubertal major depressive disorders. Arch Gen Psychiatry 42:511–517, 1985

Reinhart JB: Failure to thrive, in Basic Handbook of Child Psychiatry, Vol 2. Edited by Noshpitz J. New York, Basic Books, 1979, pp 593–599

Rie HE: Depression in childhood: a survey of some pertinent contributions. J Am Acad Child Psychiatry 5:653–685, 1966

Robertson J: Mother-infant interaction from birth to twelve months: 2 case studies, in Determinants of Infant Behaviour, Vol 3. London, Methuen, 1965, pp 111–127

Rochlin G: The loss complex: a contribution to the etiology of depression. J Am Psychoanal Assoc 7:299–316, 1959

Ryan ND, Puig-Antich J, Ambrosini P, et al: The clinical picture of major depression in children and adolescents. Arch Gen Psychiatry 44(10):854–861, 1987

Sandler J, Joffe W: Notes on obsessional manifestations in children. Psychoanal Study Child 20:425–438, 1965

Schoenbach VJ, Kaplan BH, Grimson RC, et al: Use of a symptom scale to study the prevalence of a depressive syndrome in young adolescents. Am J Epidemiology 116(5):791–800, 1982

Selye H: The general adaptation syndrome and the diseases of adaptation. J Clin Endocrinol 6:117, 1946

Selye H: The Physiology and Pathology of Exposure to Stress. Montreal, Acta, 1950

Shafii M, Shafii SL: Depression in infancy, childhood, and adolescence: failure in human contact, sadness, and withdrawal, in Pathways of Human Development. New York, Thieme-Stratton, 1982a, pp 77–95

Shafii M, Shafii SL: Self-destructive, suicidal behavior, and completed suicide, in Pathways of Human Development. New York, Thieme-Stratton, 1982b, pp 164–180

Shafii M, Whittinghill R, Healy M: The pediatric-psychiatric model for emergencies in child psychiatry: a study of 994 cases. Am J Psychiatry 136:1600–1601, 1979

Shafii M, Whittinghill JR, Dolen DC, et al: Psychological reconstruction of completed suicide in childhood and adolescents, in Suicide in the Young. Edited by Sudak H, Ford AB, Rushforth NB. Boston, MA, John Wright PSG, 1984, pp 271–294

Shafii M, Carrigan SP, Whittinghill JR, et al: Psychological autopsy of completed suicide in children and adolescents. Am J Psychiatry 142:1061–1064, 1985

Shafii M, Steltz-Lenarksky J, Derrick AM, et al: Comorbidity of mental disorders in the postmortem diagnosis of completed suicide in children and adolescents. J Affective Disord 15:227–233, 1988

Shafii M, Foster MB, Greenberg RA, et al: Pineal gland and depressive disorders in children and adolescents, in Biological Rhythms, Mood Disorders, Light Therapy, and the Pineal Gland. Edited by Shafii M, Shafii SL. Washington, DC, American Psychiatric Press, 1990, pp 97–116

Smart MS, Taylor RW: Depression and recovery at 9 weeks of age. J Am Acad Child Psychiatry 12:506–510, 1973

Spitz RA: Hospitalism. Psychoanal Study Child 1:53–74, 1945

Spitz RA: Anaclitic depression: an inquiry into the genesis of psychiatric conditions in early childhood, II. Psychoanal Study Child 2:313–342, 1946

Spitz RA: The First Year of Life. New York, International Universities Press, 1965

Spitz RA, Wolf K: The smiling response: a contribution to the ontogenesis of social relations. Genet Psychol Monogr 34:57–125, 1946

Sroufe LA, Rutter M: The domain of developmental psychology. Child Dev 55:17–29, 1984

Teri L: The use of the Beck Depression Inventory with adolescents. J Abnorm Child Psychol 10(2):277–284, 1982

Trad PV: Infant Depression: Paradigms and Paradoxes. New York, Springer-Verlag, 1986

Tronick E, Als H, Adamson L, et al: The infant's response to entrapment between contradictory messages in face-to-face interaction. J Am Acad Child Psychiatry 17:1–13, 1978

Weinberg WA, Rutman J, Sullivan L, et al: Depression in children referred to an education diagnostic center: diagnosis and treatment. J Pediatr 83:1065–1072, 1973

Weller EB, Weller RA, Fristad MA, et al: The dexamethasone suppression test in hospitalized prepubertal depressed children. Am J Psychiatry 141:290–291, 1984

Weller EB, Weller RA, Fristad MA, et al: Dexamethasone suppression test and clinical outcome. Am J Psychiatry 143:1469–1470, 1986

Welner A, Welner Z, Fishman R: Psychiatric adolescent inpatients—eight-to-ten-year follow-up. Arch Gen Psychiatry 36:698–700, 1979

Wisdom JO: A phase of depression in a six-months-old boy. Int J Psychoanal 58:375–377, 1977

CHAPTER 2

Epidemiology and Etiology of Depressive Disorders

Javad H. Kashani, M.D.
Lynette S. Schmid, M.D.

The use of epidemiology in psychiatry is rapidly evolving into a complex field with far-reaching ramifications for the future. Simply put, epidemiologists try to identify who gets which disease where, when, and why. Possible etiologic risk factors are generated and used to form hypotheses that in turn are tested in research studies for their potential validity. Ultimately, the conclusions drawn from epidemiological research become the basis for primary, secondary, and tertiary prevention.

The development of reliable diagnostic criteria for depressive disorders in children and adolescents has made it possible to carry out meaningful epidemiological studies in this area. From the National Institute of Mental Health Epidemiologic Catchment Area Studies, we know that the 6-month prevalence of depressive disorders in adults ages 18 years and older is 5.7% (Myers et al. 1984; Weissman and Myers 1978). This makes depression one of the most common psychiatric disorders in adults. We need to look at depression and other mood disorders in children and adolescents to determine what, if any, relationship they hold to adult depression.

In this chapter we will review epidemiological research on childhood and adolescent depressive disorders, including prevalence, possible risk factors, completed longitudinal follow-up studies, and the implications that these findings have for prevention, treatment strategies, and future research studies.

PREVALENCE

One of the basic building blocks of epidemiology is the measurement of how frequently a disease occurs. This measurement is expressed in terms of incidence or prevalence. Prevalence is a measurement of the number of actual cases present either at a particular point in time (point prevalence) or over a specified time period (period prevalence). Incidence, on the other hand, is concerned with the number of new cases occurring over a period of time. Studies looking at the prevalence and incidence of mental disorders are important in facilitating our understanding of the natural course of these illnesses and in generating potential risk factors that may have causal links.

The study of the epidemiological aspects of childhood and adolescent mood disorders has lagged behind that of adults. In earlier literature, most studies reported overall emotional and behavioral impairment (Kashani 1982). In the current literature, the prevalence of mood disorders varies depending on the criteria used and the population studied.

Mood disorders may be divided into two broad categories: bipolar disorders and depressive disorders. Bipolar disorders consist of mania or hypomania alternating with depressive symptoms; a milder form is cyclothymia, consisting of hypomania alternating with periods of depressed mood of at least 1 year's duration. Depressive disorders include major depressive disorder (five symptoms of at least 2 weeks' duration) and dysthymia (three depressive symptoms of at least 1 year's duration). (See Chapter 1.)

To date, no studies have been published utilizing DSM-III (American Psychiatric Association 1980) or DSM-III-R (American Psychiatric Association 1987) criteria applied to infants; this remains a largely unexplored area. When adult criteria are used, depression is rarely found among preschoolers. A prevalence of 0.3% was found by Kashani et al. (1986) in a general population of preschoolers. In a clinically referred sample, less than 1% met the criteria for a major depressive disorder (Kashani and Carlson 1987).

The frequency of major depression in the preadolescent group is also relatively low among the general population. When DSM-III criteria are used, the rate of major depression in local studies was 1.9% and 1.8% in prepubertal children in the United States and New Zealand, respectively (Kashani et al. 1979, 1983). Kashani et al. (1982) and Kazdin et al. (1983a) found that, in clinically referred samples in an inpatient setting, the rate increases significantly to between 13% and 15%.

In the adolescent age group, rates for depressive disorders continue to increase in both the general population and in clinically referred samples. In a general population study of 14- to 16-year-olds, Kashani et al. (1987) found that 4.7% met the DSM-III criteria for major depression, were functioning on an impaired level, and were in need of treatment. Robbins et al. (1982a) found that 28% of hospitalized adolescents had a major depressive disorder.

Little has been written about dysthymia in the child and adolescent psychiatric literature. Kashani et al. (1983) found that 2.5% of their sample of 9-year-olds had minor depression (dysthymia) and 1.8% had major depression. Anderson et al. (1987) found that dysthymia overlapped with major depression in the majority of those 11-year-olds who were judged to be depressed with a combined prevalence of 1.8%. Of the 14 children in this sample diagnosed as depressed, 3 had only one of the depression diagnoses. (See Chapter 1.)

The prevalence of bipolar disorder has not been systematically studied in children and adolescents. Strober et al. (1981) and Strober and Carlson (1982) did show that the adult DSM-III criteria for bipolar disorder were reliable and applicable to the adolescent population. (See Chapter 12.) However, mania and hypomania appear to be rare in prepubertal children (Akiskal et al. 1985; Anthony and Scott 1960; Kuyler et al. 1980). Mania and hypomania become much more frequent during later adolescent and young adult years. Carlson and Kashani (1988) found that four or more symptoms of mania of at least 2 days' duration occurred in 13.3% of a nonreferred population of 150 adolescents ages 14–16 years. Further work is needed to determine the prevalence of cyclothymia and bipolar disorder in this age group.

ETIOLOGY

Determining the etiology of mood disorders is an arduous and painstaking process involving numerous hypotheses, some of which ultimately flounder and fail. What is held as today's currently accepted theory is modified and expanded upon in tomorrow's never-ending search for the answers to the questions of what causes mental disorders and how they can be prevented. In this search, child and adolescent psychiatric research is in its infancy. At first glance, it is tempting to look for a single causative agent, but it is becoming increasingly clear that multifactorial analyses are needed to carefully assess the biological, psychological, and sociocultural factors that may contribute to these disorders.

RISK FACTORS

In this section we will describe biological, psychological, and social approaches to determining the risk factors of depressive disorders. Earls (1989) proposes that the term *risk factor* be specifically applied to causes of a disorder and not to correlates or consequences of a disorder. He also makes a distinction between risk factors and attributes, stating that "risk factors are modifiable premorbid conditions, while attributes are fixed and not changeable. . . . True risk factors are conditions that are external to the child. They interact with the internal milieu of the child and in doing so, operate upon sex-related and age-dependent vulnerabilities in producing psychiatric disorder." In his opinion, then, such sociodemographic variables as age, sex, race, and perhaps socioeconomic status fall into the category of an attribute rather than a risk factor, as they are "fixed and not changeable."

However, most epidemiological studies have considered age, sex, race, socioeconomic status, and other sociodemographic data to be important variables in the incidence and prevalence of disease.

Sociodemographic Factors

Age. In general, the prevalence of mood disorders increases with age. In infants, mood disorders have not been well studied. Bowlby (1969, 1980) reported a series of reactions consisting of protest, despair, and detachment in institutionalized infants, which in his view represent "depressive equivalents." (See Chapter 1.) Epidemiological studies by Kashani and Carlson (1987), Kashani and Simonds (1979), and Kashani et al. (1983, 1986, 1987) have clearly shown that the prevalence of major depression increases with age in children and adolescents. In the Isle of Wight study, subsequent reinterviews of the 10-year-olds 4 years later showed a threefold increase in depressive disorders (Rutter 1986a). Rutter (1980a, 1980b, 1986b, 1989) states, however, that the increase in depressive feelings in adolescents is more a function of puberty than of age.

The prevalence rates of dysthymia (minor depression) also seem to follow the trend of increasing with age. Kashani et al. (1983) found that 2.5% of their sample of 9-year-olds had minor depression. In a sample composed of 14- to 16-year-olds, 8% met the criteria for dysthymia (Kashani et al. 1987). However, only 3.3% had pure dysthymia without an accompanying major depressive disorder.

Though manic episodes before puberty are rare, affective symptoms not fully meeting the criteria for mania or hypomania may be experienced prior to puberty (Loranger and Levine 1978; Perris 1966). Carlson and Kashani (1988) found that 20 of 150 14- to 16-year-olds had four or more manic symptoms of at least 2 days' duration, but they cautioned the reader about interpreting these data because of the varying criteria used in diagnosing bipolar disorder and the poor concordance between child and parent interviews. (See Chapters 12 and 13.)

Sex. Some studies have reported a preponderance of depressive disorders in males prior to puberty and in females after puberty. An example is Anderson et al. (1987), who found a male-to-female ratio of 5:1 for depressive disorder at age 11 years. At age 13 years, the male-to-female ratio was 4:1 (McGee and Williams 1988). In contrast, Kovacs (1985) found the sex distribution of referred children ages 8–13 years to be roughly equal for major depression, dysthymia, and adjustment disorder with depressed mood. Kashani et al. (1987) found a female-to-male ratio of 5:1 for depressive disorders meeting the DSM-III criteria in a sample of 150 14- to 16-year-olds. Kandel and Davies (1982) also found that adolescent females ages 14–18 years had more depressive symptomatology than males. This is consistent with the predominance of depressive disorders in females that is seen in the adult population (Boyd and Weissman 1981; Boyd et al. 1982).

In adult studies, there is a preponderance of women with bipolar disorder, although this preponderance is not as striking as it is in major depression (Clayton 1981).

Race. Some authors have found the prevalence of mood disorders to be similar for all races (Raft et al. 1977; Steele 1978). Others, however, have found differences (Adebimpe et al. 1982; Comstock and Helsing 1976; Faden 1977; Roberts et al. 1981; Warheit et al. 1973). Zung et al. (1988) found no difference in the prevalence of depressive symptoms in black and white adult patients in an outpatient setting. Childhood depression is found in different races, although no systematic studies have been performed to determine whether race is really a significant factor. Kandel and Davies (1982) found that race had no effect on the rate of depressive mood in 14- to 18-year-olds.

Socioeconomic status. The effects of socioeconomic status have not been thoroughly studied in childhood and adolescent mood disorders. Some authors suggest that in adults mood disorders, especially bipolar disorder, are more prevalent in higher socioeconomic classes (Bebbington 1978; Ripley 1977). Weissman and Myers (1978) found that major depressive disorder had no strong relationship to social class. However, rates of bipolar disorders were highest in the upper socioeconomic classes, whereas rates of minor depression were highest in the lower socioeconomic classes.

Kovacs et al. (1984a, 1984b) found that depressed children ages 8–13 years were more likely to be from the lower socioeconomic class, but this was a referred sample. In contrast, Kandel and Davies (1982) found that socioeconomic status had no effect on the rates of depressive mood in 14- to 18-year-olds.

Biological Factors

Neurochemical factors. The monoamine neurotransmitters, such as norepinephrine and serotonin, are among the most studied in determining the neurobiological etiologies of depressive disorders. Relative deficiencies of these two neurotransmitters are presumed to result in certain types of depression. The monoamine hypothesis suggests that antidepressants relieve depression by blocking the reuptake of these neurotransmitters from the synaptic cleft in the central nervous system.

In animal studies, chronic treatment with antidepressants has shown that a decrease in the number of postsynaptic β-adrenergic receptors and a decreased responsiveness of serotonergic receptors result in decreased sensitivity in both of these receptors; however, this occurs only after a latency interval. This correlation is one possible reason that clinical improvement with antidepressant therapy is not seen until 1–3 weeks after initiation of treatment. However, the exact action of antidepressant medication remains largely unknown. Many studies have also reported abnormalities in the metabolites of these neurotransmitters in individuals with depressive disorders. However, Cytryn et al. (1974) reported that these metabolite changes are somewhat age dependent. (See Chapters 3 and 10.)

Other neurotransmitters may play a role in the development of mood disorders. Homovanillic acid, a metabolite of dopamine, is decreased in unipolar but not bipolar depression in adults (Van Praag and Krof 1971). Lower levels of γ-aminobutyric acid (GABA) are found in depressed individuals (Gold et al. 1980; Petty and Schlesser 1981), whereas individuals with bipolar depression and secondary depression have levels similar to those in normal individuals. Manic individuals have higher levels of GABA. The endogenous opioids, second messenger systems, and vasopressin are also implicated in the development of mood disorders (Schildkraut et al. 1989).

Some research shows abnormalities of lithium transport across red blood cell membranes in family members of bipolar patients. It is suggested that these abnormalities may be a biological marker of bipolar illness (Dorus et al. 1979, 1983). Lithium is thought to work in bipolar disorder by altering sodium transport in nerve cells, effecting a shift toward the intraneuronal metabolism of catecholamines. One hypothesis suggests that lithium's specific action is to block the enzyme inositol-1-phosphatase within neurons, thereby reducing the formation of phosphatidylinositol. This would result in decreased cellular responses to neurotransmitters that are linked to this second messenger system. However, the exact mechanism of action of lithium remains unknown. (See Chapters 12 and 13.)

Acetylcholine is thought to play a role in higher cognitive functions, especially memory (Coyle et al. 1983). Overactivity of cholinergic systems is suggested in mood and sleep disorders (Janowsky et al. 1980). There may be increased receptor sensitivity to acetylcholine in individuals who are at risk for developing a mood disorder (Gershon et al. 1989; Janowsky et al. 1972, 1980; Schildkraut et al. 1989; Sitaram et al. 1982). Fibroblasts grown in vitro from these individuals show an increased density of muscarinic cholinergic receptors sensitive to acetylcholine, but further research needs to be done to replicate these findings (Nadi et al. 1984). Studies utilizing brain imaging and other specialized techniques, such as evoked potentials, have thus far provided limited and inconclusive data on adult mood disorders. Overall, it seems that mood disorders are accompanied by heterogeneous dysfunctions of the neurochemical system.

Neuroendocrine factors. In the neuroendocrine system, the hypothalamus receives input from various portions of the cerebral cortex and limbic system, and the hypothalamus in turn affects the pituitary gland and its target organs. Feedback can occur from any of the various components. Individuals with mood disorders have dysfunctions in this system.

The hypersecretion of cortisol found in some depressed individuals is the underlying basis for the dexamethasone suppression test (DST). In normal individuals, dexamethasone suppresses the blood level of cortisol, but this suppression does not occur in approximately 70% of depressed hospitalized children (Weller et al. 1984). In hospitalized adolescents, there is a 30–70% rate of nonsuppression (Robbins et al. 1982b; Puig-Antich 1986). However, this is a nonspecific finding that is also seen in patients with alcoholism, eating disorders, Alzheimer's disease, schizophrenia, and other conditions.

Casat et al. (1989) recently reviewed 13 prospective studies on the use of the DST in children and adolescents. In children with major depression, the sensitivity of the DST was 69.6% and the specificity was 69.7%. In adolescents with major depression, however, the sensitivity was 47.1% and the specificity was 80.2%. On the other hand, Puig-Antich et al. (1989a) found essentially no differences between the cortisol secretion of prepubertal children with major depression and that of normal controls and children with nonaffective psychiatric disorders in a "nonstressful environment." They argue that cortisol hypersecretion occurs infrequently in prepubertal children with major depression and that the results are influenced by both age effects and the lack of stressors in their study. (See Chapter 3.)

Other biological markers have been studied, including a blunted thyroid-stimulating hormone response to thyrotropin-releasing hormone stimulation (Schildkraut et al. 1989), a decreased release of growth hormone in response to noradrenergic stimulation (Schildkraut et al. 1989), decreased basal levels of follicle-stimulating hormone and luteinizing hormone (Reus 1989), and decreased testosterone levels in males (Reus 1989). Prepubertal children with major depression secrete an increased amount of growth hormone during their sleep compared with other children with and without psychiatric disorders and have a decreased growth hormone response to insulin-induced hypoglycemia (Puig-Antich et al. 1984a, 1984b, 1984c, 1984d). These abnormalities persist even after treatment for the depression; in contrast, the hypersecretion of cortisol often normalizes after treatment (Puig-Antich et al. 1979, 1981). However, the results of research studies have been disappointing regarding the sensitivity and specificity of most of these biological markers. From a clinical standpoint, they have limited applicability.

Neuroimmunology. In the adult literature, immunological abnormalities are reported in individuals with mood disorders. Possible mechanisms for an immunological role in the development of mood disorders include either immunological suppression, leading to a central nervous system infection, or immunological overactivity, resulting in a damaged central nervous system or endocrine tissues. In animal studies, lesions made in the central nervous system resulted in immunological dysfunction. It is not known whether immunological abnormalities are causal in nature, a coeffect, or a consequence of the mood disorder.

In humans, studies of bereaved spouses and individuals with major depression have shown a decrease in T-cell proliferation (Bartrop et al. 1977; Kronfol et al. 1983). Also, there is an overall decrease in the number of lymphocytes in individuals with major depression (Kronfol et al. 1984; Schleifer et al. 1984). Munck et al. (1984) found that glucocorticoid secretion suppresses the immune system and that in times of stress there is an association between the endocrine and immune systems. Many other hormones have a modulating effect, either positive or negative, on the immune system.

Calabrese et al. (1987), in a review of this subject, state that no firm conclusions can be made regarding the clinical significance of the data suggesting compromise of the immune system in times of stress, bereavement, or depression. Well-designed prospective studies are needed. Schleifer et al. (1989) proposed that altered immunity is not a specific biological correlate of major depressive disorder. Immune system differences may be related to age and symptom severity. Therefore, changes in immune status may occur only in subgroups of depressed patients. This area remains relatively unexplored in children and adolescents.

Chronobiology. Chronobiology is the study of biological rhythms in living organisms. In humans, rhythms help govern body temperature, various hormone levels, menstruation, sleep, and wakefulness. When a rhythm is out of phase, it may be advanced (begin earlier than usual) or be delayed (begin later than usual) producing a "disease state." Chronobiology is significant in the study of mood disorders. Depression is thought to be a phase-advanced disorder, as evidenced by the biological changes in the neuroendocrine system and sleep (Jarrett 1989; Lewy et al. 1990). Wehr and Rosenthal (1989) reviewed the literature on seasonality and affective illness and found strong support for a link between changes in the physical environment and changes in the biological systems for human adaptation. (See Chapter 4.)

Sleep abnormalities. Depressed adults have abnormalities of sleep on polysomnography, including a shortened rapid eye movement (REM) latency, an increased amount of time spent in the first REM period, a decreased amount of delta-wave sleep, a shortened amount of time spent in stages III and IV of sleep, and an increased amount of REM sleep early in the sleep period accompanied by both frequent nocturnal awakenings and early morning awakening. Manic adults also have abnormalities of sleep on polysomnography, including hyposomnia and REM changes similar to those seen in depressed patients, with the exception of preservation of delta-wave sleep (Hudson et al. 1988). The authors suggest that mood disorders have pathophysiological mechanisms in common. Various factors appear to precipitate mania by their capacity to cause sleep deprivation (Wehr et al. 1987).

In polysomnographic studies of prepubertal children, there is some evidence of age sensitivity and maturational effects (Ryan and Puig-Antich 1986). Prepubertal children with major depression essentially show no abnormalities in their polysomnogram, although adolescents with major depression have a shortened REM latency.

Genetics. Research in genetic studies of mood disorders is limited and inconclusive. It appears that both unipolar and bipolar depression can cluster in some families; a genetic basis might be suspected (Gershon et al. 1983). Children of depressed parents are at greater risk for psychopathology, particularly major depression (Weissman et al. 1984b). For mood disorders there is a 76% concordance rate in monozygotic twins reared together, a 67% concordance rate in monozygotic twins reared apart, and a 19% concordance rate in dizygotic twins (Tsuang 1978). Puig-Antich (1980) found a lifetime morbidity risk for major depression of 0.42 in first-degree relatives of depressed adolescents at least 16 years of age. A later study by the same author and colleagues found higher familial rates of psychopathology, especially major depressive disorder, alcoholism, and anxiety disorders in both the first- and second-degree relatives of prepubertal children with a major depressive disorder (Puig-Antich et al. 1989b).

There is a 27% chance that an adult offspring will have a mood disorder if one parent has a mood disorder and a 50–74% chance if both parents are afflicted with a mood disorder (Cummins and Robson 1986; Gershon et al. 1982). Most family studies show that the rates of both bipolar and unipolar disorders are increased among the relatives of individuals with bipolar disorder, whereas the rate of unipolar depression is increased among the relatives of individuals with unipolar depression (Gershon et al. 1982; Weissman et al. 1984b).

The evidence for a genetic role in bipolar disorders is even stronger than that in unipolar depression (Winokur 1978). First-degree relatives of patients with bipolar disorder are at least 24 times more likely to develop bipolar disorder than are relatives of control subjects (Weissman et al. 1984a). Approximately one-half of bipolar patients have a parent with a mood disorder, usually unipolar depression (Clayton 1981). Egeland et al. (1987) found that an Amish family with a long history of bipolar disorder had a dominant gene on the short arm of chromosome 11 that predisposes them to bipolar illness. Another family predisposed to bipolar disorder was found to have a gene defect on the X chromosome (Baron et al. 1987). However, many others afflicted with bipolar illness do not have these genes or defects, lending support to the notion that bipolar disorders are heterogeneous in nature (Detera-

Wadleigh et al. 1987; Hodgkinson et al. 1987; Mendlewicz et al. 1979). (See Chapters 12 and 13.) .

Psychological Factors

Psychoanalytic and psychodynamic models. Freud (1917) and Abraham (1927) made significant contributions to the psychoanalytic and psychodynamic models of depression, including factors such as the loss of a libidinal object, the ambivalent introjection of a lost object, aggression turned inward toward the self, narcissistic injury, and masochism. Denial of depressive symptoms resulted in a release of energy leading to mania and its symptoms. Bibring (1953) suggests that "object loss" at various stages of development contributes to a disturbance of self-esteem and results in depression. Kohut (Silber 1989), in the study of narcissistic personality disorder, stressed the importance of differentiating this disorder from bipolar illness. In narcissistic personality disorder, the individual has brief periods of euphoria followed by self-deprecation and depression. Alternatively, Sandler and Joffe (1965) suggested that depression results from an individual's loss of a sense of well-being and that object loss is important only insofar as it affects this sense of well-being. On the other hand, Jacobson (1971) sees self-evaluation as the basis of self-esteem—the degree of similarity or discrepancy between the idealized self and the actual self-representation. Low self-esteem may lead to depression. (See Chapter 7.)

Cognitive-behavioral model. Beck (1974) describes a negative self-concept, a negative interpretation of life experiences, and a negative expectation for the future as a triad of cognitions experienced by those who are depressed, resulting in feelings of helplessness and hopelessness. In theory, these negative cognitions develop in childhood, when failure is not adequately prepared for or when its importance is overestimated. Studies utilizing cognitive-behavioral techniques to alter mood and depression support this model. Depressed individuals report an increased sensitivity to the quality of neutral and negative life experiences. They distort perceptions and overestimate the frequency of negative self-evaluations. (See Chapter 9.)

The child and adolescent literature shows that nondepressed children have different self-concepts than depressed children (Strauss et al. 1984). Depressed hospitalized children have negative worldviews (Asarnow et al. 1987). They also have a negative expectation for the future (Kazdin et al. 1983b). Kashani et al. (1989a, 1989b), in a community sample of 8-, 12-, and 17-year-olds, found that hopelessness did not increase with age and that children and adolescents with a high hopelessness score reported significantly more school problems and were at greater risk for overall psychopathology, including depression and suicide.

Coyne and Gotlib (1983) suggested that depressed individuals are actually more accurate than their nondepressed counterparts in their judgments of negative stimuli that are relevant to the self. The depressed individuals studied by the researchers investigating the cognitive triad theory may have been able to decipher the underlying hypotheses from the experimental situation and conform their behavior accordingly. In summation, it is not clear whether distorted cognitions are a cause of depression, a coexisting entity, or a consequence of the depression.

Learned helplessness model. The learned helplessness model developed from observing that when animals were repeatedly given an electrical shock in a situation from which they could not escape, they eventually gave up trying and were rendered "helpless." When humans experience events over which they have no control, they are led to believe that they will have no control over future events, resulting in motivational and cognitive deficits and emotional helplessness (Seligman 1975). Therefore, depression is improved when the individual regains his or her sense of control over the environment. In support of this model, Breier et al. (1987) found that in healthy adults lack of control over an aversive stimulus (i.e., noise level) resulted in alterations of mood and changes in the neuroendocrine and autonomic nervous systems with higher self-ratings of helplessness, lack of control, tension, stress, unhappiness, anxiety, and depression. These individuals also had elevated levels of plasma adrenocorticotropic hormone, epinephrine, and electrodermal activity.

Abramson et al. (1978) proposed additionally that the individual's attributional style, or way of explaining things, is important. For example, if an individual experiences a negative outcome and then explains that negative outcome by referring to internal, stable, and global causes, that person is then at risk for depression. (See Chapter 9.) Seligman et al. (1984) found that a community sample of children with depressive symptoms more frequently endorsed internal, stable, and global explanations for negative outcomes compared with children without depressive symptoms. They also found that the mother's attributional style correlated with the child's, lending support to the belief that this may be a learned process wherein the mother and child reinforced each others' attributional styles and symptoms. In another community sample of children found to be depressed on results of psychometric testing, Nolen-Hoeksema et al. (1986) found that a dysfunctional explanatory style correlated with the depression and could predict a future depression.

Family systems model. Family systems theory is a transactional model with an underlying premise that the family is a dynamic organization of interconnected parts forming a whole. Psychiatric problems in any member of the family are seen as manifestations of dysfunctional relationships within the family. In therapy, these problems are considered within the context of the family system. Interventions within the system (i.e., those aspects of the system that serve to maintain the symptom) hopefully lead to effective treatment.

Self-control model. Rehm's (1977) model of depression is based on Kanfer's (1970) work on self-control. In this model, depressed individuals are seen as being deficient in one or more of the following areas: self-monitoring, self-evaluation, and self-reinforcement. This deficiency may include a disproportionate focus on negative events, emphasis on the immediate consequences of actions rather than the delayed ones, setting of unrealistic goals, distorted perceptions of personal success and failure, a decreased amount of positive self-feedback, and excessive self-abasement. In support of this model, Cole and Rehm (1986) found that fewer rewards were given by mothers of depressed adolescents and that high standards distinguished a clinical sample of depressed children from nondepressed ones, but not from normal controls.

Personality factors. In adults, no one personality trait or type is a predisposing factor to depression. Certain personality types (e.g., the obsessive-compulsive, borderline, histrionic, and antisocial), however, are at greater risk for depression. In children, the relationship between personality type and depression has not been as well studied. However, Chess et al. (1983) found that their patients with depressive syndrome did not consistently show an earlier life tendency toward a temperamentally negative mood and that there was no evidence from longitudinal data that any temperamental characteristics played a role in the etiology or development of the disorder. These findings should be considered preliminary, due to the very small sample size. Kashani et al. (1990) reported that 7- to 12-year-old depressed, hospitalized children had lower self-concepts, greater hopelessness, and higher scores on the withdrawal and depression subscales of the Personality Inventory for Children than did the nondepressed group. Further investigation of personality traits and factors in depressed children and adolescents is clearly needed.

Social Factors

Life events and stress. Stress from life events was thought to be an etiological factor contributing to the development of depression. Most of the literature on adults, however, indicates that stressful life events pave the way for and sustain depression rather than cause it, although the research data are inconclusive. For example, the literature does not support a link between the death of a parent during childhood and later adult depression (Crook and Eliot 1980; Roy 1983; Tennant et al. 1980). On the other hand, families of preschoolers with depressive symptoms reported more stressful life events than did control families (Kashani et al. 1986). Another study showed that depressed, hospitalized children ages 7–12 years reported more negative life events than did the rest of the sample (Kashani et al. 1990).

Social skills deficits. Lewinsohn and Hoberman (1982) hypothesized that depression is caused and/or maintained by a decrease in positive social reinforcement secondary to deficits in social skills. Youngren and Lewinsohn (1980) also state that these deficits may be a consequence of depression impairing normal developmental tasks, rather than a cause of it.

Ambrosini and Puig-Antich (1985) report that children with major depression have impaired relationships with their mothers and peers and that only the mother-child relationship improved after the depression cleared. Puig-Antich et al. (1985a, 1985b) found that prepubertal children with major depressive disorder regularly present with social relation deficits and that these deficits in intra- and extrafamilial relationships only partially improved after recovery from the depressive episode. Research has also demonstrated that peers rate depressed children as less popular (Lewinsohn and Hoberman 1982; Youngren and Lewinsohn 1980). Teachers evaluate depressed children as less socially competent (Lefkowitz and Tesiny 1980; Vosk et al. 1982).

Childhood depression can be predicted by social withdrawal, decreased social competence, and negative social behavior (Reaven 1986). Social skills training has been utilized successfully to treat childhood depression (Kaslow et al. 1984), but its etiological significance remains unclear.

FOLLOW-UP OF LONGITUDINAL STUDIES

Longitudinal studies are carried out over a long period of time and provide information about causal factors and risk of illness, the validity and predictive nature of the diagnosis, the nature and course of the illness, and the impact of treatment measures on the illness. However, these studies are expensive and time-consuming. Only a limited number of longitudinal studies have been carried out in children and adolescents with mood disorders.

Poznanski et al. (1976) studied 10 children who had been affectively depressed in childhood. On follow-up, an average of 6½ years later, they found psychopathology in all subjects and 50% were thought to be experiencing a clinical depression. (See Chapter 1.)

Kovacs et al. (1984a, 1984b) studied referred children ages 8–13 years who had various psychiatric diagnoses singly or in combination (e.g., major depressive disorder, dysthymic disorder, or adjustment disorder with depressed mood) and a nondepressed psychiatric control group for 5 years. The children were evaluated at various points in time. They found that children who had an adjustment disorder with depressed mood had a relatively benign course, with the illness lasting an average of 5½ months and with better than 50/50 odds that no other psychiatric disorder would be present at the time of the illness and that no other depressive disorder would develop during the follow-up course. However, children with a major depressive disorder were afflicted for an average of 7½ months and were likely to have concomitant diagnoses of dysthymic disorder and/or anxiety disorders. The rate of recurrence of a major depressive disorder within 5 years of the onset of the first episode was 72%. A companion diagnosis of dysthymia increased the risk for recurrence. Kovacs et al. also found that dysthymia was indeed a chronic illness, lasting on average 3 years, and that it was likely to be accompanied by other psychiatric conditions, especially major depression and anxiety disorder. For both the major depressive group and the dysthymic group, the more prolonged episodes occurred in younger children.

As part of an ongoing longitudinal study, Kashani et al. (1983) originally studied a cohort of 9-year-old New Zealand children enrolled in the Dunedin Multidisciplinary Health and Development Research Unit. Based on this screening, 251 children were interviewed for the presence of past or current episodes of major and/or minor depression. A past depressive disorder was found in 23 children, and 17 were found to be suffering from a current depressive disorder.

The entire sample was followed up when the children were 11 and 13 years of age. McGee and Williams (1988) divided these children into three groups: those with a current depressive episode, those with a past depressive episode, and those with no previous depressive episode. As in the Kovacs study, depressive symptoms were reported more frequently in those children who had had a depressive disorder at or before age 9 years. Accompanying behavioral and emotional problems were also noted in these children, and comorbidity was a frequent finding. There was some evidence that depression was more persistent and accompanied by antisocial behaviors in boys, but not in girls.

Garber et al. (1988) followed up on adolescents who had been hospitalized 8 years previously. Those who had depressive symptoms consistent with a major depressive disorder had a high probability of having one or more episodes of major depression during the follow-up period compared with the nondepressed control group.

In summary, the literature indicates that, with the exception of an adjustment disorder with depressed mood, the diagnosis of a specific depressive disorder in childhood carries with it a high probability of the presence of another depressive disorder or anxiety disorder and a high likelihood of subsequent recurrence of depressive symptoms.

FUTURE RESEARCH DIRECTIONS

Further progress in research on mood disorders in children and adolescents depends upon the agreement to use standardized criteria throughout the scientific community. This would provide for a more accurate means of establishing the incidence and prevalence of these disorders worldwide.

A large epidemiological survey of the general population of children and adolescents, similar to the National Institute of Mental Health Epidemiological Catchment Area survey of the adult general population, should be done utilizing structured interviews and standardized criteria. With this survey, one could gather information on sociodemographic characteristics in relationship to mood disorders, the relationship of these disorders to each other and to other psychiatric disorders, the possible risk factors involved in developing and maintaining these disorders, and the possible protective factors that spare vulnerable individuals from developing a mood disorder. One possible risk factor that should be looked at specifically is the effect of temperament and personality on the development and/or maintenance of mood disorders. Also important is the impact of these disorders on afflicted individuals throughout life. Studies are needed on the efficacy of various treatment modalities for mood disorders, including pharmacological and psychosocial interventions alone and in various combinations. (See Chapters 7, 8, 9, and 10.)

REFERENCES

Abraham K: A short study of the development of the libido viewed in the light of mental disorders, in Selected Papers of Karl Abraham, M.D. London, Hogarth Press, 1927, pp 480–502

Abramson LY, Seligman MEP, Teasdale JD: Learned helplessness in humans: critique and reformulation. J Abnorm Psychol 87:4947, 1978

Adebimpe VR, Hedlund JL, Cho DW, et al: Symptomatology of depression in black and white patients. J Natl Med Assoc 74:185–190, 1982

Akiskal HS, Downs J, Jordan P, et al: Affective disorders in referred children and younger siblings of manic-depressives: mode of onset and prospective course. Arch Gen Psychiatry 42:996–1003, 1985

Ambrosini PJ, Puig-Antich J: Major depression in children and adolescents, in The Clinical Guide to Child Psychiatry. Edited by Shaffer D, Ehrhardt AA, Greenhill LL. New York, Free Press; London, Collier Macmillan, 1985, pp 182–191

American Psychiatric Association: Diagnostic and Statistical Manual of Mental Disorders, 3rd Edition. Washington, DC, American Psychiatric Association, 1980

American Psychiatric Association: Diagnostic and Statistical Manual of Mental Disorders, 3rd Edition, Revised. Washington, DC, American Psychiatric Association, 1987

Anderson JC, Williams S, McGee R, et al: DSM-III disorders in preadolescent children. Arch Gen Psychiatry 44:69–76, 1987

Anthony EJ, Scott P: Manic-depressive psychosis in childhood. J Child Psychol Psychiatry 1:53–72, 1960

Asarnow JR, Carlson GA, Guthrie D: Coping strategies, self-perceptions, hopelessness, and perceived family environments in depressed and suicidal children. J Consult Clin Psychol 55:361–366, 1987

Baron M, Risch N, Hamburger R, et al: Genetic linkage between X-chromosome markers and bipolar affective illness. Nature 326:289–292, 1987

Bartrop RW, Luckhurst E, Lazarus L, et al: Depressed lymphocyte function after bereavement. Lancet 1:834–836, 1977

Bebbington PE: The epidemiology of depressive disorders. Cult Med Psychiatry 2:297–341, 1978

Beck AT: The development of depression: a cognitive model, in The Psychology of Depression: Contemporary Theory and Research. Edited by Friedman RJ, Katz MM. New York, John Wiley, 1974, pp 3–20

Bibring E: Affective Disorders: The Mechanisms of Depression. Edited by Greenacre P. New York, International Universities Press, 1953

Bowlby J: Attachment and Loss, Vol I. Attachment. London, Hogarth Press, 1969

Bowlby J: Attachment and Loss, Vol III. Loss, Sadness and Depression. New York, Basic Books, 1980

Boyd JH, Weissman MM: Epidemiology of affective disorders: a reexamination and future directions. Arch Gen Psychiatry 38:1039–1046, 1981

Boyd JH, Weissman MM, Thompson WD, et al: Screening for depression in a community sample. Arch Gen Psychiatry 39:1195–1204, 1982

Breier A, Albus M, Pickar D, et al: Controllable and uncontrollable stress in humans: alterations in mood and neuroendocrine and psychophysiological function. Am J Psychiatry 144:1419–1425, 1987

Calabrese JR, Kling MA, Gold PW: Alterations in immunocompetence during stress, bereavement, and depression: focus on neuroendocrine function. Am J Psychiatry 144:1123–1134, 1987

Carlson GA, Kashani JH: Manic symptoms in a non-referred adolescent population. J Affective Disord 15:219–226, 1988

Casat CD, Arana GW, Powell K: The DST in children and adolescents with major depressive disorder. Am J Psychiatry 146:503–507, 1989

Chess S, Thomas A, Hassibi M: Depression in childhood and adolescence: a prospective study of six cases. J Nerv Ment Dis 171(7):411–420, 1983

Clayton PJ: The epidemiology of bipolar affective disorder. Compr Psychiatry 22(1):31–43, 1981

Cole DA, Rehm LP: Family interaction patterns and childhood depression. J Abnorm Child Psychol 14:297–314, 1986

Comstock GW, Helsing KJ: Symptoms of depression in two communities. Psychol Med 6:551–563, 1976

Coyle JT, Price D, Delong MR: Alzheimer's disease: a disorder of cortical cholinergic innervation. Science 219:1184–1190, 1983

Coyne JC, Gotlib IH: The role of cognition in depression: a critical appraisal. Psychol Bull 94:472–505, 1983

Crook T, Eliot J: Parental death during childhood and adult depression: a critical review of the literature. Psychol Bull 87:252–259, 1980

Cummins BD, Robson KS: Genetic issues in child psychiatry, in Manual of Clinical Child Psychiatry. Edited by Robson KS. Washington, DC, American Psychiatric Press, 1986, pp 303–312

Cytryn L, McKnew DH Jr, Logue M, et al: Biochemical correlates of affective disorders in children. Arch Gen Psychiatry 31:659–661, 1974

Detera-Wadleigh SD, Berrettini WH, Goldin LR, et al: Close linkage of c-Harvey-ras-1 and the insulin gene to affective disorder is ruled out in three North American pedigrees. Nature 325:806–808, 1987

Dorus E, Pandey GN, Shaughnessey R, et al: Lithium transport across the red cell membrane: a cell membrane abnormality in manic-depressive illness. Science 205:932–934, 1979

Dorus E, Cox NJ, Gibbons RD, et al: Lithium ion transport and affective disorders within families of bipolar patients. Arch Gen Psychiatry 40:545–552, 1983

Earls F: Epidemiology and child psychiatry: entering the second phase. Am J Orthopsychiatry 59(2):279–283, 1989

Egeland JA, Gerhard DS, Pauls DL, et al: Bipolar affective disorders linked to DNA markers on chromosome 11. Nature 325:783–787, 1987

Faden VB: Primary diagnosis of discharges from non-federal general hospital psychiatric inpatient units, in United States 1975: Mental Health Statistical Note 137. Rockville, MD, National Institute of Mental Health, 1977

Freud S: Mourning and melancholia (1917), in The Standard Edition of the Complete Psychological Works of Sigmund Freud, Vol 14. Translated and edited by Strachey J. London, Hogarth Press, 1957, p 243

Garber J, Kriss MR, Koch M, et al: Recurrent depression in adolescents: a follow-up study. J Am Acad Child Adolesc Psychiatry 27(1):49–54, 1988

Gershon ES, Hamovit J, Guroff JJ, et al: A family study of schizoaffective, bipolar I, bipolar II, unipolar probands and normal controls. Arch Gen Psychiatry 39:1157–1167, 1982

Gershon ES, Nurnberger J, Nadi NS, et al: The Origins of Depression: Current Concepts and Approaches. Berlin, Dahlemkonferenzen, 1982; New York, Springer-Verlag, 1983

Gershon ES, Berrettini WH, Goldin LR: Mood disorders: genetic aspects, in Comprehensive Textbook of Psychiatry, 5th Edition. Edited by Kaplan HI, Sadock BJ. Baltimore, MD, Williams & Wilkins, 1989, pp 879–888

Gold BI, Bowers MB, Roth RH, et al: GABA levels in CSF of patients with psychiatric disorders. Am J Psychiatry 137:362–364, 1980

Hodgkinson S, Sherrington R, Gurling H, et al: Molecular genetic evidence for heterogeneity in manic depression. Nature 325:805–806, 1987

Hudson JI, Lipinski JF, Frankenburg FR, et al: Electroencephalographic sleep in mania. Arch Gen Psychiatry 45:267–273, 1988

Jacobson E: Depression. New York, International Universities Press, 1971

Janowsky DS, El-Yousef MK, David JM: A cholinergic-adrenergic hypothesis of mania and depression. Lancet 2:632–635, 1972

Janowsky DS, Risch CD, Parker D, et al: Increased vulnerability to cholinergic stimulation in affective-disorder patients. Psychopharmacol Bull 16:29–31, 1980

Jarrett DB: Chronobiology, in Comprehensive Textbook of Psychiatry, 5th Edition. Edited by Kaplan HI, Sadock BJ. Baltimore, MD, Williams & Wilkins, 1989, pp 125–131

Kandel DB, Davies M: Epidemiology of depressive mood in adolescents. Arch Gen Psychiatry 39:1205–1212, 1982

Kanfer FH: Self-monitoring: methodological limitations and clinical applications. J Consult Clin Psychol 35:148–152, 1970

Kashani JH: The epidemiology of childhood depression, in Psychiatry 1982: The American Psychiatric Association Annual Review, Vol 1. Edited by Grinspoon L. Washington, DC, American Psychiatric Press, 1982, pp 281–288

Kashani JH, Carlson GA: Seriously depressed preschoolers. Am J Psychiatry 144:348–350, 1987

Kashani JH, Simonds JF: The incidence of depression in children. Am J Psychiatry 136:1203–1205, 1979

Kashani JH, Cantwell DP, Shekim WO, et al: Major depressive disorder in children admitted to an inpatient community mental health center. Am J Psychiatry 139:671–672, 1982

Kashani JH, McGee RO, Clarkson SE, et al: Depression in a sample of 9-year-old children. Arch Gen Psychiatry 40:1217–1223, 1983

Kashani JH, Holcomb WR, Orvaschel H: Depression and depressive symptomatology in preschool children from the general population. Am J Psychiatry 143:1138–1143, 1986

Kashani JH, Carlson GA, Beck NC, et al: Depression, depressive symptoms, and depressed mood among a community sample of adolescents. Am J Psychiatry 144:932–934, 1987

Kashani JH, Reid JC, Rosenberg TK: Levels of hopelessness in children and adolescents: a developmental perspective. J Consult Clin Psychol 57(4):496–499, 1989a

Kashani JH, Rosenberg TK, Reid JC: Developmental perspectives in child and adolescent depressive symptoms in a community sample. Am J Psychiatry 146:871–875, 1989b

Kashani JH, Dandoy AC, Reid JC: Life events and depression in an inpatient sample. Compr Psychiatry 31:266–274, 1990

Kaslow NJ, Rehm LP, Siegel AW: Social-cognitive and cognitive correlates of depression in children. J Abnorm Child Psychol 12:605–620, 1984

Kazdin AE, French NH, Unis AS, et al: Assessment of childhood depression: correspondence of child and parent rating. J Am Acad Child Psychiatry 22(2):157–164, 1983a

Kazdin AE, French NH, Unis AS, et al: Hopelessness, depression, and suicidal intent among psychiatrically disturbed inpatient children. J Consult Clin Psychol 51(4):504–510, 1983b

Kovacs M: The natural history and course of depressive disorders in childhood. Psychiatric Annals 15(6):387–389, 1985

Kovacs M, Feinberg TL, Crouse-Novak MA, et al: Depressive disorders in childhood, I: a longitudinal prospective study of characteristics and recovery. Arch Gen Psychiatry 41:229–237, 1984a

Kovacs M, Feinberg TL, Crouse-Novak MA, et al: Depressive disorders in childhood, II: a longitudinal study of the risk for a subsequent major depression. Arch Gen Psychiatry 41:643–649, 1984b

Kronfol Z, Silva J, Greden J, et al: Impaired lymphocyte function in depressive illness. Life Sci 33:241–247, 1983

Kronfol Z, Turner R, Nasrallah H, et al: Leukocyte regulation in depression and schizophrenia. Psychiatry Res 13:13–18, 1984

Kuyler PL, Rosenthal L, Igel G, et al: Psychopathology among children of manic-depressive patients. Biol Psychiatry 15:589–597, 1980

Lefkowitz MM, Tesiny EP: Assessment of childhood depression. J Consult Clin Psychol 48(1):43–50, 1980

Lewinsohn PM, Hoberman HM: Depression, in International Handbook of Behavior Modification and Therapy. Edited by Bellack AS, Hersen M, Kazdin AE. New York, Plenum, 1982, pp 397–431

Lewy AJ, Sack RL, Singer CM: Bright light, melatonin, and winter depression: the phase-shift hypothesis, in Biological Rhythms, Mood Disorders, Light Therapy, and the Pineal Gland. Edited by Shafii MS, Shafii SL. Washington, DC, American Psychiatric Press, 1990, pp 141–173

Loranger AW, Levine P: Age of onset of bipolar affective illness. Arch Gen Psychiatry 35:1345–1348, 1978

McGee R, Williams S: A longitudinal study of depression in nine-year-old children. J Am Acad Child Adolesc Psychiatry 27(3):342–348, 1988

Mendlewicz J, Linkowski P, Guroff JJ, et al: Color blindness linkage to bipolar manic-depressive illness. Arch Gen Psychiatry 36:1442–1449, 1979

Munck A, Guyre PM, Holbrook NJ: Physiological functions of glucocorticoids in stress and their relation to pharmacological actions. Endocr Rev 5:25–44, 1984

Myers JK, Weissman MM, Tischler GL, et al: Six-month prevalence of psychiatric disorders in three communities. Arch Gen Psychiatry 41:959–967, 1984

Nadi NS, Nurnberger JI, Gershon ES: Muscarinic cholinergic receptors on skin fibroblasts in familial affective disorder. N Engl J Med 311:225–230, 1984

Nolen-Hoeksema S, Girgus JS, Seligman MEP: Learned helplessness in children: a longitudinal study of depression, achievement, and explanatory style. J Pers Soc Psychol 51:435–552, 1986

Perris G (ed): A study of bipolar (manic depressive) and unipolar recurrent depressive psychoses. Acta Psychiatr Scand Suppl 42:194, 1966

Petty F, Schlesser MA: Plasma GABA in affective illness: a preliminary investigation. J Affective Disord 3(4):339–343, 1981

Poznanski EO, Krahenbuhl V, Zrull JP: Childhood depression: a longitudinal perspective. J Am Acad Child Psychiatry 15:491–501, 1976

Puig-Antich J: Affective disorders in childhood: a review and perspective. Psychiatr Clin North Am 3:403–424, 1980

Puig-Antich J: Psychobiological markers: effects of age and puberty, in Depression in Young People. Edited by Rutter M, Izard CE, Read PB. New York, Guilford, 1986, pp 341–381

Puig-Antich J, Chambers WJ, Halpern F, et al: Cortisol hypersecretion in prepubertal depressive illness: a preliminary report. Psychoneuroendocrinology 4:191–197, 1979

Puig-Antich J, Tabrizi MA, Davies MA, et al: Prepubertal endogenous major depressives hyposecrete growth hormone in response to insulin-induced hypoglycemia. Journal of Biological Psychiatry 16:801–818, 1981

Puig-Antich J, Goetz R, Davies M, et al: Growth hormone secretion in prepubertal children with major depression, II: sleep-related plasma concentrations during a depressive episode. Arch Gen Psychiatry 41:463–466, 1984a

Puig-Antich J, Goetz R, Davies M, et al: Growth hormone secretion in prepubertal children with major depression, IV: sleep-related plasma concentrations in a drug-free, fully recovered clinical state. Arch Gen Psychiatry 41:479–483, 1984b

Puig-Antich J, Novacenko H, Davies M, et al: Growth hormone secretion in prepubertal children with major depression, I: final report on response to insulin-induced hypoglycemia during a depressive episode. Arch Gen Psychiatry 41:455–460, 1984c

Puig-Antich J, Novacenko H, Davies M, et al: Growth hormone secretion in prepubertal children with major depression, III: response to insulin-induced hypoglycemia after recovery from a depressive episode and in a drug-free state. Arch Gen Psychiatry 41:471–475, 1984d

Puig-Antich J, Lukens E, Davies M, et al: Psychosocial functioning in prepubertal major depressive disorders, I: interpersonal relationships during the depressive episode. Arch Gen Psychiatry 42:500–507, 1985a

Puig-Antich J, Lukens E, Davies M, et al: Psychosocial functioning in prepubertal major depressive disorders, II: interpersonal relationships after sustained recovery from affective episode. Arch Gen Psychiatry 42:511–517, 1985b

Puig-Antich J, Dahl R, Ryan N, et al: Cortisol secretion in prepubertal children with major depressive disorder. Arch Gen Psychiatry 46:801–809, 1989a

Puig-Antich J, Goetz D, Davies M, et al: A controlled family history of prepubertal major depressive disorder. Arch Gen Psychiatry 46:406–418, 1989b

Raft D, Spencer R, Toomey T, et al: Depression in medical outpatients: use of the Zung scale. Diseases of the Nervous System 38:999–1004, 1977

Reaven N: Depression and social functioning in children. Unpublished doctoral dissertation, University of Missouri, Columbia, 1986

Rehm LP: A self-control model of depression. Behavior Therapy 8:787–804, 1977

Reus VI: Psychoneuroendocrinology, in Comprehensive Textbook of Psychiatry, 5th Edition. Edited by Kaplan HI, Sadock BJ. Baltimore, MD, Williams & Wilkins, 1989, pp 105–111

Ripley HS: Depression and life span: epidemiology in depression, in Depression: Clinical, Biological, and Psychological Perspectives. Edited by Usdin G. New York, Brunner/Mazel, 1977, pp 1–27

Robbins DR, Alessi NE, Cook SC, et al: The use of the Research Diagnostic Criteria (RDC) for depression in adolescent psychiatric inpatients. J Am Acad Child Psychiatry 21(3):251–255, 1982a

Robbins DR, Alessi NE, Yanchyshyn GW, et al: Preliminary report on the dexamethasone suppression test in adolescents. Am J Psychiatry 139:942–943, 1982b

Roberts RE, Stevenson JM, Breslow L: Symptoms of depression among blacks and whites in an urban community. J Nerv Ment Dis 169:774–779, 1981

Roy A: Early parental death and adult depression. Psychol Med 13:861–865, 1983

Rutter M: Attachment and the development of social relationships, in Scientific Foundations of Developmental Psychiatry. Edited by Rutter M. London, Heinemann, 1980a, pp 267–279

Rutter M: Changing Youth in a Changing Society: Patterns of Adolescent Development and Disorder. London, Nuffield Provincial Hospitals Trust, 1979; Cambridge, MA, Harvard University Press, 1980b

Rutter M: Child psychiatry: the interface between clinical and developmental research. Psychol Med 16:151–169, 1986a

Rutter M: Depressive feelings, cognitions, and disorders: a research postscript, in Depression in Young People. Edited by Rutter M, Izard CE, Read PB. New York, Guilford, 1986b, pp 491–519

Rutter M: Isle of Wight revisited: twenty-five years of child psychiatric epidemiology. J Am Acad Child Adolesc Psychiatry 28(5):633–653, 1989

Ryan ND, Puig-Antich J: Affective illness in adolescents, in Psychiatry Update: American Psychiatric Association Annual Review, Vol 5. Edited by Frances AJ, Hales RE. Washington, DC, American Psychiatric Press, 1986, pp 420–450

Sandler J, Joffe WG: Notes on childhood depression. Int J Psychoanal 46:88–96, 1965

Schildkraut JJ, Green AI, Mooney JJ: Mood disorders: biochemical aspects, in Comprehensive Textbook of Psychiatry, 5th Edition. Edited by Kaplan HI, Sadock BJ. Baltimore, MD, Williams & Wilkins, 1989, pp 868–879

Schleifer SJ, Keller SE, Meyerson AT, et al: Lymphocyte function in major depressive disorder. Arch Gen Psychiatry 41:484–486, 1984

Schleifer SJ, Keller SE, Bond RN, et al: Major depressive disorder and immunity. Arch Gen Psychiatry 46:81–87, 1989

Seligman MEP: Helplessness: On Depression, Development, and Death. San Francisco, CA, Freeman & Company, 1975

Seligman MEP, Peterson C, Kaslow NJ, et al: Attributional style and depressive symptoms among children. J Abnorm Psychol 93:235–238, 1984

Silber A: Mood disorders: psychodynamic etiology, in Comprehensive Textbook of Psychiatry, 5th Edition. Edited by Kaplan HI, Sadock BJ. Baltimore, MD, Williams & Wilkins, 1989, pp 888–892

Sitaram N, Nurnberger JI, Gershon ES, et al: Cholinergic regulation of mood and REM sleep: a potential model and marker for vulnerability to depression. Am J Psychiatry 139:571–576, 1982

Steele RE: Relationship of race, sex, social class, and social mobility to depression in normal adults. J Soc Psychol 104:37–47, 1978

Strauss CC, Forehand R, Frame C, et al: Characteristics of children with extreme scores on the children's depression inventory. Journal of Clinical Child Psychology 13:227–231, 1984

Strober M, Carlson G: Bipolar illness in adolescents: clinical, genetic, and pharmacologic predictors in a three- to four-year prospective follow-up. Arch Gen Psychiatry 39:549–555, 1982

Strober M, Green J, Carlson G: Reliability of psychiatric diagnosis in hospitalized adolescents: interrater agreement using DSM-III. Arch Gen Psychiatry 38:141–145, 1981

Tennant C, Bebbington P, Hurry J: Parental death in childhood and risk of adult depressive disorders. Psychol Med 10:289–299, 1980

Tsuang MT: Genetic counseling for psychiatric patients and their families. Am J Psychiatry 135:1465–1475, 1978

Van Praag HM, Krof J: Endogenous depressions with and without disturbances in 5-hydroxy-tryptamine metabolism: a biochemical classification. Psychopharmacology 19:148–152, 1971

Vosk B, Forehand R, Parker JB, et al: A multimethod comparison of popular and unpopular children. Developmental Psychology 18:571–575, 1982

Warheit GJ, Holzer CE, Schwab JJ: An analysis of social class and racial differences in depressive symptomatology: a community study. J Health Soc Behav 14:291–299, 1973

Wehr TA, Sack DA, Rosenthal NE: Sleep reduction as a final common pathway in the genesis of mania. Am J Psychiatry 144:201–204, 1987

Wehr TA, Rosenthal NE: Seasonality and affective illness. Am J Psychiatry 146:829–839, 1989

Weissman MM, Myers JK: Affective disorders in a U.S. urban community. Arch Gen Psychiatry 35:1304–1311, 1978

Weissman MM, Gershon ES, Kidd KK, et al: Psychiatric disorders in the relatives of probands with affective disorders: the Yale University–National Institute of Mental Health collaborative study. Arch Gen Psychiatry 41:13–21, 1984a

Weissman MM, Prusoff BA, Gammon GD, et al: Psychopathology in the children (ages 6–18) of depressed and normal parents. J Am Acad Child Adolesc Psychiatry 23:78–84, 1984b

Weller EB, Weller RA, Fristad MA, et al: The dexamethasone suppression test in hospitalized prepubertal depressed children. Am J Psychiatry 141:290–291, 1984

Winokur G: Mania and depression: family studies and genetics in relation to treatment, in Psychopharmacology: A Generation of Progress. Edited by Lipton MA, DiMascio A, Killam KF. New York, Raven, 1978, pp 1213–1221

Youngren MA, Lewinsohn PM: The functional relationship between depression and problematic interpersonal behavior. J Abnorm Psychol 89:333–341, 1980

Zung WWK, MacDonald J, Zung EM: Prevalence of clinically significant depressive symptoms in black and white patients in family practice settings. Am J Psychiatry 145:882–883, 1988

CHAPTER 3

Neurobiology of Depression

Shahnour Yaylayan, M.D.
Elizabeth B. Weller, M.D.
Ronald A. Weller, M.D.

Childhood depression is similar to adult depression and can be diagnosed using adult-type criteria (American Psychiatric Association 1980; American Psychiatric Association 1987). This view is also supported by numerous researchers, including Weinberg et al. (1973), Poznanski et al. (1979), Puig-Antich et al. (1979), Carlson and Cantwell (1980), and Weller and Weller (1984), who have used adult-type criteria to diagnose depression in children. According to DSM-III-R, a diagnosis of major depressive disorder requires five or more of the following signs and symptoms: depressed mood, loss of interest or pleasure, significant weight loss or weight gain, insomnia or hypersomnia, psychomotor agitation or retardation, fatigue or loss of energy, feelings of worthlessness or excessive guilt, diminished concentration, recurrent thoughts of death, suicidal ideation, and suicide attempt. These features should be present concurrently for at least 2 weeks. Melancholia is a subtype of depression that indicates more severe psychopathology. (See Chapter 1.)

Despite the fact that children and adults have similar diagnostic criteria for major depression, the form of expression in children, depending on the developmental level, may be different from that in adults (Poznanski et al. 1982). Because children are at various developmental stages with respect to cognitive and language skills, both structured and unstructured questions need to be asked for diagnostic assessment. (See Chapter 6.) Some depressed children have other psychiatric disorders (comorbidity) as a presenting problem, so careful diagnostic interviews should be conducted to make accurate diagnoses (Weller et al. 1986). A variety of sources (parents, teachers, friends) should be utilized before making a diagnosis. As children become older, they can communicate better and are more adept in the use of language. At this point, children should be interviewed individually because they will be able to report internal experiences of sadness, suicidal thoughts, and sleep disturbances that might not be known to their parents. However, parents are good sources of information regarding the child's interest level, social functioning, and behavior.

Since childhood depression is clinically similar to adult depression, biological correlates observed in adult depression may also be found in children who are depressed. Evidence for this is provided by the "biological markers" that have been studied in both adults and children. Studies searching for such biological markers have involved the areas of neuroendocrinology, polysomnography, and biochemical abnormalities.

Biological markers are of two types: state and trait markers. A state marker is a characteristic or an abnormality that is absent prior to the onset of a major depressive episode. This marker is present only during an episode, and it disappears or returns to normal after an episode has ended. A trait marker is a characteristic or abnormality that is present long before a depressive episode begins. A trait marker remains abnormal after the episode is over, even in a fully recovered drug-free state. Biological markers may be of clinical importance by predicting which individuals are predisposed to developing future depressive episodes. They may also be important in assessing adequacy or determining duration of treatment in some patients with depression.

THE HYPOTHALAMIC-PITUITARY-ADRENOCORTICAL AXIS

Abnormalities in neuroendocrine function are associated with major depressive disorders, especially "endogenous" disorders. Sachar et al. (1980) suggest two reasons for this connection: 1) Major depressive disorders are associated with disturbances in sex drive, sleep, appetite, mood, autonomic activity, and diurnal variation of symptoms—all of which suggest hypothalamic dysfunction. 2) The same neurotransmitters (norepinephrine, serotonin) that regulate the hypothalamic neuroendocrine cells are also thought to be involved in mood disorders.

Stokes and Sikes (1988), in a review of the hypothalamic-pituitary-adrenocortical (HPA) axis function in major depression, reported that the production and release of cortisol from the adrenal glands are part of a very complex system. At the central nervous system (CNS) level, different neurotransmitter pathways synapse on hypothalamic cells, which in turn release corticotropin-releasing hormone (CRH). In response to stimulation by CRH, the anterior pituitary releases adrenocorticotropic hormone (ACTH). Three mechanisms have been implicated in the secretion of ACTH and hence the regulation of cortisol release: 1) Endogenous rhythms in the CNS cause the release of ACTH and cortisol that produces the observed circadian pattern. 2) Psychological and physical stresses can increase ACTH and cortisol release above the spontaneous pattern. 3) The HPA axis has feedback loops that maintain the homeostasis of the system.

Plasma Measures

Measurements of total plasma cortisol represent both free (active) and protein-bound (inactive) cortisol and hence are inaccurate reflections of physiological cortisol. However, almost all studies looking at HPA axis activity in depressed subjects have measured total plasma cortisol, which is determined by either radioimmunoassay (RIA) or competitive protein binding (CPB) (Stokes and Sikes 1988). To investigate the effect of the cortisol assay method on test outcome, Arana and Mossman (1988) looked at 44 studies. Of these, 11 studies involving a total of 738 depressed patients used CPB and 33 studies involving a total of 1,438 patients used RIA. The rates of nonsuppression were similar—50% with the CPB method and 46% with RIA. The authors recommended that all assays be standardized in each medical center and that standardization should be particularly accurate in the range between 1 and 10 μg/dl, which is most critical to the dexamethasone suppression test (DST).

Urine Measures

Cortisol and its metabolites are excreted via the urine and are measured as 17-hydroxycorticosteroids, 17-ketogenic steroids, and unchanged cortisol. Urinary measurements of cortisol and its metabolites are done over a 24-hour period, hence eliminating the problems associated with episodic release that may affect the results of plasma determinations (Stokes and Sikes 1988).

Saliva Measures

The DST can be useful in assessing major depression in children, but it requires blood sampling, which is unpleasant to most children. Obtaining saliva samples, however, is noninvasive; these samples also can be obtained frequently and do not require skilled technicians. In preliminary work in adults, Climko et al. (1987) suggested that salivary cortisol levels could be used in place of serum cortisol levels in performing the DST without loss of sensitivity or specificity.

Woolston et al. (1983) studied 18 pediatric patients (age range, 1.5–15 years) with significant endocrinological problems who underwent the DST. A strong correlation between serum and saliva cortisol levels ($r = .82$, $P < .001$) was obtained using 59 paired samples.

Bober et al. (1988) studied 15 prepubertal children. Baseline serum and saliva samples were collected at 8:00 A.M. and 4:00 P.M. Serum samples were always obtained first. Dexamethasone, 0.5 mg orally, was administered at

11:00 P.M. that same evening. Serum and saliva samples were then collected the following day at 8:00 A.M. and 4:00 P.M. Serum and salivary cortisol concentrations were determined by RIA. The overall correlation for all paired samples ($n = 53$) was .90.

Cortisol

About 50% of adults with endogenous major depression hypersecrete cortisol. This cortisol hypersecretion appears to be secondary to increased secretion of ACTH. Cortisol secretion returns to normal upon recovery from the depressive syndrome (Sachar 1975; Sachar et al. 1973). Subsequently, multiple studies of depressed adults have also reported cortisol hypersecretion (Nuller and Ostroumova 1980; Schlesser et al. 1980). In children, there are fewer studies.

Puig-Antich et al. (1979) measured plasma cortisol every 20 minutes for 10–24 hours in four prepubertal children fitting the Research Diagnostic Criteria (RDC; Spitzer et al. 1978) for major depressive disorder, endogenous subtype. Two subjects had cortisol hypersecretion during their illness, which subsided after clinical recovery.

In a later study, Puig-Antich et al. (1983) studied 20 prepubertal children who met RDC for major depressive disorder. Fifteen had a possible or definite diagnosis of endogenous subtype and 5 did not. None of the children in the nonendogenous group hypersecreted cortisol over a 24-hour period, whereas 20% of the children in the endogenous group did. This is approximately half the reported rate in endogenously depressed adults (Sachar 1975; Sachar et al. 1973). These differences were attributed to age, possible preponderance of patients who will ultimately fit criteria for depressive spectrum disease, or other unknown factors.

Other studies have indicated that baseline cortisol levels may be elevated in depressed children. Doherty et al. (1986) found that only 5% of depressed hospitalized children ages 3–16 years failed to maintain a diurnal variation in their cortisol secretion. In the same study, elevated basal cortisol levels were a nonspecific finding in some depressed children and nondepressed controls. Weller et al. (1985a) studied 50 hospitalized prepubertal children who met DSM-III criteria for major depressive episode, 18 hospitalized controls with other psychiatric disorders, and 18 nonhospitalized normal controls. Baseline and post-DST cortisol levels were measured at 8:00 A.M. and 4:00 P.M. The depressed children had consistently higher cortisol levels than the controls at baseline.

DEXAMETHASONE SUPPRESSION TEST

The DST has become one of the most extensively investigated biological tests in psychiatry. It has been suggested that a positive DST is diagnostic for the melancholic subtype of major depressive disorder (Carroll et al. 1981). In reading about the DST, one should be aware of the definitions of sensitivity and specificity. Sensitivity is defined as the proportion of subjects with the disease who have a positive test. It indicates how good a test is at identifying the disease. Specificity is defined as the proportion of subjects without the disease who have a negative test. It indicates how good a test is at identifying nondiseased individuals. Arana and Mossman (1988) reviewed the use of the DST in adults. They found variations in the diagnostic criteria, sampling time, dose of dexamethasone, and plasma cortisol level used to define DST nonsuppression. The studies reviewed included a total of 4,400 subjects with major depressive disorder. Of these, 43% had a positive DST. Of 2,000 nondepressed controls, 86.5% had a negative DST.

Poznanski et al. (1982) studied the DST in 18 children ages 6–12 years. Nine depressed (according to RDC) outpatients and nine psychiatric controls were each given 0.5 mg of dexamethasone at 11:00 P.M. The next day, plasma cortisol levels were determined by the CPB method. The DST sensitivity was 55.6%, and the specificity was 88.9%.

Geller et al. (1983) studied the DST in 14 outpatients ages 5–12 years who met both RDC and DSM-III criteria for depression. Ten children met RDC criteria for endogenous depression, and 9 met DSM-III criteria for melancholia. They were given a dexamethasone dose of 20 µg/kg. Cortisol levels were assayed by both RIA (11 subjects) and CPB (3 subjects). Two different laboratories were utilized. The sensitivity of the DST was 10% and its specificity was 75%.

Livingston et al. (1984) studied 15 hospitalized children ages 6–12 years. Although standard structured diagnostic interviews were not used, subjects met DSM-III criteria for major depressive disorder or separation anxiety disorder. Children were given 0.5 mg of dexamethasone in the evening. Plasma concentrations were determined by RIA. Sensitivity was 75% and specificity was 63%. These authors concluded that the DST may be nonspecific for depression.

In the same study that documented elevated baseline cortisol levels in depressed children (Weller et al. 1985a), the DST was also studied in 50 hospitalized prepubertal children who met DSM-III criteria for major depressive disorder, 18 hospitalized controls with other psychiatric disorders, and 18 nonhospitalized normal controls. Children were given 0.5 mg of dexamethasone at 11:00 P.M. Plasma cortisol levels were determined by RIA. The sensitivity of the DST was 82%, and the specificity was 72% in the psychiatric controls and 89% in the normal controls.

Petty et al. (1985) studied 30 hospitalized children ages 5–12 years who met DSM-III criteria for major depressive disorder or dysthymia (depressed group) or who definitely did not meet criteria for these diagnoses (control group). Subjects were given 0.5 mg of dexamethasone. Cortisol levels were determined by RIA. In this study, the sensitivity was 86% percent and the specificity was 53%.

To assess the effect of the dexamethasone dose on DST results, Puig-Antich (1987) studied outpatient endogenously depressed children, non-endogenously depressed children, and normal children. Two doses of dexamethasone were used: 0.25 mg and 0.5 mg. The three groups did not differ significantly with respect to their 24-hour integrated plasma cortisol levels either at baseline or after either 0.25 mg or 0.5 mg of dexamethasone.

Pfeffer et al. (1989) also examined the effect of dexamethasone administered to 51 prepubertal inpatients ages 6–12 years (39.2% with major depression, 58.8% with separation anxiety disorder, 70.6% with dysthymia, 58.8% with conduct disorder, 17.6% with schizophrenia or schizoaffective disorder). Diagnoses were made using DSM-III criteria and the Schedule for Affective Disorders and Schizophrenia—Children's Version for the evaluation of the current state or present episode. Plasma cortisol measurements were done by RIA. Each child was given both 0.5 mg (average dose, 0.012 mg/kg) and 1.0 mg (average dose, 0.025 mg/kg). The second dose of dexamethasone was given no sooner than 72 hours and no later than 7 days after the first dose. The order in which the two doses were given was counterbalanced among subjects.

Results of this study suggested a plasma cortisol level of 5 μg/dl was the best cutoff for determining nonsuppression for the 0.5-mg dose of dexamethasone. Furthermore, no optimal cutoff plasma cortisol level for nonsuppression that had acceptable sensitivity, specificity, and adequate predictive value could be established for the 1.0-mg dose of dexamethasone. The DST sensitivity was 52.9% at 8:00 A.M. after the 0.5 mg of dexamethasone, and the specificity was 87.1% when children who had major depressive disorder were compared with children who had other disorders. They concluded that both 8:00 A.M. and 4:00 P.M. cortisol levels after 0.5 mg of dexamethasone can help confirm the diagnosis of major depressive disorder.

Adolescents

The DST has also been performed in adolescents. The dose of dexamethasone used in adolescents is typically 1.0 mg, which is the dose used in adults but is more than that used in most child studies. Results are similar to those in children. A brief summary of individual studies follows.

Extein et al. (1982) administered the DST to 27 adolescent inpatients ages 13–18 years. Fifteen subjects met DSM-III criteria and RDC for major depression. The 12 control subjects were patients with schizophrenia or conduct disorder. Cortisol blood levels were measured by RIA. The dexamethasone dose was 1.0 mg. The sensitivity of the DST was 53%, and the specificity was 92%.

Robbins et al. (1982) studied the DST in nine inpatient adolescents ages 12–18 years. Four adolescents met RDC criteria for major depression, and five were psychiatric controls. Of the four patients with major depressive disorder, two had abnormal DSTs (sensitivity, 50%). None of the five controls had an abnormal DST (specificity, 100%). Cortisol levels were determined by RIA. The dexamethasone dose was 1.0 mg.

Targum and colleagues (1983a) administered the DST to 120 adolescent psychiatric inpatients ages 13–19 years. Seventeen patients met DSM-III criteria for major depressive disorder. One hundred and three patients had "other" diagnoses. Seven of the 17 depressed patients had abnormal DSTs (sensitivity, 41.2%). Specificity of the DST was 82.5%. Serum cortisol levels were measured by RIA. The dexamethasone dose was 1.0 mg.

Hsu et al. (1983) administered the DST to 110 adolescent inpatients ages 13–19 years. Fourteen met DSM-III criteria for major depression. Of these, nine (64%) showed nonsuppression. Specificity of the DST in the psychiatric controls was 68.1%. Cortisol levels were measured by RIA. The dexamethasone dose was 1.0 mg.

Ha et al. (1984) administered the DST to 42 adolescent psychiatric inpatients ages 13–17 years. Of the 26 adolescents diagnosed as depressed, 9 (34.6%) failed to suppress cortisol. Of the 16 nondepressed adolescents, 3 (18.8%) also failed to suppress cortisol. Diagnoses were made according to RDC. Cortisol levels were measured by using CPB. The dexamethasone dose was 1.0 mg.

Klee and Garfinkel (1984) studied 33 inpatient children and adolescents ages 11.2–17.4 years. They used RDC to make the diagnosis of depression. Dexamethasone 1 mg was given at 11:00 P.M., and plasma cortisol levels were determined by CPB. The DST was found to have a 40% sensitivity and a 92% specificity.

Khan (1987) administered the DST to 84 inpatient adolescents ages 13–17 years. Thirty-three patients satisfied DSM-III criteria for major depression. Of the depressed patients, 23 (70%) had positive DSTs, and 82% of the nondepressed group had negative DSTs. Cortisol levels were measured by RIA. The dexamethasone dose was 1 mg.

Casat et al. (1989) reviewed 13 studies of DST in children and adolescents and found numerous differences in methodology, such as the cortisol assay method (RIA or CPB), the time of serum sampling for cortisol assay, diagnostic methods and criteria (structured or unstructured interviews, DSM-III, or RDC), and patient status (inpatient or outpatient). Furthermore, many studies had small patient samples. Of 79 children with major depressive disorder, 55 were nonsuppressors, yielding a DST sensitivity of 69.6%

and a DST specificity of 69.7%. Of 157 adolescents with major depressive disorder, 74 failed to suppress cortisol, yielding a sensitivity of 47.1% and a specificity of 80.2%. These results compare to a sensitivity of 43.1% and a specificity of 86.5% in adults (Arana and Mossman 1988). Thus, the sensitivity of the DST is higher in children (69.9%) than in adolescents (47.1%) or adults (43.1%). However, the specificity was higher in adolescents (80.2%) than in adults (76.5%) or children (69.7%).

In their review paper, Casat et al. (1989) discussed some of the factors that may account for the high rate of DST nonsuppression in depressed children. For example, the cortisol cutoff value of greater than or equal to 5 µg/dl selected for DST nonsuppression may not be appropriate. Also, the HPA axis response to stress in children may be different than that in adults. Finally, dexamethasone pharmacokinetics, higher basal levels of plasma cortisol in children, and familial loading of major depression in children who are depressed may account for differences. Future research that addresses these factors may lead to better understanding of HPA axis dysfunction in children and adolescents.

Suicide and the DST

Suicide is now the second leading cause of death among adolescents ages 15–19 years. It accounts for 12% of the deaths in the adolescent/young adult age group (Centers for Disease Control 1985). If there were a link between DST results and suicidality, it would have important clinical implications. The DST has been studied in adults and adolescents who have made serious suicide attempts. Some prospective studies examining DST results and suicidality in adults found that DST nonsuppressors were more likely to attempt and complete suicide at a later date (Yehuda et al. 1988). Another study by Coryell and Schlesser (1981) reported that 4 of 96 depressed DST nonsuppressors subsequently committed suicide, whereas only 1 of 142 depressed patients who had normal DST results later committed suicide. Others have observed no relationship between DST nonsuppression and suicide (Brown et al. 1986; Secunda et al. 1986).

Although there are no published studies on prepubertal children that relate DST results to suicide, two studies have addressed this issue in adolescents. Chabrol et al. (1983) evaluated 20 nondepressed (diagnoses not specified) adolescents who made a suicide attempt. Of these, 20% had positive DSTs. Robbins and Alessi (1985) studied 45 inpatient adolescents ages 13–18 years, of whom 23 had attempted suicide. Six adolescents who had attempted suicide (26%) had positive DSTs. None of those with a normal DST had made a serious attempt. Four of the 6 suicidal nonsuppressors had made a potentially lethal attempt.

Treatment Response and the DST

Arana and Mossman (1988) reviewed studies of adults that assessed the DST as a predictor of treatment response. There were considerable differences among studies as to treatment response rates between nonsuppressors and suppressors. The overall difference in response to treatment was not statistically significant.

Georgotas et al. (1983) reported that elderly endogenously depressed outpatients with abnormal DSTs did not respond to placebo and supportive treatment. Nonendogenously depressed patients with normal DSTs had a high response rate to placebo. The endogenously depressed patients who failed to respond to placebo subsequently responded to nortriptyline. However, nonendogenously depressed patients who did not respond to placebo also did not respond to nortriptyline.

Preskorn et al. (1987) did a double-blind, placebo-controlled, imipramine treatment study in 22 hospitalized prepubertal children ages 6–12 years. All met DSM-III criteria for major depressive disorder and had been depressed at least 30 days. All were treated with imipramine and had a DST performed prior to drug treatment. DST nonsuppression was defined as postdexamethasone (0.5 mg) cortisol levels at both 8:00 A.M. and 4:00 P.M. that were greater than 5 μg/dl. The DST nonsuppressors showed the best response to imipramine and the poorest response to placebo. There was no difference between the responses to imipramine or placebo in the DST suppressor group. (See Chapter 10.)

Some studies report that as depressed adults improve with treatment, their DST results gradually return to normal. Albala et al. (1981) and Carroll (1985) report that when the DST results become normal before significant clinical change is evident, this is usually a good prognostic sign that the patient will eventually respond. Such information may be helpful in avoiding premature changes of treatment. Conversely, some patients who improve clinically will continue to show abnormal test results and will often have early relapse if treatment is stopped (APA Task Force on Laboratory Tests in Psychiatry 1987). Peselow et al. (1987) evaluated the DST as an aid in monitoring clinical recovery. Subjects included 127 outpatient adults with major depression who received the DST during and after recovery from major depression. The DST status did not predict 6-month relapse.

Yerevanian et al. (1983) studied 14 patients with positive DSTs who were treated with antidepressants and/or electroconvulsive therapy. After recovery, a repeat DST showed that 10 of the 14 continued to have positive DSTs. All 10 with persistently positive DSTs relapsed, while 3 of the 4 with normalized DSTs remained in remission.

To date there are few studies in children or adolescents that examine the DST as a predictor of response or relapse. Weller et al. (1986) studied hospitalized prepubertal children ages 6–12 years who met DSM-III criteria for major depression and had abnormal DST results. Children were treated and given repeated DSTs at 6 weeks (*n* = 21) and 5 months (*n* = 14). DST results were significantly correlated with clinical status at 5 months but not at 6 weeks.

At the American Psychiatric Association annual meeting in 1983, Targum et al. (1983b) presented follow-up data on 18 adolescents with abnormal DSTs. These subjects were matched with adolescents with normal DSTs. Upon follow-up, 12–15 months later, no differences were found between the two groups as to the rate of rehospitalization or ongoing treatment. Further follow-up studies of depressed children and adolescents who have been given the DST will be needed to determine the value of the DST in predicting outcome.

DST Versus Cortisol Suppression Index

Bernstein et al. (1982) have proposed the cortisol suppression index (CSI) as an alternative to the standard DST for determining cortisol nonsuppression. The CSI is the ratio of the predexamethasone cortisol level to the postdexamethasone cortisol level, both measured at the same time on consecutive days. If this ratio is less than 4.0 at 8:00 A.M., nonsuppression has occurred. In a later study, Bernstein et al. redefined an 8:00 A.M. CSI of less than 7.0 or a 4:00 P.M. CSI of less than 2.5 as nonsuppression, and these values increased sensitivity and specificity.

Weller et al. (1985b) compared the results of the DST and the CSI in 50 depressed inpatient prepubertal children, 36 control subjects (hospitalized psychiatric controls), and 18 normal subjects. The 4:00 P.M. DST, the two-point DST (both 8:00 A.M. and 4:00 P.M. cortisol levels greater than 5 µg/dl), and the 8:00 A.M. revised-criterion CSI (CSI of less than 7.0) yielded the best results and had similar clinical utility and diagnostic confidence.

DST Versus Children's Depression Inventory

As depression in children has become more frequently recognized and diagnosed, self-report inventories and biological markers have been increasingly used in this age group. The Children's Depression Inventory (CDI) is a 27-item, self-report questionnaire completed by the child. It is patterned after the Beck Depression Inventory. (See Chapter 6.) Fristad et al. (1988) compared the CDI and DST in three groups of prepubertal children ages 6–12 years: 63 hospitalized depressed children who met DSM-III criteria for depression, 14 hospitalized psychiatric controls, and 21 nonhospitalized normal volunteers. Sixty-two percent of depressed children had positive DSTs and CDI scores indicating significant depression. Seven percent of psychiatric controls had positive results on both tests, whereas none of the normal controls had positive results on both tests. Results suggested that scores equal to or greater than 15 on the CDI obtained from either a parent or the child provide a good screening instrument (sensitivity, 89%). If the DST was administered to all children with elevated CDI scores, diagnostic confidence was 97.5%. The authors concluded that the CDI should not be used to diagnose childhood depression but rather as a general screening test.

DST Status and Blood Chemistries

Tollefson et al. (1986) reported that pre-DST serum sodium levels were significantly correlated with post-DST cortisol levels in depressed adults. Yaylayan et al. (1989) also looked at serum sodium levels, as well as levels of potassium, glucose, and cholesterol, to determine whether they predicted DST results in prepubertal hospitalized patients ages 6–12 years. None of these blood chemistries alone or in combination could predict DST suppressor status.

GROWTH HORMONE

Abnormalities in growth hormone (GH) secretion have been reported in depressed adults (Sachar et al. 1973). GH is secreted by somatotrophs, which comprise about 50% of the cells in the anterior pituitary. GH may have a direct effect as an insulin antagonist. Patients with GH deficiency are sensitive to insulin-induced hypoglycemia (Daniels and Martin 1987).

Researchers have implicated serotonin in the release of GH and cortisol. Some have reported that GH response to clonidine is impaired in adult patients with endogenous depression. Others found that patients with recurrent depression had a significant reduction in GH secretion during sleep. This reduction persisted throughout treatment and into the recovered drug-free state. The reduction in GH may thus be considered a trait marker in adult patients with recurrent depression (Jarrett et al. 1990).

GH Response to Insulin Tolerance Test

To assess GH abnormalities in depression, Puig-Antich et al. (1984a) carried out insulin tolerance tests (ITTs) in three groups of drug-free prepubertal children: 1) 13 children with major depressive disorder, endogenous type (according to RDC); 2) 17 children with nonendogenous major depressive disorder (according to RDC); and 3) 16 children with nondepressed neurotic disorders according to DSM-III criteria. Children with endogenous depression had significant hyposecretion of GH compared with the other groups. Therefore, prepubertal children may hyposecrete GH in response to insulin-induced hypoglycemia during an episode of endogenous major depression. These studies need to be duplicated.

GH Secretion During Sleep

Kutcher et al. (1988) studied nocturnal GH secretion in nine depressed adolescents (according to DSM-III criteria) and nine normal controls matched for age (16–19 years), sex, menstrual phase, and Tanner stages of pubescence (stage V). The nocturnal GH profile showed that the depressed group had significantly greater secretory amplitudes at 2400 and 0100 hours. Secretion at other times did not differ between the two groups.

Prepubertal children with major depression, regardless of endogenous features, were found to hypersecrete GH during sleep compared with normal and psychiatric controls. Puig-Antich et al. (1984b) studied 22 children with endogenous major depression, 20 children with nonendogenous major depressive disorder, 21 children with nondepressed neurotic disorders, and 8 normal children. GH concentrations were measured every 20 minutes during sleep. They found that both endogenous and nonendogenous depressed groups secreted significantly more GH during sleep than did normal controls or those with neurotic disorders.

GH Response to Desmethylimipramine

GH response to desmethylimipramine, a relatively pure presynaptic norepinephrine reuptake blocker, has been studied by Puig-Antich et al. (unpublished data) in both prepubertal children with major depressive disorder and in controls. The dose of desmethylimipramine was either 50 mg or 75 mg, depending on the child's weight, to approximate a dose of 2 mg/kg. The total amount of GH secretion, as well as the maximum peak increase of GH (compared with baseline), did not differ significantly between the groups.

GH Responses to Clonidine Challenge

The GH response to clonidine (an α_2-adrenergic receptor agonist) has been proposed as a useful and potentially safer test than the ITT for children. It has been used as a standard test of GH release in children being evaluated for GH deficiency (Gil-Ad et al. 1979; Salti et al. 1981). However, this is the only published study of its use in depressed children.

Meyer et al. (1985) studied five boys ages 7–13 years who were at Tanner stages I–III. All met RDC for major depressive disorder. The endocrine evaluation consisted of determining the total secretion of GH and cortisol over a 24-hour period. Also, the rise in GH in response to a clonidine challenge was measured. Controls were 17 males, similar in age and pubertal development. Some controls had normal stature, but others had either genetically short stature or constitutional delay of puberty. Controls had no signs or symptoms of depression. Depressed children had significantly less GH secretion over 24 hours than controls. GH was consistently decreased during the day, night, and sleep. The highest hourly integrated concentration of GH during the 24-hour period was also lower in children with major depression. GH response to clonidine was assessed in the following manner. Clonidine was given orally at a dose of 0.15 mg/m². Blood was drawn for GH at time 0 and every 30 minutes for 180 minutes. GH was measured by RIA. The peak GH responses after administration of clonidine were significantly decreased compared with those of the controls.

GH Secretion in Recovered Prepubertal Depressed Children

Puig-Antich et al. (1984c) found that prepubertal children experiencing an episode of major depression had increased GH secretion during sleep. These subjects were tested when they were in a fully recovered state (for at least 3 months) and were drug free (for at least 1 month). Increased GH secretion during sleep was unchanged.

GH and Suicidal Ideation

Ryan et al. (1987) looked at the relationship between GH and suicidal ideation. The study was done at two different sites with two samples. One sample included 13 suicidal depressed, 14 nonsuicidal depressed, and 28 normal adolescents. A second sample included 21 suicidal depressed, 26 nonsuicidal depressed, and 38 normal adolescents. All subjects were at Tanner stage III. Normal adolescents had the highest GH secretion, nonsuicidal depressed subjects were intermediate, and the depressed suicidal adolescents had the lowest age-corrected mean sleep GH secretion.

MELATONIN

Endogenously depressed adults may have decreased nighttime melatonin secretion (Beck-Friis et al. 1984; Wetterberg 1983). This low nighttime melatonin secretion may remain abnormal even after recovery from major depression (Beck-Friis et al. 1985; Wetterberg 1983). If these findings are confirmed, melatonin secretion could be a potential trait marker for major depression in adults.

Cavallo et al. (1987) examined circadian rhythms of melatonin in depressed children ages 7–13 years. Subjects were 9 males with various types of depressive disorders, and controls were 10 males similar to the subjects in age and pubertal development who had normal stature, genetically short stature, or constitutional delay of puberty. The mean 24-hour and mean overnight melatonin concentrations were significantly lower in the depressed males. Shafii et al. (1990) studied 96 children and adolescents ages 6–16 years. The children and adolescents were divided into three groups. Group I (n = 21) had primary depression: major depression, major depression with dysthymia, or dysthymia. Group II (n = 36) had secondary depression: depression with coexisting psychiatric problems, including conduct disorder, identity disorder, adjustment disorder, or attention-deficit disorder as the primary diagnosis but with some symptoms of depression. Group III (n = 39) was the control group; diagnoses included conduct disorder and/or oppositional disorders. Overnight melatonin secretion in the urine of these children was significantly higher in the primary depressed group than in either the secondary depressed group or the control group. Adjustments for age, sex, race, height, weight, season of the year, and Tanner staging did not affect this finding.

THYROID-STIMULATING HORMONE RESPONSE TO THYROTROPIN-RELEASING HORMONE

The thyrotropin-releasing hormone (TRH) test involves the measurement of serum thyroid-stimulating hormone (TSH) following TRH administration. TRH is secreted from axons of cell bodies in the median eminence of the hypothalamus, binds to membrane receptors, and induces the release of TSH (Grant et al. 1972). The TRH stimulation test is performed by injecting TRH (0.5 mg) at 9:00 A.M. after an overnight fast. TSH levels are taken at baseline and 15, 30, and 60 minutes later (Loosen 1988).

Some depressed patients have a grossly deficient rise in TSH concentration after administration of TRH (Mendlewicz et al. 1979; Prange et al. 1972). Loosen and Prange (1982) reported that 25–30% of depressed patients had a "blunted" increase of TSH in response to TRH. Puig-Antich (1987) found no differences in TSH response to TRH between prepubertal depressed children and controls. Greenberg et al. (1985) also reported similar negative results for depressed adolescents. Thus, the results have been mixed, and additional studies will be necessary to clarify the usefulness of this test in children and adolescents.

POLYSOMNOGRAPHIC FINDINGS DURING A MAJOR DEPRESSIVE EPISODE

Sleep abnormalities reported in endogenously depressed adults include reduced delta (slow-wave) sleep, increased rapid eye movement (REM) density in the early REM periods during the night, short REM latency, and disturbances in sleep continuity (Kupfer et al. 1985; Rush et al. 1982). Studies of sleep abnormalities in depressed children and adolescents have also been performed.

Puig-Antich et al. (1982) studied 54 prepubertal (ages 6–12 years) depressed children (according to RDC) and two groups of controls (11 healthy and 25 with emotional disorders). The polysomnographies of the depressed children were not any different from those of the two control groups.

Young et al. (1982) studied 12 inpatients ages 7–13 years who met Weinberg's criteria for childhood depression (Weinberg et al. 1973). Controls were 12 psychiatrically well children who were matched for sex and age. None of the all-night sleep measures discriminated the depressed patients from their age-matched normal controls.

Goetz et al. (1985) studied 39 children with major depression according to RDC (21 had the endogenous subtype) and 14 children who had emotional disorders but who were not depressed. All subjects were studied in the sleep laboratory for three consecutive nights. There were no differences between the groups for REM signs.

Emslie et al. (1987) performed polysomnography on 17 inpatients ages 9–14 years who had major depression according to DSM-III criteria, 13 of whom met criteria for the melancholic subtype. The researchers did not collect their own control group, but used age-matched published data on normal control subjects from Coble et al. (1984). There were no significant differences between the pre- and postpubertal groups on any sleep EEG measures. When the depressed subjects were compared with the controls, the subjects had a significantly greater number of arousals, shorter REM latency, and greater REM density. Lahmeyer et al. (1983) found that 13 depressed adolescents had significantly greater REM density and shorter REM latency than age-matched normal controls.

In another report, Emslie et al. (1990) studied 25 hospitalized depressed children (according to DSM-III criteria) and 20 age-matched healthy controls. All were at Tanner stages I–III. The depressed subjects had decreased REM latencies. The most sensitive discriminator between depressed patients and controls was the shortest single-night REM latency recorded for each subject. Also, depressed children had increased sleep latency and REM sleep time. However, there were no differences in stage IV sleep.

EEG Findings After Recovery From Major Depressive Episodes

Puig-Antich et al. (1983) studied 28 fully recovered, drug-free, prepubertal children with major depressive disorder. All subjects were scheduled to sleep for three consecutive nights in the laboratory. The EEG sleep measures of the recovered subjects were compared with their own EEG sleep measures during the depressive episode and with the baseline sleep measures of two control groups: nondepressed psychiatrically ill children and normal controls. The recovered prepubertal children had significantly shorter first REM period latency and a higher number of REM periods.

Goetz et al. (1985) studied 19 fully recovered (at least 4 months in remission) depressed children who were drug free for at least 30 days. Controls were 19 nondepressed children with emotional disorders and 9 normal subjects. No significant differences were found among the groups in slow-wave sleep, sleep efficiency, REM density, or temporal distribution of REM sleep during the night. No EEG sleep data are available from adolescents who have recovered from an episode of major depression.

Knowles et al. (1982) conducted an informal survey and found the definition of REM latency to be idiosyncratic. They identified seven definitions of REM latency. Each definition was applied to 70 records taken from five normal subjects, five previously depressed subjects currently in remission, and 14 currently depressed patients. In all three groups, REM latencies calculated on the basis of the seven definitions differed significantly. The authors recommended adopting a common definition to facilitate communication and interpretation of findings from various investigators.

BIOCHEMICAL CORRELATES OF DEPRESSION

Strom-Olson and Weil-Malherbe (1958) reported decreased catecholamine excretion in the urine of depressed patients. However, not all depressed adults exhibit low urinary 3-methoxy-4-hydroxyphenylethylene glycol (MHPG). Similar studies of urinary catecholamine secretion have been conducted in children.

McKnew and Cytryn (1979) examined three chronically depressed inpatients, orthopedic patients screened for affective disorders and found to be free of psychopathology, and a control group of physically and emotionally healthy children. Norepinephrine, vanillylmandelic acid, and MHPG were measured in the urine. Only MHPG concentrations varied significantly among the three study groups. MHPG excretion was highest in the control group, intermediate in the depressed group, and the lowest in the orthopedic group. Khan (1987) studied 84 hospitalized depressed adolescents and 51 nondepressed adolescents ages 13–17 years. Urinary MHPG did not significantly differentiate the two groups.

SUMMARY

During the last decade major strides have been made in investigating neurobiological correlates of major depressive disorder in adults, adolescents, and children. Because of changes in vasovegetative signs such as increase or decrease in sleep or appetite, decrease in sexual function and energy, and diurnal variation in mood, the neuroendocrine system, particularly the HPA axis, has been studied extensively by measuring serum cortisol or its derivative in the urine, or by challenging the HPA axis with dexamethasone, a synthetic steroid.

If a normal adult is given 1.0 mg of dexamethasone orally at 11:00 P.M.

and a blood sample is taken at 8:00 A.M., 4:00 P.M., and 11:00 P.M. the next day, a significant suppression of serum cortisol will occur to the level of less than or equal to 5 µg/dl. This test is called the dexamethasone suppression test. In approximately 50% of adults with major depression, dexamethasone does not suppress serum cortisol. After recovery from major depression, these patients return to a normal DST response.

After the initial enthusiasm about the possible diagnostic value of DST in depression, we have become aware of its limited sensitivity, although the specificity is somewhat better. Sensitivity is defined as the proportion of the subjects with the disorder who have a positive test. It indicates how good a test is at identifying the disorder. Specificity is defined as the proportion of subjects without the disease who have a negative test. It indicates how good a test is at identifying nondiseased individuals. In a review of a number of studies involving a total of 4,400 adult patients with major depression, 43% had a positive DST. Of 2,000 nondepressed controls, 86.5% had a negative DST. DST sensitivity appears to be poor, but the specificity is acceptable in diagnosing major depression in adults.

In several studies of prepubertal children with major depression, 0.5 mg of dexamethasone was given at 11:00 P.M., and blood samples were taken at 8:00 A.M. and 4:00 P.M. the next day. The DST sensitivity was 52–70% and the specificity was 70–87% at 8:00 A.M. Like adults, adolescents usually received 1.0 mg of dexamethasone the night before, and blood samples were taken at 8:00 A.M. and 4:00 P.M. the next day. DST sensitivity in adolescents was 47% and specificity was 80%. This compares with a sensitivity of 43% and a specificity of 86% in adults. It appears that the sensitivity of DST is higher in children than in adolescents and adults.

Other biological markers, such as GH, have also been studied in children. GH has been reported to be significantly higher during sleep in prepubertal children with major depression than in the control group. When these depressed children were divided into endogenous versus nonendogenous subtypes and were given a challenge dose of insulin (ITT), the prepubertal children with major depression endogenous subtype secreted significantly less GH. In place of insulin, a safer drug, clonidine, was given to another group of endogenously depressed children. These children had significantly less GH secretion over a 24-hour period than the controls. Further studies need to be completed to confirm these findings.

In some depressed adult patients with a positive DST, serum melatonin (a hormone of the pineal gland) was reported to be lower than in the nondepressed population. In a study of a mixed group of depressed children and adolescents, serum melatonin was also reported to be lower. However, in a larger study, overnight urinary melatonin was higher in children and adolescents with primary depression (mostly major depression) compared with patients in the same age group who had secondary depression and/or other psychiatric disorders. Further studies are needed in this area.

TSH was lower (blunted) in adult depressed patients following the injection of TRH. In children and adolescents the results were mixed.

Sleep abnormalities such as increased REM density, short REM latency, reduced delta (slow-wave) sleep (stage IV sleep), and disturbance in sleep continuity and efficiency have been reported in adults with major depression. In a number of sleep studies in prepubertal children, the aforementioned findings were not observed. However, some authors have noticed shortened REM latency, greater REM density, and an increased number of arousals in depressed children. No differences in stage IV sleep have been found.

CONCLUSION

Depression in children and adolescents is clinically similar to that in adults. Now there is accumulating evidence that it might be biologically similar as well. Much of this evidence is provided by the fact that some of the biological markers that are present in depressed adults are also present in depressed children. However, most of this research is preliminary, and there is still much to be learned about the neurobiology of childhood depression as well as other childhood disorders.

Most studies in childhood depression are done in the areas of neuroendocrinology, polysomnography, and biochemical changes. To date, the DST has been the most extensively studied biological marker. It appears that the sensitivity of the DST is highest in depressed children (69.9%) and that adolescents have a DST sensitivity comparable to that of adults (47.1% versus 43.1%). However, the specificity was lowest in children (69.7%). There are numerous speculations as to why these differences exist.

Investigators have studied GH response to ITT, desmethylimipramine, or clonidine. Others have studied GH secretion during sleep and examined GH secretion and suicidality. Results of GH studies are somewhat more varied and need replication.

Sleep EEG findings are also mixed. Some investigators have found no significant sleep changes in depressed children. Others have reported findings similar to those observed in depressed adults. Studies on biochemical correlates of childhood depression are few in number, and results must be considered preliminary.

To draw a meaningful conclusion from these neurobiological studies, replication of findings by other investigators is needed. Studies involving a greater number of subjects will also be necessary. To facilitate communication and replication of findings, it may be necessary to adopt common definitions, methods of measurement, and diagnostic classification. If such measures are undertaken, progress can be made in assessing the neurobiology of depression in children and adolescents.

REFERENCES

Albala AA, Greden FJ, Tarika J, et al: Changes in serial dexamethasone suppression test among unipolar depressives receiving electroconvulsive treatment. Biol Psychiatry 16:551–560, 1981

American Psychiatric Association: Diagnostic and Statistical Manual of Mental Disorders, 3rd Edition. Washington, DC, American Psychiatric Association, 1980

American Psychiatric Association: Diagnostic and Statistical Manual of Mental Disorders, 3rd Edition, Revised. Washington, DC, American Psychiatric Association, 1987

APA Task Force on Laboratory Tests in Psychiatry: The dexamethasone suppression test: an overview of its current status in psychiatry. Am J Psychiatry 144:1253–1262, 1987

Arana GW, Mossman D: The dexamethasone suppression test and depression. Approaches to the use of a laboratory test in psychiatry. Endocrinol Metab Clin North Am 17(1):21–39, 1988

Beck-Friis J, Von Rosen D, Kjellman BF, et al: Melatonin in relation to body measures, sex, age, season and the use of drugs in patients with major depressive disorders and healthy subjects. Psychoneuroendocrinology 10:261–277, 1984

Beck-Friis J, Kjellman BF, Aperia B, et al: Serum melatonin in relation to clinical variables in patients with major depressive disorder and a hypothesis of low melatonin syndrome. Acta Psychiatr Scand 71:319–330, 1985

Bernstein JP, Chung SY, Avila KSM, et al: Cortisol suppression index: a new approach to interpreting the DST in depression. J Clin Psychiatry 43:476–478, 1982

Bober JF, Weller EB, Weller RA, et al: Correlation of serum and salivary cortisol levels in prepubertal school-aged children. J Am Acad Child Adolesc Psychiatry 27(6):748–750, 1988

Brown RP, Mason B, Stoll P, et al: Adrenocortisol function and suicidal behavior in depressive disorders. Psychiatry Res 17:317–323, 1986

Carlson GA, Cantwell DP: A survey of depressive symptoms, syndrome and disorder in a child psychiatric population. J Child Psychol Psychiatry 21:19–25, 1980

Carroll BJ: Dexamethasone suppression test: a review of contemporary confusion. J Clin Psychiatry 46:13–24, 1985

Carroll BJ, Feinberg M, Greden JF, et al: A specific laboratory test for the diagnosis of melancholia. Arch Gen Psychiatry 38:15–22, 1981

Casat CD, Arana GW, Powell K: The DST in children and adolescents with major depressive disorder. Am J Psychiatry 146:503–507, 1989

Cavallo A, Holt K, Hejazi MS, et al: Melatonin circadian rhythm in childhood depression. J Am Acad Child Adolesc Psychiatry 26(3):395–399, 1987

Centers for Disease Control: Suicide Surveillance 1970–1980. Atlanta, GA, U.S.

Department of Health and Human Services, Public Health Service, Violent Epidemiology Branch, Center for Health Promotion and Education, 1985

Chabrol H, Chaverie J, Moron P, et al: DST, TRH test and adolescent suicide attempts. Am J Psychiatry 140:265, 1983

Climko RP, Martin D, Bonsall EK: Salivary and serum cortisol levels in the DST. Paper presented at the annual meeting of the American Psychiatric Association, Chicago, IL, May 1987

Coble PA, Kupfer DJ, Taska LS, et al: EEG sleep of normal healthy children, part I: findings using standard measurement methods. Sleep 7:289–303, 1984

Coryell W, Schlesser MA: Suicide and DST in unipolar depression. Am J Psychiatry 138:1120–1121, 1981

Daniels GH, Martin JB: Harrison's Principles of Internal Medicine, 11th Edition. New York, McGraw-Hill, 1987

Doherty MB, Mandansky D, Kraft J, et al: Cortisol dynamics and test performance of the dexamethasone suppression test in 97 psychiatrically hospitalized children aged 3–16 years. J Am Acad Child Psychiatry 25(3):400–408, 1986

Emslie GJ, Roffwarg HP, Rush AJ, et al: Sleep EEG findings in depressed children and adolescents. Am J Psychiatry 144:668–670, 1987

Emslie GJ, Rush AJ, Weinberg WA, et al: Children with major depression show reduced rapid eye movement latencies. Arch Gen Psychiatry 47:119–124, 1990

Extein I, Rosenberg G, Pottash ALC, et al: The dexamethasone suppression test in depressed adolescents. Am J Psychiatry 139:1617–1619, 1982

Fristad MA, Weller EB, Weller RA, et al: Self-report versus biological markers in assessment of childhood depression. J Affective Disord 15:339–345, 1988

Geller B, Rogol AD, Knitter EF, et al: Preliminary data on the dexamethasone suppression test in children with major depressive disorder. Am J Psychiatry 140:602–622, 1983

Georgotas A, Stokes P, Cooper T, et al: Dexamethasone suppression in the elderly: diagnostic and treatment implications. Paper presented at the 33rd annual meeting of the Society of Biological Psychiatry, New York, May 1983

Gil-Ad I, Topper E, Laron Z: Oral clonidine as a growth hormone stimulation test. Lancet 2:278–279, 1979

Goetz RR, Hanlon C, Puig-Antich J, et al: Signs of REM prior to the first REM period in prepubertal children. Sleep 8:1–10, 1985

Grant G, Vale W, Guillemin R: Interaction of thyrotropin-releasing factor with membrane receptors of pituitary cells. Biochem Biophys Res Commun 46:28–34, 1972

Greenberg R, Rosenberg G, Weisberg L, et al: The dexamethasone suppression test and the thyrotropin-releasing hormone test in adolescent major depressive disorder. Paper presented at the New Research Section of the 32nd annual meeting of the American Academy of Child Psychiatry, San Antonio, TX, October 1985

Ha H, Kaplan S, Foley C: The dexamethasone suppression test in adolescent psychiatric patients. Am J Psychiatry 141:421–423, 1984

Hsu LK, Molcan K, Cashman MA, et al: The dexamethasone suppression test in adolescent depression. J Am Acad Child Psychiatry 22(5):470–473, 1983

Jarrett DB, Miewald JM, Kupfer DJ: Recurrent depression is associated with a persistent reduction in sleep-related GH secretion. Arch Gen Psychiatry 47:113–118, 1990

Khan AU: Biochemical profile of depressed adolescents. J Am Acad Child Adolesc Psychiatry 26(6):873–878, 1987

Klee SJ, Garfinkel BD: Identification of depression in children and adolescents: the role of the dexamethasone suppression test. J Am Acad Child Adolesc Psychiatry 23(4):410–415, 1984

Knowles JB, MacLean AW, Cairns J: Definitions of REM latency: some comparisons with particular reference to depression. Biol Psychiatry 17:993–1002, 1982

Kupfer DJ, Ulrich RF, Coble PA, et al: Electroencephalographic sleep of young depressives. Arch Gen Psychiatry 42:806–810, 1985

Kutcher SP, Williamson P, Silverberg J, et al: Nocturnal growth hormone secretion in depressed older adolescents. J Am Acad Child Adolesc Psychiatry 27(6):751–754, 1988

Lahmeyer HW, Poznanski EO, Bellur SN: Sleep in depressed adolescents. Am J Psychiatry 140:1150–1153, 1983

Livingston R, Reis CJ, Ringdahl IC: Abnormal dexamethasone suppression test results in depressed and nondepressed children. Am J Psychiatry 141:106–108, 1984

Loosen PT: Thyroid function in affective disorders and alcoholism. Endocrinol Metab Clin North Am 17(1):55–82, 1988

Loosen PT, Prange AJ Jr: The serum thyrotropin (TSH) response to thyrotropin-releasing hormone (TRH) in depression: a review. Am J Psychiatry 139:405–416, 1982

McKnew DH, Cytryn L: Urinary metabolites in chronically depressed children. J Am Acad Child Adolesc Psychiatry 18(4):608–615, 1979

Mendlewicz J, Linowski P, Brauman H: TSH response to TRH in women with unipolar and bipolar depression. Lancet 2:1079–1080, 1979

Meyer WJ, Richards GE, Cavallo A, et al: Growth hormone and cortisol secretion dynamics in children with major depressive disorder. Paper presented at the annual meeting of the American Academy of Child Psychiatry, San Antonio, TX, October 1985

Nuller JL, Ostroumova MN: Resistance to inhibiting effect of dexamethasone in patients with endogenous depression. Acta Psychiatr Scand 61:169–177, 1980

Peselow ED, Baxter N, Fieve PR, et al: The dexamethasone suppression test as a monitor of clinical recovery. Am J Psychiatry 144:30–35, 1987

Petty LK, Asarnow JR, Carlson GA, et al: The dexamethasone suppression test in depressed, dysthymic, and nondepressed children. Am J Psychiatry 142:631–633, 1985

Pfeffer CR, Stokes P, Weiner A, et al: Psychopathology and plasma cortisol responses to dexamethasone in prepubertal psychiatric inpatients. Biol Psychiatry 26:677–689, 1989

Poznanski EO, Cook SC, Carroll BJ, et al: A depression rating scale for children. Pediatrics 64:442–450, 1979

Poznanski EO, Carroll BJ, Banegas MC, et al: The dexamethasone suppression test in prepubertal depressed children. Am J Psychiatry 139:321–324, 1982

Prange AJ Jr, Wilson IC, Lara PO, et al: Effects of thyrotropin-releasing hormone in depression. Lancet 2:999–1002, 1972

Preskorn SH, Weller EB, Hughes CW, et al: Depression in prepubertal children: DST nonsuppression predicts differential response to imipramine versus placebo. Psychopharmacol Bull 23:128–133, 1987

Puig-Antich J: Affective disorder in children and adolescents: diagnosis, validity and psychobiology, in Psychopharmacology: The Third Generation of Progress. Edited by Meltzer HY. New York, Raven, 1987, pp 843–859

Puig-Antich B, Blau S, Marx N, et al: Prepubertal major depressive disorder. J Am Acad Child Psychiatry 17:695–707, 1978

Puig-Antich J, Chambers W, Halpern F, et al: Cortisol hypersecretion in prepubertal depressive illness: a preliminary report. Psychoneuroendocrinology 4:191–197, 1979

Puig-Antich J, Goetz R, Hanlon C, et al: Sleep architecture and REM sleep measures in prepubertal children with major depression: a controlled study. Arch Gen Psychiatry 39:932–939, 1982

Puig-Antich J, Raymond G, Hanlon C, et al: Sleep architecture and REM sleep measures in prepubertal major depressives: studies during recovery from the depressive episode in a drug-free state. Arch Gen Psychiatry 40:187–192, 1983

Puig-Antich J, Novacenko H, Davies M, et al: Growth hormone secretion in prepubertal children with major depression, I: final report on response to insulin-induced hypoglycemia during a depressive episode. Arch Gen Psychiatry 41:455–460, 1984a

Puig-Antich J, Goetz R, Davies M, et al: Growth hormone secretion in prepubertal children with major depression, II: sleep-related plasma concentrations during a depressive episode. Arch Gen Psychiatry 41:463–466, 1984b

Puig-Antich J, Goetz R, Davies M, et al: Growth hormone secretion in prepubertal children with major depression, IV: sleep-related plasma concentrations in a drug-free fully recovered clinical state. Arch Gen Psychiatry 41:479–483, 1984c

Robbins DR, Alessi NE: Suicide and the dexamethasone suppression test in adolescence. Biol Psychiatry 20:94–119, 1985

Robbins DR, Alessi NE, Yanchyshyn GW, et al: Preliminary report on the dexamethasone suppression test in adolescents. Am J Psychiatry 139:942–943, 1982

Rush AJ, Griles DE, Roffwarg HP, et al: Sleep EEG and dexamethasone suppression test findings in outpatients with unipolar major depressive disorders. Biol Psychiatry 17:327–341, 1982

Ryan ND, Puig-Antich J, Meyer V, et al: Growth hormone secretion during sleep in depressed adolescents. Paper presented at the Consortium on Affective Disorders in Children, Boston, MA, September 1987

Sachar EJ: Neuroendocrine abnormalities in depressive illness, in Topics in Psychoneuroendocrinology. Edited by Sachar EJ. New York, Grune & Stratton, 1975, pp 135–156

Sachar EJ, Hellman L, Roffwarg HP: Disrupted 24-hour patterns of cortisol secretion in psychotic depression. Arch Gen Psychiatry 28:19–24, 1973

Sachar EJ, Asnis G, Halbreich V, et al: Recent studies in the neuroendocrinology of major depressive disorders: advances in psychoneuroendocrinology. Psychiatric Clin North Am 3(2):313–327, 1980

Salti R, Galluzzi F, Becherucci P, et al: Oral clonidine: an effective provocative test of growth hormone release. Helv Paediatr Acta 36:527–531, 1981

Schlesser MA, Winokur G, Sherman BM: Hypothalamic-pituitary-adrenal axis activity in depressive illness: its relationship to classification. Arch Gen Psychiatry 37:737–743, 1980

Secunda SK, Cross CK, Koslow S, et al: Biochemistry and suicidal behavior in depressed patients. Biol Psychiatry 21:756, 1986

Shafii M, Foster MB, Greenberg RA, et al: The pineal gland and depressive disorders in children and adolescents, in Biological Rhythms, Mood Disorders, Light Therapy, and the Pineal Gland. Edited by Shafii M, Shafii SL. Washington, DC, American Psychiatric Press, 1990, pp 99–116

Spitzer RL, Endicott J, Robins E: Research Diagnostic Criteria: rationale and reliability. Arch Gen Psychiatry 35:773–782, 1978

Stokes PE, Sikes CR: The hypothalamic-pituitary-adrenal axis in major depression. Endocrinol Metab Clin North Am 17(1):1–19, 1988

Strom-Olson R, Weil-Malherbe H: Humeral changes in manic-depressive psychosis with particular references to the excretion of catecholamines in urine. Journal of Mental Sciences 104:696–704, 1958

Targum SD, Rosen L, Capodanno AE: The dexamethasone suppression test in suicidal patients with unipolar depression. Am J Psychiatry 140:7, 1983a

Targum SD, Capodanno AE, Unger S: The DST in adolescents: a matched follow-up study. Paper presented at the annual meeting of the American Psychiatric Association, New York, May 1983b

Tollefson GD, Zander J, Luxenberg M: Prediction of post-dexamethasone cortisol levels by serum sodium levels in patients with major depression. Am J Psychiatry 143:81–84, 1986

Weinberg WA, Rutman J, Sullivan L, et al: Depression in children referred to an educational diagnostic center: diagnosis and treatment. Behavioral Pediatrics 83:1065–1072, 1973

Weller EB, Weller RA: Current Perspectives on Major Depressive Disorders in Children. Washington, DC, American Psychiatric Press Monograph Series, 1984

Weller EB, Weller RA, Fristad MA, et al: The dexamethasone suppression test in prepubertal depressed children. J Clin Psychiatry 46:511–513, 1985a

Weller RA, Weller EB, Fristad MA, et al: A comparison of the cortisol suppression index and the dexamethasone suppression test in prepubertal children. Am J Psychiatry 142:1370–1372, 1985b

Weller EB, Weller RA, Fristad MA, et al: Dexamethasone suppression test and clinical outcome in prepubertal depressed children. Am J Psychiatry 143:1469–1470, 1986

Wetterberg L: The relationship between the pineal gland and the pituitary-adrenal axis in health, endocrine, and psychiatric conditions. Psychoneuroendocrinology 8:75–80, 1983

Woolston JL, Gianfredi S, Gertner JM, et al: Salivary cortisol: a nontraumatic sampling technique for assaying cortisol dynamics. J Am Acad Child Psychiatry 22:474–476, 1983

Yaylayan SK, Weller EB, Weller RA, et al: DST status and blood chemistries in prepubertal children. Psychiatry Res 29:215–219, 1989

Yehuda R, Southwick SM, Ostroff RB, et al: Neuroendocrine aspect of suicidal behavior. Endocrinol Metab Clin North Am 17(1):83–102, 1988

Yerevanian BI, Olafsdottir H, Milanese E, et al: Normalization of dexamethasone suppression tests at discharge from hospital: its prognostic value. J Affective Disord 5:191–197, 1983

Young W, Knowles JB, MacLean AW, et al: The sleep of childhood depressives: comparison with age-matched controls. Biol Psychiatry 17:1163–1168, 1982

CHAPTER 4

Chronobiology of
Seasonal Mood Disorders

William A. Sonis, M.D.

Geophysical periodicity is a ubiquitous part of life. Given the daily, monthly, and yearly changes that occur around us, it is not surprising that geophysical rhythms influence our lives. For thousands of years, physicians and other observers of the human condition have noted a relationship between geophysical periodicity and seasonal changes in mood, activity, and energy. In this chapter, I will review concepts used to describe and understand rhythms; the ontogeny of biologic rhythms; the chronobiological hypothesis of mood disorders; links between geophysical and biopsychosocial seasonal rhythms; and the current knowledge about recurrent winter depression, also known as seasonal affective disorder (SAD).

Present knowledge of chronobiology and its relationship to SAD is based on studies in animals and adult humans. Careful clinical observations and data-based studies in children and adolescents are very limited. Specific references to SAD in children and adolescents are found at the end of this chapter in the section titled "Seasonal Affective Disorder in Children and Adolescents."

DESCRIPTION OF RHYTHMS

A rhythm is the organization of a phenomenon in time. It is the arrangement of regularly occurring sequences of a process in relationship to specific time markers. Regularly observable examples include geophysical rhythms, such as the tides, light and dark cycles, and lunar and seasonal cycles; biological rhythms, such as heart rate and respiratory cycles; and behavioral rhythms, such as sleep-wake cycles, hibernation, and seasonal reproduction cycles.

I wish to thank Peter Whybrow, M.D., and Kristina Rask for their critical comments and helpful suggestions in preparing this manuscript. The author is supported by NIMH Child and Adolescent Mental Health Academic Award 1 K07 MH00769-01.

Chronobiology is the objective, quantitative description of biological time structures (Carandente 1984).

SPECIFIC TERMS USED IN CHRONOBIOLOGY

Period, Frequency, Phase, and Amplitude

Specific terms used to describe the measurable parameters of a biological rhythm are period, frequency, phase, and amplitude (see Figure 4–1). Period (t) is the time needed for the rhythm to complete one full cycle, frequency (f) is the inverse of the period and is expressed as cycles per specific unit of time, and the amplitude is half the difference between the peak and the trough value. Rhythms that have different periods when isolated from external time cues are said to be disassociated. Phase is the location of any particular point in the wave form or the timing of the wave form relative to an extrinsic marker, such as time. The acrophase (0) is the time of the rhythm peak. Thus, the phase of a rhythm describes the relationships between either a specific rhythm and a marker not associated with the rhythm (external phase rela-

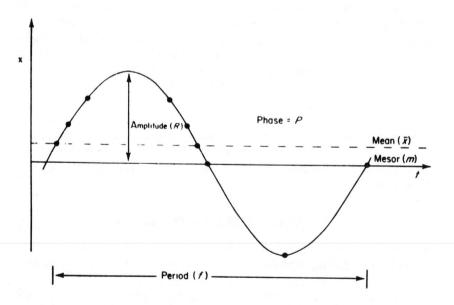

Figure 4–1. The five major parameters of a rhythm. Note that when sampling is irregular, the mean and mesor may not coincide. Reproduced from TH Monk: Research methods of chronobiology, in Biological Rhythms, Sleep and Performance. Edited by Webb WB. New York, John Wiley, 1982, p. 130. Copyright 1982 John Wiley & Sons, Ltd. Reprinted by permission of John Wiley & Sons, Ltd.

tionship) or between two or more rhythms in the same organism (internal phase relationships). Two or more rhythms are described as either synchronized (that is, they maintain the same phase relationship) or desynchronized (indicating a difference in the phase relationships). Desynchronized rhythms can be either advanced (one rhythm occurs earlier relative to a specific marker) or delayed (one rhythm occurs later relative to a specific marker).

Ultradian, Circadian, and Infradian Rhythms

A rhythm can be also described by the number of cycles that occur in a 24-hour period (frequency), the shape of the wave modality, and the type of process involved. Rhythms that occur more than once in a 24-hour period are designated as ultradian rhythms. Examples of human ultradian rhythms include EEG rhythms, cardiac rhythms, and the rapid eye movement (REM)–nonrapid eye movement (NREM) cycle. Rhythms that occur once in a 24-hour period are designated as circadian (from the Latin *circa* = "about," *dies* = "day") rhythms. Examples of human circadian rhythms include the sleep-wake cycle, cortisol secretion, and core body temperature. Cycles that occur less than once in a 24-hour period are designated as infradian. Specific human infradian rhythms are described by their period and include circaseptan (weekly), circatrigintan (monthly), and circannual (yearly) rhythms. Examples of human infradian rhythms include menstrual cycles (circatrigintan) and seasonal (circannual) rhythms in mortality, conception, and children's growth rate (Aschoff 1981).

Shape and Process of Rhythms

The shape of the wave and the type of process involved are also used to describe a rhythm. Wave shape is described by both the number of peaks (unimodal, bimodal, or multimodal) and the deviation of the curve from a normal distribution. Rhythms are also described by the type of process involved. Some rhythms, such as oxygen saturation, are functions with multiple values that form a continuous curve, while others are relatively discontinuous, such as the sleep-wake cycle.

Entrainment of Rhythms

Period, phase, amplitude, shape, and process are all used to describe both physical and biological rhythms. Geophysical rhythms originate from the interaction of multiple physical systems. For example, light-dark, tidal, and seasonal temperature cycles are all geophysical rhythms that arise from the interaction between planets, atmosphere, and the stars. Biological rhythms originate from specific types of cells that serve as timekeepers (clocks or oscillators) for the organism (Moore-Ede et al. 1982). These timekeepers serve as pacemakers for the timing of other rhythmic biological events, such as alertness, feeding, sleeping, and hibernation.

Although oscillators serve an important function in biology, their output is rarely directly observed. An observed or measured rhythm may reflect the output of the oscillator and modifications imposed by external or internal events that may or may not be intrinsically rhythmic. Changes in the periodicity of a biological rhythm may be caused by periodic factors in the environment. Rhythms in biological organisms can be synchronized to a periodic input from outside the biological unit (exogenous) or from within the biological unit (endogenous). The ability of periodic environmental factors (also known as synchronizers or zeitgebers) to modify the period of an endogenous oscillator is called entrainment.

The same terminology used to characterize a rhythm (period, frequency, phase, and amplitude) is also used to describe the characteristics of synchronizers or zeitgebers. Zeitgebers may be either physical or social. For example, human sleep rhythms can be entrained to external synchronizers that vary greatly from a 24-hour cycle. Human growth hormone secretion is entrained to sleep onset, which is an internal rhythm, but it can be desynchronized relative to an external zeitgeber (time) when sleep onset is phase-shifted relative to the external environment. In humans, light-dark cycles entrain sleep-wake cycles, as do social and environmental cues. However, some oscillators are so strong that they cannot be entrained. Despite shifts in sleep-wake, the rhythm of core body temperature continues to cycle with a 24-hour rhythm (Wever 1983).

Masking

The distortion of an endogenous wave form by external events is called "masking." Masking may change the phase and shape of a rhythm but does not change the frequency or period of the rhythm. Masking occurs less often with ultradian rhythms but is more evident in circadian and infradian rhythms. For example, strenuous exercise at the time of the circadian nadir of body temperature increases core body temperature, causing spikes in the temperature curve and thus distorting or masking the normal sinusoidal shape of the circadian temperature rhythm (Wever 1983).

Oscillators in Humans

Biological oscillators can be isolated from masking rhythms in experimental studies in which external events or "masking elements" are systematically controlled to eliminate externally generated rhythmicity. Cells or tissues whose rhythmicity continues when isolated from masking rhythms are called pacemakers or oscillators. It is currently believed that there are two oscillators in the human central nervous system: a strong oscillator (X), which controls core temperature, cortisol secretion, REM sleep, and urinary potassium, and a weak oscillator (Y), which controls slow-wave sleep, skin temperature, growth hormone, and urinary calcium (Moore-Ede et al. 1982). The notion of "strong" versus "weak" relates to the degree to which these oscillators can be phase-shifted by changes in external synchronizers. For example, the circadian rhythm of temperature (governed by a strong oscillator) does not phase-shift when an individual's sleep onset is changed; however, the onset of growth hormone (governed by a weak oscillator) does change (Moore-Ede et al. 1982).

Chronobiological research in psychiatry has focused on the identification and description of circadian rhythms in psychiatric disorders. This work has been followed by the study of drug-rhythm interactions and ultradian and infradian rhythms (Monk 1982). Although ultradian and circadian rhythms have been experimentally demonstrated since the early 18th century (Moore-Ede et al. 1982), circannual rhythms were first validated experimentally in the late 1950s and early 1960s (Gwinner 1981). Seasonality, or the study of the relationship between infradian geophysical rhythms and psychobiological phenomena, is a relatively new area of chronobiological research (Gwinner 1981).

ONTOGENY OF PSYCHOBIOLOGICAL RHYTHMS

Oscillating biological systems begin, mature, and age throughout the life span of the organism. Changes in these systems during development account for some of the differences between the rhythmic patterns observed in neonates, children, adolescents, and adults.

Development of Rhythms in Humans

Two generalizations can be made about the development of rhythms in humans: 1) different rhythms appear at different ages, and 2) most of these rhythms pass through some period of maturation. In general, the amplitude of a rhythm increases as the organism matures. The increase can occur as an outgrowth of one or both of the following dichotomous processes: 1) a rise in peak values, a decline in trough values, or both simultaneously; and 2) a simultaneous decrease in amplitude at one time of day and an increase at another. The second process represents a selective increase of specific ultradian rhythms at a specific time of day. In contrast to the increased amplitude seen with maturation, as an organism ages, rhythms decrease in amplitude and occurrence of spontaneous desynchronization increases (Davis 1981).

To describe the ontogeny of a rhythm, the rhythm itself must be measurable. Measurability is related to both the frequency with which the function is sampled and the maturation of the function being sampled. This is particularly true when an overt or secondary rhythm, different from a pacemaker rhythm, is measured in an already rhythmic environment. This environment (sample time) may simply impose a rhythm on the overt function. Thus, infrequent sampling of an immature rhythm will provide a distortion of the oscillatory pattern. For example, sampling a neonate's sleep every 8 hours would provide an entirely different "picture" of the sleep-wake rhythm than would samples obtained every 4 hours. In contrast, sampling an adolescent's sleep every 8 hours would provide a more representative picture of the actual sleep-wake pattern.

Sleep and temperature rhythms. Despite these problems with measurement, many biological rhythms (sleep-wake, temperature, and various neurohormones) have demonstrated a specific ontogeny. Sleep-wake rhythmicity appears during the second month of postnatal life, with diurnal variation in sleep-wake cycles appearing by the 3rd month. Shifts in the timing and duration of REM-NREM episodes continue to change throughout the life span. The shift in the timing and duration of REM-NREM episodes across the life span may account for the lack of reported REM latency in depressed children and adolescents and the presence of this finding in adults (Anders 1982; Puig-Antich 1987). Core body temperature does not demonstrate a rhythmic variation in the first week of life, but a clearly defined adult-shaped circadian rhythm develops by the 10th month of life. The amplitude of the core temperature rhythm continues to increase during childhood, reaching a maximum at 7 years of age. After the age of 7 years, there is an overall decrease in the amplitude during the remainder of life (Abe et al. 1978).

Neuroendocrine rhythms. During neonatal life, the adrenocorticotropic hormone (ACTH)–cortisol circadian rhythm is multimodal (two to four equal peaks during each 24-hour period), with the adult biphasic ACTH-cortisol curve taking 2 years to emerge. While human growth hormone (GH) is secreted in a random episodic pattern in high concentration throughout the day in newborns, the nocturnal pulsatility of human GH does not begin to emerge until about 4 months of age. Additional pulsatile episodes begin to appear again during prepuberty and adolescence, and human GH secretion then declines to almost undetectable levels during the fifth decade of life. Gonadotropins and gonadal steroids demonstrate sex dimorphic patterns that also change throughout development (Miller et al. 1982; Sizonenko 1978).

Mood changes throughout the life cycle. In addition to the ontogeny of biological rhythms, psychobiological mood rhythms also demonstrate specific ontogeny. Templer et al. (1981–1982) studied diurnal mood variation and age in 230 subjects ages 13–89 years. The authors found that older individuals reported feeling better in the morning than in the evening. Abe and Suzuki (1985) found an inverse curvilinear relationship among self-report of early morning waking, feeling worse in the morning, and age in 6,034 subjects ages 9–60 years. Early morning awakening was least prevalent in teenagers, whereas feeling worse in the morning was most prevalent in young adults. Thus, the older the individual, the more likely one is to have a positive mood in the morning.

Larson et al. (1980) found that 76 high school students had a wider range of moods that switched more rapidly compared to 107 adult volunteers ages 19–65 years. Thus, there appears to be both a decrease in the amplitude and the frequency of mood shifts as an individual ages. Although there may be alternative hypotheses to explain these age-related differences in mood, these observed trends may be an indication of maturational changes in oscillators controlling mood regulation, thereby providing important information about the etiology of mood disorders.

CHRONOBIOLOGICAL HYPOTHESIS OF MOOD DISORDERS IN ADULTS

There are specific clinical associations between mood disorders and putative disturbances in chronobiology. These associations include episodes of illness itself (periodic exacerbations and remissions), symptom presentation (diurnal variation in mood and early morning awakening), and the seasonal pattern of mood disturbance (seasonal peaks in hospital admissions and suicide) (Wehr and Goodwin 1983).

Phase Dyssynchrony

The phase dyssynchrony hypothesis is an integration of several chronobiological hypotheses. These hypotheses posit that depressive and manic symptoms occur because of changes in biological rhythms, which assume abnormal phase positions in relation to each other (internal phase disorder) and because of entraining geophysical and social cycles (external phase disorder) (Kripke 1983; Wehr and Goodwin 1983). The specific precipitant that initiates the phase dyssynchrony is presumed to be either an internal response to an external stressor (Ehlers et al. 1988) or, as in the case of recurrent winter depression, a photoperiodic event. There are also different types of phase dyssynchronies that often correspond to subtypes of depression. For example, patients with winter depression exhibit a phase delay in dim-light melatonin onset (DLMO), while patients with nonwinter depression exhibit a phase advance in DLMO (Lewy and Sack 1987; Lewy et al. 1990).

Evidence in support of the phase dyssynchrony hypothesis is emerging from three areas of study: the relationship between sleep and mood, phase shifts in neuroendocrine functions and mood, and the biological manipulation of circadian rhythms.

Initially, shortened REM latency (Kupfer and Foster 1972) was believed to be pathognomonic of depression and indicated a phase advance of the sleep-wake cycle. However, this finding has since been observed in multiple disorders (for example, schizophrenia [Stern et al. 1969], obsessive-compulsive disorder [Insel et al. 1982], and alcoholism [Spiker et al. 1977]). Sleep often dramatically changes the symptoms of depression, and many of the biological disturbances observed in depression are intimately linked with evidence of disturbed hypothalamic function (Halbreich 1987). Bipolar patients, in a depressive phase, often become manic when deprived of sleep, and depressed patients tend to improve when they are deprived of sleep (Wehr 1988).

The changes in neuroendocrine function observed in depressive patients (decreased thyroid-stimulating hormone pulsatility, decreased hypothalamic-pituitary-thyroid and adrenal rhythm amplitude) are mediated by pacemaker cells in the hypothalamus that are sensitive to changes in sleep-wake cycling (Krieger 1988; Wehr 1988). Phase shifts in 3-methoxy-4-hydroxyphenylethylene glycol (MHPG) excretion, as well as an increased ultradian amplitude of MHPG excretion, have been observed in depressed patients and reflect circadian shifts in noradrenergic function (Halaris 1987). Other evidence in support of the phase dyssynchrony hypothesis is provided by day-night reversal studies of normal individuals that include changes in REM and cortisol rhythmicity that are found in depressed patients (Wehr and Goodwin 1983); phase changes in the circadian rhythms of temperature, motor activity, serotonin, cortisol, prolactin, salivary flow rate, and DLMO in depressed patients (Lewy and Sack et al. 1987; Wehr and Goodwin 1983); and clinical response to chronobiological treatment.

Treatment Strategies

These treatment strategies have developed from the phase dyssynchrony hypothesis: phototherapy, which involves the use of bright light to shift aberrant rhythms; sleep deprivation, which changes the phase relationship between sleep onset-offset and other internal rhythms; and psychopharmacology, which uses chemical mediators to change and reorder internal rhythms.

Light therapy. Light has been used to treat medical and psychiatric conditions for thousands of years (Wehr 1989). The current era of phototherapy began with a single case study reporting the use of bright full-spectrum light (2,500 lux) to successfully treat a patient with recurrent winter depression (Lewy et al. 1982, 1990). To date, at least 562 patients have been treated with phototherapy at multiple centers using different types of experimental designs. Using pooled data, Terman (1989) found that all regimens of bright light exposure yielded similar mean posttreatment scores on the Hamilton Depression Rating Scale (HDRS) (Hamilton 1960). There is, however, a difference in response when morning phototherapy is compared with evening or midday phototherapy. If a score reduction of at least 50% in the HDRS is used as the criterion for determining improvement, 66% of patients with SAD improved when morning light was presented by itself or in combination with evening light, compared to 50% who improved when midday or evening light was presented alone. If a posttreatment score of less than 8 (nondepressed) on the HDRS is used as the criteria for improvement, 52% of SAD patients improved using morning light and 43% improved when exposed to midday or evening light. When these two measures (50% reduction in score and a score of less than 8) are used as the criteria of improvement, a remission rate of 51% is obtained when morning light is used either alone or in combination with evening light, and a 38% remission rate is obtained when midday or evening light is used alone. Terman also found that this proportional difference was statistically significant.

Although the specific type of light used (white or full spectrum) does not appear to be crucial to the therapeutic effect, the intensity of illumination is crucial. Between 2,000 and 2,500 lux at eye level is required for a therapeutic effect (Lewy and Sack 1989; Zucker 1988). In comparison to the 2,000 lux needed for a therapeutic effect, ordinary room lighting is about 200 lux, while illumination outside on a sunny summer day is 110,000 lux. Treatment regimens studied have generally used 2 hours (at 2,500 lux) to 30 minutes (at 10,000 lux) per day. In general, the higher the intensity of light, the shorter the duration of treatment (Terman 1989). Intensities above 10,000 lux have not been used in treatment studies.

There is conflicting evidence on the efficacy of bright light (1,500–2,500 lux) for the treatment of nonwinter depression. Kripke et al. (1989), in their study involving over 100 patients, found that treatment with bright white light over a period of 1 week had a mild antidepressant effect. Some studies have shown that bright white light had significant antidepressant effects compared with either baseline or red light, whereas other studies failed to show the same therapeutic effect. Additional studies are in progress comparing bright white light phototherapy with imipramine therapy; the long-term efficacy of bright white light in the treatment of nonwinter depression is also being tested (Kripke et al. 1987, 1989).

Sleep deprivation. Sleep deprivation has also been a powerful tool in understanding the role of circadian rhythms in depression. Gillin (1983), reporting studies of over 1,000 depressed patients, found that 70% of depressed bipolar patients, 60% of endogenously unipolar patients, and 40% of reactive or neurotically depressed unipolar patients improved in response to total sleep deprivation. The component of sleep deprivation that accounts for the therapeutic effect and alleviation of depressive symptoms is not clear. Sleep deprivation treatment consists of several interventions, including deprivation of sleep; exposure to light; changes in body heat, temperature, and posture; physical activity; and social stimuli (Wehr 1988). Several investigators have attempted to pinpoint the specific intervention responsible for the therapeutic effect of sleep deprivation. Exposure to light is not necessary for the therapeutic effect (Wehr et al. 1985).

Partial sleep deprivation in the second half of the night is as effective an antidepressant as total sleep deprivation (Schilgen and Tolle 1980) and is more effective than partial sleep deprivation in the first half of the night (Goetze and Tolle 1981). Shifts in sleep onset have also been capable of inducing remission in depressed patients; changing the time of sleep onset from the usual 11:00 P.M. to 7:00 A.M. period to a 5:00 P.M. to 1:00 A.M. schedule has induced remission in depressed patients (Sack et al. 1985; Wehr et al. 1979). The antidepressant effect of wakefulness in the last half of the night lends additional evidence to the hypothesis that the relationship between sleep-wake cycles and other biological circadian rhythms is important to the genesis of depression.

Pharmacotherapy. Studies of effective pharmacological interventions used to treat mood disorders have shed additional light on the relationship between circadian pacemakers, measurable rhythms, and depression. Lithium slows circadian pacemakers (which means that the period of the rhythm increases) in many different organisms from unicellulars through mammals and has been the most widely studied chronotropic psychopharmacological agent to date (Engelmann 1987). In humans, lithium delays the sleep cycle by 14.2 minutes in healthy subjects under entrained conditions. In free-running conditions, the period interval of human core body temperature, activity, and sleep-wake cycles were increased with the use of lithium by 1.2 hours in four of eight healthy students (Engelmann 1987). The phase shifts observed with lithium administration may be responsible for its therapeutic efficacy. Manic-depressive patients who demonstrate abnormally shortened circadian rhythms are lithium responders, whereas patients with prolonged circadian rhythms are lithium nonresponders (Kripke et al. 1979).

Thus, the phase dyssynchrony hypothesis is a central, integrative, and controlling mechanism that provides a hierarchical framework across multiple systems for understanding the neurotransmitter, neuroendocrine, and behavioral disturbances observed in mood disorders. The developmental aspects of chronobiology have yet to be integrated into this model. However, much of the accumulated data to date remain contradictory and incomplete.

GEOPHYSICAL AND BIOLOGICAL SEASONAL RHYTHMS AND MOOD VARIATION IN ADULTS

The recognition that seasonal rhythms influence our moods has been a theme in medicine and literature for almost 2,500 years. Wehr (1989) found numerous historical references to the intimate relationship between the seasons, mood, and light:

> Hippocrates noted that melancholia appears in the spring. Posidonius in the 4th century A.D. also noted the seasonal occurrence of mood disorder and stated "Melancholy occurs in the autumn whereas mania occurs in the summer. . . ." Aretaeus (2nd century A.D.) and Caelius Aurelianus (250–320 A.D.) both prescribed light for depression. . . . Chaucer in the Knights Tale stated that "For May wol have no sluggardye anight . . . And maketh out of his sleep to sterte. . . ." T.S. Eliot in the Wasteland observed, "April is the cruelest month, breeding lilacs out of the dead land," while Emily Dickinson stated, "There's a certain slant of light on winter afternoons, that oppresses, like the weight of cathedral tunes." (pp. 14, 26, 13)

Seasonal and Latitudinal Effects

These observations on the relationship between season and mood have been validated by epidemiological studies that demonstrate that depression and mania evidence latitudinal and seasonal variation. Aschoff (1981) analyzed a 100-year span of world mortality (all causes of death), suicide, and conceptions and found definite seasonal rhythms in all three sets of statistics. The mortality and suicide acrophases (peak) were independent of latitude; that is, the time (season) of the peak did not vary with latitude and the peak occurred at roughly the same time each year. In the northern hemisphere, the mortality rate peaked in January, whereas in the southern hemisphere it peaked in July. Suicide in the northern hemisphere peaked in May. Data on suicides in the southern hemisphere are limited, and only tentative conclusions can be drawn. Two authors (Gaedeken 1911; Krapf 1937) have published seasonal analyses of suicides in the southern hemisphere (Buenos Aires). These authors found a bimodal distribution of suicides: November (spring) and April (fall).

   Sunshine and heat. The amplitude (or the height of the peak) of mortality and suicide did vary with latitude, reaching a maximum at about 40° north latitude. The relative amplitude in mortality was more closely correlated with the amplitude of the average duration of sunshine than with temperature across the globe (Aschoff 1981). Both the ambient monthly temperature and monthly duration of sunshine reach maximal value at about 40° latitude. There was also a steady decline in the amplitude of all three data sets during the past 100 years, despite the consistency of the acrophase timing. This pattern suggests either a decrease in the effectiveness of the synchronizing environmental factors or a decrease in the sensitivity of the human organisms to these synchronizers (Ashoff 1981).

   In support of Ashoff's interpretation, seasonal peaks in suicide have been repeatedly confirmed with different samples by multiple investigators

(DeMaio et al. 1982; Kevan 1980; Lester 1971; Meares et al. 1981; Nayah 1982; Parker and Walter 1982; Warren et al. 1983). Those researchers who included adolescents in their sample (DeMaio et al. 1982; Kevan 1980) discovered that this subpopulation followed the same general seasonal patterns that were followed by adults. There are no seasonal data on suicide trends for prepubertal children.

Hospital admissions. Studies of hospital admissions for mood disorders have also consistently demonstrated seasonal peaks. Depending upon the criteria, different subgroups of mood-disordered patients demonstrate differences in seasonal hospital admissions. To understand the effect of latitude (climatic variation) on psychiatric hospital admissions, the effect of time lag must be taken into account. That is, the time between the onset of symptoms and presentation for treatment can be months for depression, but it is often much shorter for manic episodes. Thus, the ability to associate specific climatic factors that may account for the seasonal peaks of hospital admissions is weaker for depression than for mania. In general, studies of bipolar depressed patients have demonstrated a bimodal peak (spring and fall) for hospital admissions (Frangos et al. 1980; Rihmer 1980). Studies of unipolar depressed populations show a primary unimodal distribution with a predominant spring peak and a smaller peak later on in the fall (Frangos et al. 1980). Endogenous depressed patients were admitted most frequently in the spring, whereas neurotic depressed patients were most frequently admitted in the fall (Eastwood and Stiasny 1978).

Summer peaks for admissions of manic patients were found by Symonds and Williams (1976), Myers and Davies (1978), and Carney et al. (1988). A 50-year sample of manic admissions to one state hospital in Greece (Frangos et al. 1980) found a bimodal distribution (spring and fall peak) similar to that reported by the authors for bipolar depression. Myers and Davies (1978) investigated acute manic episodes and demonstrated a significant correlation between admissions and the current month's mean temperature, along with the previous month's mean amount of daylight. They concluded that light appeared to be a coarse adjuster and heat was a fine adjuster for the precipitation of manic episodes. In contrast to Myers and Davis's (1978) 1-month lag, Carney et al. (1988) found a stronger correlation between monthly total hours of sunshine and admissions and suggested that proximal rather than distal factors accounted for manic episodes. No data are available about the seasonal distribution of child or adolescent psychiatric hospital admissions for depression or mania.

Normal Variation of Mood

Individual differences in nonpathological seasonal mood variation have also been discovered. For example, seasonal variation of normal mood was reported by Cason (1931), who studied the retrospective estimation of daily, weekly, and monthly feelings in 900 subjects ages 15–85 years. His subjects reported feeling lowest in January and best in June. Springer and Roslow (1935) replicated Cason's findings in 133 male college students, but also demonstrated the low test-retest reliability of retrospective recall. Nelson (1971), in a prospective survey of college students, found that cheer reached its nadir and unhappiness and depression reached the maximum toward the end of each quarter. Although Nelson concluded that this rhythm was related to the demands of finals, the design of this study actually demonstrated an infradian (70-day) mood rhythm.

Whitton (1978) studied 18 subjects over a minimum of 320 days, using a self-report diary measure of health, sleep, anxiety, clarity of thinking, and mood. Sixty-one percent of his subjects reported cycles in at least three of the variables, with 56% of the subjects reporting periods between 3 and 8 weeks. Eastwood et al. (1985) compared mood, sleep, and energy rhythms over 18 months in 30 bipolar patients and 34 controls matched for age, sex, marital status, and socioeconomic status who had no psychiatric diagnosis. Independent of diagnosis and sex, 35% of the subjects reported seasonal periodicity (greater than 85 days), 15% reported monthly periodicities, and 14% had weekly periodicities. Compared with matched controls, individuals with bipolar illness reported a greater amplitude across all periodicities. Unfortunately, family history of mood disorders was not controlled in this study and thus may have been responsible for the findings of multiple periodicities in some of the controls.

Random Survey of Seasonal Pattern of Mood

Other evidence supporting the seasonal variation of mood comes from a random general population survey conducted by Terman (1989) in New York City. Terman used the Seasonal Pattern Assessment Questionnaire (SPAQ), a self-report of seasonal symptoms (Rosenthal et al. 1984). He found that 25% of his sample ($n = 200$) complained of mood, sleep, and appetite changes that caused personal problems in the winter; another 35% of the sample noted seasonal symptoms but did not complain that the changes interfered with their function. Of the 25% of the sample classified as "complainers," 80% reported lowered energy, 61% reported increased weight, 53% reported increased sleep, 53% reported decreased social activity, and 41% reported feeling worst in the winter. Further analysis of these data demonstrated an extremely strong correlation ($r = .97$) between seasonal changes in length of sleep and changes in the time of sunrise.

Psychiatrists have long noted seasonal patterns of clinically significant mood variations in individual patients. This was particularly true of the 18th and 19th century descriptive psychiatrists, such as Pinel, Esquirol, Griesinger, Ballarger, Plicz, and Kraepelin, but it has also been true of psychiatrists in the late 20th century (Wehr 1989).

SEASONAL AFFECTIVE DISORDER IN ADULTS

In an attempt to understand more about individual differences in the seasonal pattern of recurrent depressive episodes, Rosenthal and his colleagues at the National Institute of Mental Health began to recruit subjects who experienced recurrent winter depression followed by spring and summer remission. They named this pattern seasonal affective disorder, or SAD (Rosenthal et al. 1984). During the past decade, several other centers for the study of SAD have developed. Using pooled subject data ($n = 496$) from research centers in Maryland, Switzerland, Pennsylvania, Oregon, New York, and Alaska, Hellekson (1989) found the mean subject age to be 40.6 years; the mean age at onset of symptoms was 21.3 years. Most subjects (83.3%) were female. The symptoms reported by individuals with SAD frequently include decreased activity, sadness, anxiety, and increased appetite and weight. Sleep duration was increased in these individuals as well (Table 4–1) (Hellekson 1989).

SAD, Bipolar Disorder II, and Major Depressive Disorder

There are marked diagnostic differences in SAD subjects across centers. Sites in Maryland, Switzerland, and Alaska found bipolar disorder II (winter depression, spring and summer hypomania) to be the most common diagnosis, whereas centers in Oregon, New York, and Pennsylvania diagnosed major depressive disorder (winter depression only) most frequently. The discrepancy between the major diagnostic groupings at each center was whether the increased energy component in the summer met the criteria for hypomania (Hellekson 1989).

Other forms of nonwinter seasonal mood disorders exist and are currently being researched. These include summer depression and mixed seasonal depression. Individuals with summer depression present a picture opposite to that of patients with winter depression. Rather than an anergic, hyperphagic, hypersomnic, depressive picture, patients with summer depression presented with an agitated, hypophagic, hyposomnic, depressive clinical picture (Wehr 1989). Heat may be the triggering environmental factor in summer depression. A few patients with this disorder improved after being isolated from heat and exposed to the cold in uncontrolled studies (Wehr 1989). Mixed types of seasonal disorder may be represented by 6.6% of Terman's (1989) New York population survey. This group has not been clinically studied.

Table 4–1. Symptoms reported by adult patients with seasonal affective disorder during winter at Bethesda (BE), Maryland, and Basel (BA), Switzerland

		Percentage of patients	
Variables	Symptoms reported	BE (n = 246)	BA (n = 63)
Activity	Decreased	95	98
Affect	Sadness	96	92
	Irritability	86	73
	Anxiety	87	85
Appetite	Increase	71	45
	Decrease	18	32
	Mixed	1	2
	No change	11	21
	Carbohydrate craving	72	73
Weight	Increase	76	52
	Decrease	10	21
	Mixed	1	0
	No change	13	25
Libido	Decrease	59	
Sleep	Increased duration	83	64
	Earlier onset	69	
	Change in quality	64	79
	Daytime drowsiness	73	
Other	Symptoms milder near equator	89 (n = 100)	
	Menstrual difficulties	58 (n = 185)	
	Work difficulties	86	95
	Interpersonal difficulties	93	84

Source. Modified from Hellekson 1989.

Unimodal and Bimodal Seasonal Rhythms

The epidemiological and individual seasonal variation in mood, energy, and sleep observed in humans may have biological roots in the multiple physiologic seasonal changes known to occur in humans. In their review of seasonal psychobiological variation in normal subjects, Lacoste and Wirz-Justice (1989) provide strong evidence for seasonal variation in multiple regulatory and metabolic functions. Numerous physiological measures demonstrate unimodal seasonal rhythms (platelet imipramine binding, thyroid function, cortisol, blood pressure, glucose, and insulin), whereas others demonstrate a bimodal seasonal rhythm (melatonin, fatigue, and depression).

These seasonal rhythms are modified by age and sex. Touitou et al.

(1984) found that the amplitude of the seasonal cortisol rhythm decreases with age. In opposition to this general trend, the seasonal blood pressure rhythm increases with age (Brennan et al. 1982). Sex differences in seasonal psychobiological function also occur; females exhibit seasonal rhythms in both prolactin secretion and acral thermoregulatory warming, while males do not (Lacoste and Wirz-Justice 1989). A few studies have addressed the issue of developmental circannual psychobiological function in normal children and found that the annual rhythms of luteinizing hormone and testosterone were similar to those found in adults (Bellastella et al. 1982).

Chronobiology and Child and Adolescent Psychobiology

The relationship between developmental psychobiological rhythmicity and psychiatric disorders is a new and emerging field. Except for the study of REM latency and neuroendocrine correlates of child and adolescent depression (Puig-Antich 1986), there has been little systematic investigation of the chronobiological correlates of child and adolescent psychopathology. There are, however, occasional reports about chronobiological correlates of psychopathology. These reports include disturbed amplitude of core temperature rhythms in autistic children (Yamazaki et al. 1976); a decrease in behavior problems in third-grade boys and an increase in behavior problems in girls following the change from daylight savings time to standard time (Hicks et al. 1980); evidence of desynchronized rhythmic components (a 24-hour component and a free-running component) of the rest-activity cycle in a 17-year-old school refuser (Chiba 1984); three children with infradian cycles of behavior ratings (Taylor 1982); greater temperature amplitude than expected in four psychotic subjects (Romanczyk et al. 1980); and a case report of therapeutic sleep deprivation in a depressed child (King et al. 1987). These reports offer tantalizing insights into possible chronobiological mechanisms underlying disturbed behavior in children and adolescents.

Although the quantity and quality of the research on developmental ultradian and circadian rhythms in child and adolescent psychopathology are increasing, there remains a paucity of developmental infradian seasonal rhythm studies.

SEASONALITY IN
CHILDREN AND ADOLESCENTS

Although physicians, authors, and poets recognize the influence of seasons on adult mood, only recently has seasonality been studied in children and adolescents. Several isolated reports have appeared exploring the relationship between geophysical seasonal periodicity and mood and behavior in children and adolescents.

Meteorological Changes and Physical Complaints

Farest et al. (1974) surveyed 1,575 randomly selected subjects ages 13–29 years concerning the relationship between meteorological circumstances and physical complaints in Basel, Switzerland. Twenty-three percent of the youths claimed to be sensitive to the weather. Of these youths, more girls (29%) than boys (18%) endorsed weather sensitivity. Two-thirds of these weather-sensitive youths complained of fatigue, 50% complained of diffuse pressure sensation in the head and moods of discontent, and 33% complained of discomfort, dislike of work, increased tendency to make mistakes, insomnia, sleep disturbance, headaches, and irritability. Sex-dimorphic complaints were present in both weather-sensitive and non-weather-sensitive individuals. Significantly, more girls than boys complained of fatigue, moods of discontent, irritability, headaches, and the inability to fall asleep. Ten percent of the weather-sensitive youths used coffee, tea, and tobacco as stimulants, and 10% also used analgesics. Older subjects complained more frequently of weather sensitivity than younger subjects.

Temporal and Climatic Variability

In another study, Russell and Bernal (1977) naturalistically observed deviant, annoying, and desirable behaviors in 76 5- to 7-year-old boys and found strong support for their hypothesis that there was systematic temporal and climatic variability. Half the subjects were reported to have more discipline problems at home than the average boy, whereas the other half were reported to be no more noncompliant, disruptive, or aggressive than the average boy. There were no psychiatric evaluations or diagnoses reported. Russell and Bernal found that deviant behaviors peaked at the end of the week and were more present on days without precipitation, as well as on colder days. Desirable behaviors peaked as bedtime approached. They suggested that observational studies should control for temporal and climatic factors that may influence results.

The previous studies, although they provide examples of behavioral infradian rhythms, either concentrated on relatively short periods of time or used retrospective recall. Studies of the circannual nature of psychopathology are even more scarce than studies of circadian or ultradian rhythm.

Francezon et al. (1981) found a circannual fluctuation in the stereotyped and self-mutilating behavior of a mentally deficient adolescent. In this study, the number of blows the patient delivered to his head was recorded during 13 daily observations of 5 minutes each from 8:00 A.M. to 10:00 P.M. (except Sunday). Several categories of prominent variations were present: day-to-day variations; cyclical variations of about 1½ to 2 months; and an extensive circannual variation with a maximum in July and August and a minimum in December and January. This difference was statistically significant.

SEASONAL AFFECTIVE DISORDER
IN CHILDREN AND ADOLESCENTS

Seasonal disturbances in mood have also been reported in children and adolescents. Carlson (1983) reported a seasonal pattern of depression and mania in an 11-year-old girl with manic-depressive illness. Rosenthal et al. (1986) reported SAD, winter type, in seven children and adolescents and treated them with phototherapy. Sonis et al. (1987), in a randomly assigned, single-blind, crossover study, compared phototherapy with relaxation treatment in 5 adolescents with SAD, winter type, and 15 subjects without SAD (Rosenthal et al. 1986; Sonis et al. 1987). Phototherapy in these two studies was effective in alleviating the symptoms of the subjects with SAD. In addition, Sonis et al. (1987) found that phototherapy was significantly more effective and specific in relieving the symptoms of SAD than in relieving the symptoms of nonseasonal major depression (Table 4–2).

Although the number of children and adolescents with SAD is small, they have some important developmental similarities to and differences from adult subjects with SAD. In children and adolescents, the female-to-male ratio was closer to 1:1 rather than 4:1 as described in the adult literature (Hellekson 1989). Rosenthal's sample was younger than ours (mean age of 12.3 years versus mean age of 16.2 years), although the mean numbers of cycles expressed as duration of illness were similar (5.1 versus 6.0) (Sonis 1989). Some illustrative case studies of adolescents with SAD follow.

Table 4–2. Children's Depression Rating Scale scores

Group	Baseline[a] X	Baseline[a] SD	Light[b] X	Light[b] SD	Washout X	Washout SD	Relaxation X	Relaxation SD
Seasonal affective disorder	62.6	16.3	42.4	11.4	53.0	17.6[c]	57.4	15.2[c]
Major depression	59.9	4.9	52.3	10.4	38.3	5.9[c]	34.3	4.5
Attention-deficit disorder	33.6	6.2	22.6	5.0	24.8	8.0	24.2	8.5
No diagnosis	30.6	4.8	20.6	1.3	19.2	5.9	20.8	4.3

Note. Multivariate analysis of covariance: $F_{(6,26)} = 3.07, P < .02$.
[a]Initial and pretreatment combined.
[b]Analysis of covariance: $F_{(3,13)} = 8.81, P < .002$.
[c]Studentized maximum modulus: $df = 13, P < .05$.

Case Histories

L.C. was a 16-year-old high school junior from an intact middle-class family when she requested admission to our study. According to both L.C. and her mother, she had been experiencing problems in school, morning hypersomnia, multiple somatic complaints, decreased concentration, irritability, fatigue, and dysphoria each of the past five winters. She was known to the school nurse as a "complainer," who often reported feeling ill and tired, although no physical basis could be found. L.C. was treated with 2,500 lux of full-spectrum light for 2 hours in the evening at sundown. First her energy returned; then her sleep improved and her dysphoria resolved. She was so different that she remarked, "My friends were concerned I was on drugs." When she stopped phototherapy, her symptoms returned in the same order in which they resolved. That is, her energy decreased, her sleep pattern became disturbed, and her dysphoria returned. Her symptoms improved within 2–3 days of beginning light treatment, and she had almost complete symptom remission within a week. She has continued to use phototherapy each winter.

Another example of an adolescent with SAD was R.D., a 16-year-old male whose mother brought him to our attention. For the past 3 years, each winter he had experienced persistent dysphoria, poor school performance with decreased concentration, morning hypersomnia, and irritability. His mother, age 40 years, had been experiencing seasonal symptoms since adolescence, and there was a multigenerational history of manic-depressive illness. R.C. met criteria for SAD. He began phototherapy and reported alleviation of his depressive symptoms within 2–3 days. Symptoms reached maximum improvement by the end of a week. He used evening phototherapy for 2 hours. His mother also used the phototherapy apparatus with the successful resolution of her symptoms. The family experimented with different phototherapy regimens and found that R.C. needed 2 days of phototherapy but could skip a day without return of disabling symptoms. On the other hand, his mother only needed 1 day of phototherapy for 3 hours to maintain symptom alleviation for 2 days. Thus, until R.C. went to college, the family was able to use one phototherapy unit.

D.B. was a 9-year-old white male who was brought to the clinic because of recurrent crying episodes. According to his mother, his crying episodes occurred during the winter and were associated with persistent dysphoria, irritability, problems concentrating, restlessness, and worry. He had had two previous episodes lasting about 5 months each, one when he was 3 years old and the other at age 5 years. Each spring his symptoms would remit. His mother moved away from the area before a trial of phototherapy could be initiated.

Comparison of SAD in Adults With SAD in Children and Adolescents

As a follow-up to our initial study, we compared the symptoms of 30 subjects

(20 females and 10 males) who met criteria for SAD with the symptom profiles of adults with SAD (Rosenthal et al. 1985). The mean age of this sample was 16.4 ± 2.3 years. In comparing our SAD sample with data available on adults with SAD, we found that significantly fewer children and adolescents than adults reported changes in activity and sadness ($P < .01$), whereas significantly more of the children and adolescents reported hyposomnia ($P < .01$). In addition, fewer children and adolescents than adults with SAD reported anxiety and increased appetite, whereas more children and adolescents than adults reported irritability. These differences approached but did not reach significance (Sonis 1989).

Seasonal mood variation may also be a normally distributed population trait in children and adolescents. We surveyed 779 high school students ages 14–18 years for seasonal mood variation and depression using a child and adolescent version of the SPAQ, which has been named the Seasonal System Checklist for Children (SSCL-C) (Sonis et al. 1987). Sixteen-year-old girls scored significantly higher on the SSCL-C than any other age and sex combination. Post hoc analysis revealed that five items (fatigue, headaches, craving sweets, crying, and worrying) accounted for these significant differences. We classified 51 students (6.4% of the total sample) as "highly seasonal"; that is, their total SSCL-C scores were above the third quartile, they had experienced marked interference with activities, and they had noticed seasonal symptoms for more than 2 years. Twenty-nine percent of this sample also scored in the severely depressed range (Kaplan et al. 1984). This group (highly seasonal/severely depressed) represented 1% of the total sample. We were not able to do a second-stage interview to validate the assumption that these youngsters (highly seasonal/severely depressed) may have SAD.

FUTURE DIRECTIONS

Much work remains to be done to further identify, define, and develop treatment for specific forms of recurrent depression in children and adolescents. Recurrent winter depression, as described in the adult psychiatric literature, exists in children and adolescents. Adolescents with recurrent winter depression experience symptom relief when treated with phototherapy. Nonpathological seasonal mood variation also appears to be present in children and adolescents in roughly the same proportion as it is in randomly selected adult populations. Although the data are sparse, it is my impression that more adolescents than children experience seasonal mood variation and that entrainment and desynchronization to photoperiodic stimuli may be age dependent. This hypothesis is consistent with existing information about developmental changes in mood disorders across the peripubertal period. The changes include an increase in depressive feelings reported from childhood into adolescence; the shift in the sex ratio of major depressive disorders from a non-sex-dimorphic ratio before puberty to a female preponderance after puberty; and the emergence of mania during adolescence (Rutter 1986).

Specific areas for future psychiatric research in developmental chronobiology include the developmental aspects of entrainment, techniques to measure psychobiological circadian and infradian rhythms in children and adolescents, population-based studies of mood variation in normal and specific diagnostic groupings of children and adolescents, longitudinal studies of nondepressed and depressed prepubertal individuals, treatment studies of sleep deprivation and phototherapy as experimental probes, and family history and genetic linkage studies using specific family cell lines of winter and nonwinter depressed individuals. As these lines of investigation yield information about mood disorders across the life span, we may be able to develop methods of early identification and more effective treatment methods to minimize the psychosocial morbidity and mortality associated with child and adolescent mood disorders.

REFERENCES

Abe K, Sasaki H, Takebayaski K, et al: The development of circadian rhythm of human body temperature. Journal of Interdisciplinary Cycle Research 9(3):211–216, 1978

Abe K, Suzuki T: Age trends of early awakening and feeling worse in the morning than in the evening in apparently normal people. J Nerv Ment Dis 173(8):495–498, 1985

Anders TF: Biological rhythms in development. Psychosom Med 44(1):61–72, 1982

Aschoff J: Annual rhythms in man, in Handbook of Behavioral Neurobiology, Vol 4: Biological Rhythms. Edited by Aschoff J. New York, Plenum, 1981, pp 475–487

Bellastella A, Esposito V, Mango A, et al: Temporal relationship between circannual levels of luteinizing hormone and testosterone in prepubertal boys with constitutional short stature. Chronobiologia 9:123–125, 1982

Brennan PJ, Greenberg G, Miall WE, et al: Seasonal variation in arterial blood pressure. Br Med J 285:919–923, 1982

Carandente F: Glossary of chronobiology. Chronobiologia 11(3):313–322, 1984

Carlson GA: Bipolar affective disorders in childhood and adolescence, in Affective Disorders in Childhood and Adolescence: An Update. Edited by Cantwell DP, Carlson GA. New York, SP Medical & Scientific Books, 1983, pp 61–84

Carney PA, Fitzgerald CT, Monaghan CE: Influence of climate on the prevalence of mania. Br J Psychiatry 152:820–823, 1988

Cason H: General curves and conditions of feeling. J Appl Psychol 15:126–148, 1931

Chiba Y: A school refuser: his rest activity rhythm involved multiple circadian components. Chronobiologia 11:21–27, 1984

Davis FC: Ontogeny of circadian rhythms, in Handbook of Behavioral Neurobiology, Vol 4: Biological Rhythms. Edited by Aschoff J. New York, Plenum, 1981, pp 257–274

DeMaio D, Carandente F, Riva C: Evaluation of circadian, circaseptan, and circannual periodicity of attempted suicides. Chronobiologia 9:185–193, 1982

Eastwood MR, Stiasny S: Psychiatric disorder, hospital admission, and season. Arch Gen Psychiatry 35:769–771, 1978

Eastwood MR, Whitton JL, Kramer FM, et al: Infradian rhythms: a comparison of affective disorders and normal persons. Arch Gen Psychiatry 42:295–299, 1985

Ehlers CL, Frank E, Kupfer DJ: Social zeitgebers and biological rhythms: a unified approach to understanding the etiology of depression. Arch Gen Psychiatry 45:948–952, 1988

Engelmann W: Effects of lithium salts on circadian rhythms, in Chronobiology and Psychiatric Disorders. Edited by Halaris A. New York, Elsevier, 1987, pp 263–289

Farest V, Weidmann M, Wekner W: The influence of meteorological factors on children and youths: a 10% random selection of 16000 pupils and apprentices of Basel City (Switzerland). Acta Paedopsychiatr (Basel) 40(4):150–156, 1974

Francezon J, Visier JP, Mennesson JF: Circannual fluctuation of stereotyped behaviors with possible self-mutilation in a mentally deficient adolescent. International Journal of Chronobiology 7(3):129–140, 1981

Frangos E, Athanassenas G, Tsitourides S, et al: Seasonality of the episodes of recurrent affective psychoses, possible prophylactic intervention. J Affective Disord 2:239–247, 1980

Gaedeken P: Uber die psychophysiologishe bedeutung der atmospharischen verhlatnisse, insbesondere des lichts. Zeitschrift fur Psychotherapie III(129):126, 1911

Gillin JC: The sleep therapies of depression. Prog Neuropsychopharmacol Biol Psychiatry 7:351–364, 1983

Goetze U, Tolle R: Antidepressive wirkung des partiellen schlafentzuges wahren der 1 Halfte der nacht. Psychiatric Clinics (Basel) 14:129–149, 1981

Gwinner E: Circannual systems, in Handbook of Behavioral Neurobiology, Vol 4: Biological Rhythms. Edited by Aschoff J. New York, Plenum, 1981, pp 381–389

Halaris A: Normal and abnormal circadian patterns of noradrenergic transmission, in Chronobiology and Psychiatric Disorders. Edited by Halaris A. New York, Elsevier, 1987, pp 23–47

Halbreich U: The circadian rhythm of cortisol and MHPG in depressives and normals, in Chronobiology and Psychiatric Disorders. Edited by Halaris A. New York, Elsevier, 1987, pp 49–73

Hamilton M: A rating scale for depression. J Neurol Neurosurg Psychiatry 23:56–62, 1960

Hellekson C: Phenomenology of seasonal affective disorder: an Alaskan perspective, in Seasonal Affective Disorders and Phototherapy. Edited by Rosenthal NE, Blehar MC. New York, Guilford, 1989, pp 33–45

Hicks RA, Lawrence-Davis JR, Guynes SM: Change in the classroom deportment of children following change from daylight saving time. Percept Mot Skills 51:101–102, 1980

Insel TR, Gillin JC, Moore A, et al: The sleep of patients with obsessive-compulsive disorder. Arch Gen Psychiatry 39:1372–1377, 1982

Kaplan SI, Hong GK, Weinhold C: Epidemiology of depressive symptomatology in adolescents. J Am Acad Child Psychiatry 23(1):91–98, 1984

Kevan SM: Perspectives on season of suicide: a review. Soc Sci Med 14D:369–378, 1980

King BH, Baxter LR, Stuber M, et al: Case report: therapeutic sleep deprivation for depression in children. J Am Acad Child Adolesc Psychiatry 26(6):928–931, 1987

Krapf EE: La influencia del ritmo estacional sobre la frecuencia de las enfermedades mentales: contribucion a una meteropatologia argentina. Revista Neurologica (Buenos Aires) 2:107–135, 1937

Krieger DJ: Abnormalities in circadian periodicity in depression, in Biological Rhythms in Affective Disorders. Edited by Kupfer DJ, Monk TH, Barchas JD. New York, Guilford, 1988, pp 177–195

Kripke DF: Phase-advance theories for affective illness, in Psychobiology and Psychopathology, Vol 2: Circadian Rhythms in Psychiatry. Edited by Wehr TA, Goodwin FK. Pacific Grove, CA, Boxwood Press, 1983, pp 41–69

Kripke DF, Mullaney DJ, Atkinson ML, et al: Circadian rhythm phases in affective illness. Chronobiologia 6:365–375, 1979

Kripke DR, Gillin JC, Mullanney DJ, et al: Treatment of major depressive disorders by white light for 5 days, in Chronobiology and Psychiatric Disorders. Edited by Halaris A. New York, Elsevier, 1987, pp 207–218

Kripke DF, Mullaney DJ, Savides TJ, et al: Phototherapy for nonseasonal major depressive disorders, in Affective Disorders and Phototherapy. Edited by Rosenthal NE, Blehar MC. New York, Guilford, 1989, pp 342–356

Kupfer DJ, Foster FG: Interval between onset of sleep and rapid eye movement sleep as an indicator of depression. Lancet 2:684, 1972

Lacoste V, Wirz-Justice A: Seasonal variation in normal subjects: an update of variables current in depression research, in Affective Disorders and Phototherapy. Edited by Rosenthal NE, Blehar MC. New York, Guilford, 1989, pp 167–229

Larson R, Csikszentmihalyi M, Graef R: Mood variability and the psychosocial adjustment of adolescents. Journal of Youth and Adolescents 9(6):469–490, 1980

Lester D: Seasonal variation in suicidal deaths. Br J Psychiatry 118:627–628, 1971

Lewy AJ, Sack RL: Phase typing and bright light therapy of chronobiologic sleep and mood disorders, in Chronobiology and Psychiatric Disorders. Edited by Halaris A. New York, Elsevier, 1987, pp 181–206

Lewy AJ, Sack RL: The dim light melatonin onset as a marker for circadian phase position. Chronobiol Int 6(1):93–102, 1989

Lewy AJ, Kern HA, Rosenthal NE, et al: Bright artificial light treatment of a manic-depressive patient with a seasonal mood cycle. Am J Psychiatry 139:1496–1498, 1982

Lewy AJ, Sack RL, Singer CM: Bright light, melatonin, and winter depression: the phase-shift hypothesis, in Biological Rhythms, Mood Disorders, Light Therapy, and the Pineal Gland. Edited by Shafii MS, Shafii SL. Washington, DC, American Psychiatric Press, 1990, pp 141–173

Meares R, Medelsohn FAO, Milgrom-Freedman J: A sex difference in the seasonal variation of suicide rate: a single cycle for men, two cycles for women. Br J Psychiatry 138:321–325, 1981

Miller JD, Tannenbaum GS, Colle E, et al: Daytime pulsatile growth hormone secretion during childhood and adolescence. Journal of Endocrinology and Metabolism 55(5): 989–994, 1982

Monk TH: Research methods of chronobiology, in Biological Rhythms, Sleep and Performance. Edited by Webb WB. New York, John Wiley, 1982, pp 27–57

Moore-Ede MC, Sulzman FM, Fuller CA: A physiological system measuring time, in The Clocks That Time Us: Physiology of the Circadian Timing System. Cambridge, MA, Harvard University Press, 1982, pp 1–29

Myers DH, Davies P: The seasonal incidence of mania and its relationship to climatic variables. Psychol Med 8:433–440, 1978

Nayah S: Autumn incidence of suicides re-examined: data from Finland by sex, age, and occupation. Br J Psychiatry 141:512–517, 1982

Nelson TM: Student mood during a full academic year. J Psychosom Res 15:113–122, 1971

Parker G, Walter S: Seasonal variation in depressive disorders and suicidal deaths in New South Wales. Br J Psychiatry 140:626–632, 1982

Puig-Antich J: Psychobiological markers: effects of age and puberty, in Depression in Young People: Developmental and Clinical Perspectives. Edited by Rutter M, Izard CE, Read PB. New York, Guilford, 1986, pp 341–381

Puig-Antich J: Affective disorders in children and adolescents: diagnostic validity and psychobiology, in Psychopharmacology: The Third Generation of Progress. Edited by Meltzer HY. New York, Raven, 1987, pp 843–859

Rihmer Z: Season of birth and season of hospital admission in bipolar depressed female patients. Psychiatry Res 3:247–251, 1980

Romanczyk RG, Gordon WC, Crimmins DB: Childhood psychosis and 24-hour rhythms: a behavioral and psychophysiological analysis. Chronobiologia 7:1–14, 1980

Rosenthal NE, Sack DA, Gillin JC, et al: Seasonal affective disorder: a description of the syndrome and preliminary findings with light therapy. Arch Gen Psychiatry 41:72–80, 1984

Rosenthal NE, Sack DA, Carpenter CJ, et al: Antidepressant effects of light in seasonal affective disorder. Am J Psychiatry 142:163–170, 1985

Rosenthal NE, Carpenter CJ, James SP, et al: Seasonal affective disorder in children and adolescents. Am J Psychiatry 143:356–358, 1986

Russell MB, Bernal ME: Temporal and climactic variables in naturalistic observation. J Appl Behav Anal 10:399–405, 1977

Rutter M: Depressive feelings, cognitions and disorders: a research postscript, in Depression in Young People: Developmental and Clinical Perspectives. Edited by Rutter M, Izard CE, Read PB. New York, Guilford, 1986, pp 491–519

Sack DA, Nurnberger J, Rosenthal NE, et al: Potentiation of antidepressant medication by phase advance of the sleep-wake cycle. Am J Psychiatry 142:606–608, 1985

Schilgen B, Tolle R: Partial sleep deprivation as therapy for depression. Arch Gen Psychiatry 37:267–271, 1980

Sizonenko PC: Endocrinology of preadolescents and adolescents, I: hormonal changes during normal puberty. Am J Dis Child 132:704–712, 1978

Sonis WA: Seasonal affective disorder of childhood and adolescence: a review, in Seasonal Affective Disorders and Phototherapy. Edited by Rosenthal ME, Blehar MC. New York, Guilford, 1989, pp 46–54

Sonis WA, Yellin AM, Garfinkel BD, et al: The antidepressant effect of light in seasonal affective disorder of childhood and adolescence. Psychopharmacol Bull 23(3):360–363, 1987

Spiker DG, Foster FG, Coble DA, et al: The sleep disorder in depressed alcoholics. Sleep Research 6:161, 1977

Springer NN, Roslow S: A study in the estimation of feelings. J Appl Psychol 19:379–385, 1935

Stern M, Fram D, Wyatt RJ, et al: All-night sleep studies of acute schizophrenics. Arch Gen Psychiatry 20:470–477, 1969

Symonds RC, Williams P: Seasonal variation in the incidence of mania. Br J Psychiatry 129:45–48, 1976

Taylor WR: Several-day cycles in disturbed children's behavior. Chronobiologia 9:329–331, 1982

Templer DI, Ruff CF, Ayers JL, et al: Diurnal mood fluctuations and age. Int J Aging Hum Dev 14(3):89–193, 1981–1982

Terman M: On the question of mechanism in phototherapy for seasonal affective disorder: considerations of clinical efficacy and epidemiology, in Affective Disorders and Phototherapy. Edited by Rosenthal NE, Blehar MC. New York, Guilford, 1989, pp 357–376

Touitou Y, Fevre M, Bogdan A, et al: Patterns of plasma melatonin with aging and mental condition: stability of nyctohemeral rhythms and differences in seasonal variations. Acta Endocrinol 106:145–151, 1984

Warren CW, Smith JC, Tyler CW: Seasonal variation in suicide and homicide: a question of consistency. J Biosoc Sci 15:349–356, 1983

Wehr TA: Sleep and biological rhythms in affective illness, in Biological Rhythms and Mental Disorders. Edited by Kupfer DJ, Monk TH, Barchas JD. New York, Guilford, 1988, pp 143–175

Wehr TA: Seasonal affective disorders: a historical overview, in Seasonal Affective Disorders and Phototherapy. Edited by Rosenthal NE, Blehar MC. New York, Guilford, 1989, pp 11–32

Wehr TA, Goodwin FK: Introduction, in Psychobiology and Psychopathology, Vol 2: Circadian Rhythms in Psychiatry. Edited by Wehr TA, Goodwin FK. Pacific Grove, CA, Boxwood Press, 1983, pp 1–15

Wehr TA, Wirz-Justice A, Goodwin FK, et al: Phase advance of the circadian sleep-wake cycle as an antidepressant. Science 206:710–713, 1979

Wehr TA, Sack DA, Duncan WC, et al: Sleep and circadian rhythms in affective patients isolated from external time cues. Psychiatry Res 15:327–339, 1985

Wever RA: Organization of the human circadian system: internal interactions, in Circadian Rhythms in Psychiatry. Edited by Wehr TA, Goodwin FK. Pacific Grove, CA, Boxwood Press, 1983, pp 17–32

Whitton JL: Periodicities in self-reports of health, sleep, and mood variables. J Psychosom Res 22:111–115, 1978

Yamazaki K, Saito Y, Okada F, et al: An application of neuroendocrinological studies in autistic children and Heller's syndrome. Journal of Autism and Childhood Schizophrenia 5:232–332, 1976

Zucker I: Neuroendocrine substrates of circannual rhythms, in Biological Rhythms and Mental Disorders. Edited by Kupfer DJ, Monk TH, Barchas JC. New York, Guilford, 1988, pp 219–251

CHAPTER 5

Relationship Between Depression and Suicidal Behavior

Cynthia R. Pfeffer, M.D.

Frequently, childhood or adolescent suicidal behavior is equated with depression. An assumption is often made that if a child or adolescent is suicidal, he or she is also depressed. In fact, one DSM-III-R criterion for diagnosing a major depressive disorder in adults, children, and adolescents is the presence of suicidal ideation or acts (American Psychiatric Association 1987). However, the assumption that suicidal behavior is synonymous with depression is incorrect. Empirical research suggests that many youngsters who exhibit suicidal ideation or acts are not depressed (Pfeffer et al. 1988; Shaffer 1974). However, the majority of studies indicate that depression is a major risk factor for youth suicidal behavior (Pfeffer 1986; Robbins and Alessi 1985). This chapter specifically highlights a subgroup of suicidal children and adolescents who have depressive disorders as a significant factor in their personal or family background. The psychosocial, biological, and family aspects of depression in youngsters who commit suicide or who exhibit nonfatal suicidal behavior are described with respect to the role of depressive symptoms.

Historical Perspective

In the early to mid-1970s, systematic research on childhood and adolescent depression and suicidal behavior emerged. Before this time, psychoanalytic theory suggested that children did not become depressed or suicidal (Pfeffer 1986). The basis for this premise was that children's cognitive and psychological functioning was not sufficiently developed for them to experience the guilt necessary to produce depressive mood or to conceptualize the finality of death. Paradoxically, anaclitic depression (Spitz 1946) was described in infants as a response to the loss of consistent early nurturing. Clinical observations and systematic documentation used in recognizing and describing anaclitic depression were the forerunner of later empirical research that confirmed the existence of depression and suicidal behavior in children and adolescents. (See Chapter 1.)

GENERAL STUDIES OF YOUTH SUICIDAL BEHAVIOR

The study of the relationship between psychopathological disorders, particularly depression, and suicidal behavior employs various methodologies, such as psychological autopsy in cases of completed suicide and the exploration of risk factors for nonfatal suicidal behavior in both psychiatric and nonpsychiatric populations. Most of these studies use cross-sectional and retrospective research designs; only a few use prospective and/or follow-up assessments.

Psychological Autopsy Studies

There are five published psychological autopsy studies of youth suicide (Brent 1988; Hoberman and Garfinkel 1989; Rich et al. 1986; Shaffer 1974, 1988; Shafii et al. 1984, 1985, 1988; Shafii 1989). The earliest study, conducted by Shaffer (1974), utilized a record review of coroner, social service, and medical reports to evaluate risk factors in young adolescents who committed suicide in England and Wales between 1962 and 1968. No comparison subjects were included in this study. All youngsters who committed suicide were 12–14 years old, and 21 of the 30 suicide victims were male. Factors prevalent among these young suicide victims were a disciplinary crisis as an immediate precipitant of suicide, a history of previous suicidal behavior, the presence of psychiatric symptoms, and the presence of psychiatric disorders among first-degree relatives. Approximately 16% of these young adolescents had symptoms of depression, and 57% had both symptoms of depression and antisocial tendencies. No specific information was reported about rates of mood disorder among relatives. This study suggested that mood disorder symptoms were very prevalent among young adolescents who committed suicide.

Another psychological autopsy study of teenage suicide victims used record review to compare adolescent and young adult male and female suicide victims (Hoberman and Garfinkel 1989). This study also compared the characteristics of younger and older suicide victims. Adolescents and young adults who were 25 years of age or younger and who committed suicide between 1975 and 1985 were studied. The results indicated that males predominated and that adolescents older than 15 years were more prevalent among the suicide victims. Approximately half of the suicide victims were sad on the day of their suicide. This observation was more evident among the older adolescents. The younger adolescents more often appeared angry. With regard to psychiatric disorder, 30% had depressive disorders, 13% were alcoholic, and 15% abused other substances. The rate of mood disorders in females was twice that in males, who had a higher rate of substance abuse disorders. This study highlighted an association between depressive disorders and youth suicide.

Shafii et al. (1985) were the first to publish a comparative psychological autopsy study of children and adolescents between the ages of 11 and 19 years. These children and adolescents ($n = 20$) were compared with 17 close friends of the suicide victims for demographic features. Factors that were more prevalent among the suicide victims than the matched comparison group were use of drugs or alcohol, antisocial behavior, inhibited personality, previous psychiatric treatment, and family suicidal behavior and emotional problems. Regarding depressive disorder, 76% of the suicide victims had a primary or secondary postmortem diagnosis of depressive disorders, compared to 24% of the comparison group (Shafii et al. 1988).

The San Diego Suicide Study (Fowler et al. 1986; Rich et al. 1986) provided a developmental perspective on youth suicide and mood disorders. One hundred thirty-three suicide victims under 30 years of age were compared with 150 suicide victims over 30 years of age. Approximately 53% of the younger suicide victims abused drugs, and approximately 24% had psychiatric disorders that included atypical depression, atypical psychosis, or adjustment disorder with depressed mood. Compared with suicide victims over 30 years of age, younger suicide victims had fewer mood and organic disorders and more antisocial behavior disorders. This study suggests that, although mood disorders were evident among youthful suicide victims, there was a developmental differential, with more mood disorders and a higher incidence of suicide occurring in older groups.

Brent et al. (1988) compared 27 adolescent suicide victims with 56 adolescent suicidal psychiatric inpatients. A major finding was that the suicide victims and the suicidal psychiatric patients had similar characteristics. Specifically, both groups of adolescents had high rates of mood disorders and a family history of mood disorders, antisocial disorder, and suicide. Approximately 64% of suicide victims and 82% of suicidal inpatients had a mood disorder. However, suicide victims had a higher prevalence of bipolar disorder and affective disorders with comorbid psychiatric disorders. Approximately 44% of the suicide victims and 27% of suicidal inpatients had a comorbid nonaffective (nonmood) psychiatric disorder. The most frequent comorbid nonaffective disorders among the suicide victims were attention-deficit disorder and substance abuse, and the most frequent comorbid nonaffective disorders among the suicidal inpatients were anxiety and conduct disorders.

The largest psychological autopsy study of adolescent suicide was conducted in the New York metropolitan area (Shaffer 1988). This study involved approximately 173 adolescent suicide victims under 20 years of age.

The results suggested that a small number of adolescents were free of psychiatric symptoms at the time of their death. Furthermore, there were different trends for males and females with regard to how rates of suicide were affected by different factors. For example, for males in the general population the rate of suicide is 14 per 100,000, and for females it is 3.5 per 100,000. These rates are increased by certain risk factors for adolescent suicide. Shaffer estimated these risk factors per 100,000. In males, a prior suicide attempt increases the suicide risk to 270 per 100,000, major depression increases it to 100 per 100,000, substance abuse increases it to 70 per 100,000, antisocial behavior increases it to 40 per 100,000, and family history of suicide increases it to 35 per 100,000. In females, major depressive disorder increases suicide risk to 80 per 100,000, prior suicide attempt increases it to 20 per 100,000, antisocial behavior increases it to 8 per 100,000, family history of suicide increases it to 6 per 100,000, and substance abuse increases it to 3 per 100,000. These data support the contention that major depressive disorder in adolescent male and female suicide victims is a very significant risk factor. Major depressive disorder increases the suicide rate of adolescent males approximately 7-fold over the base rate, and it increases the suicide rate of adolescent females 23-fold over the base rate. This study provides strong evidence that major depression is an important risk factor in adolescent suicide.

Studies of Nonfatal Suicidal Behavior

Most studies of adolescent nonfatal suicidal behavior focus on patient populations such as adolescents evaluated in medical or psychiatric settings. Recent evidence suggests that there is a continuity between nonfatal suicidal behavior and suicide in youth populations (Brent et al. 1986, 1988; Pfeffer 1986). Investigation of risk factors for nonfatal suicidal behavior, therefore, can be helpful in understanding vulnerability for youth suicide.

Most reports of nonfatal suicidal behavior in youths suggest that depression is an important risk factor, although some investigations highlight the stronger influence of other factors. Brent et al. (1986) reported data obtained from a sample of 231 children and adolescents who were evaluated in a large urban psychiatric service. Children, adolescents, and their parents were interviewed with a standard research instrument, the Diagnostic Interview Schedule, which yields DSM-III diagnoses (American Psychiatric Association 1980) and quantitative ratings of symptoms (Costello and Dulcan 1985). This study determined that the severity of nonfatal suicidal tendencies was directly associated with features of depression. For example, severity of suicidal ideation was positively associated with vegetative signs of depression, affective signs of depression, overall symptoms of depression, and parents' reports of intensity of depressive symptomatology. Symptoms of other psychiatric disorders were not evaluated in this phase of the study.

Garfinkel et al. (1982) reported on an emergency room chart review of a large sample of adolescents evaluated for suicidal behavior. A total of 505 youngsters who attempted suicide were compared with a similar number of nonsuicidal youngsters evaluated for medical problems in the same emergency room. There was a significantly greater number of girls in both groups. Factors that were more prominent among the suicidal youngsters were a history of substance abuse, having a psychiatric disorder at the time of the visit, and having a medical illness. Approximately 55% of those who were suicidal had dysphoric mood, 41% had aggressive tendencies, and 34% were responding to a crisis situation. In addition, the suicidal youngsters had more family history of psychiatric or medical illness. There was a significantly greater prevalence of suicide and suicidal attempts among relatives of the suicidal youngsters. For example, 8.3% of the suicidal adolescents, compared to 1.1% of the nonsuicidal adolescents, had a family history of suicidal behavior. In the suicidal adolescent group, substance abuse was prevalent in relatives with psychiatric illness.

This study by Garfinkel et al. utilized a record review and therefore is limited by a lack of systematic assessment of the adolescents and relatives for signs of psychiatric symptoms. The lack of reported depression may be related to a lack of systematic assessment of depressive symptomatology. Nevertheless, this study represents a large group of youngsters from the general community, and the symptoms described may represent strong profile characteristics of such youngsters. It may be that depression is less evident in this selected group.

Several studies of suicidal adolescent psychiatric inpatients assessed the associations between suicidal behavior and symptoms of depression. The results of these studies differ. One report (Khan 1987) evaluated 40 adolescent psychiatric inpatients who attempted suicide just before hospitalization, 40 adolescent nonsuicidal psychiatric inpatients, and 40 adolescent nonsuicidal psychiatric outpatients. Although this study controlled for the level of psychopathology in the three groups by using psychiatric patients as controls, it was limited by failure to include a nonpatient sample. All adolescents were 14–17 years old. They were evaluated for psychiatric disorders by means of a clinical interview. Since standard research instruments were not used to evaluate the psychiatric disorders of these adolescents, the reliability of the data may be limited. The results indicated that there were no significant differences in prevalence of mood or conduct disorders in the three groups of adolescents. Each group had a wide variety of psychiatric disorders; therefore, the conclusion drawn was that there is diagnostic heterogeneity among suicidal adolescents.

A systematic assessment of 140 consecutively hospitalized adolescent psychiatric patients was conducted (Apter et al. 1988) using the Kiddie

Schedule for Affective Disorders and Schizophrenia (K-SADS), a standard research instrument. This instrument rates symptoms and behaviors on individual scales that can be quantitatively compared. The results indicated that ratings of suicidal ideation and behavior were highest among adolescents with conduct disorder and lowest among adolescents with schizophrenia. Furthermore, the statistical differences in ratings of suicidal behavior for adolescents with conduct disorder and adolescents with major depressive disorder were significant. Conduct disorder was more significantly associated with suicidal behavior than was depression. In addition, ratings on the suicidal ideation and behavior scale did not correlate with other scales that measured symptoms of anxiety, mania, delusions, hallucinations, and thought disorder. This study suggested that, although symptoms of depression are correlated with suicidal tendencies, symptoms of antisocial behavior had a stronger association with suicidal tendencies in these adolescent inpatients.

A detailed analysis of the relationship between depressive symptoms and suicidal behavior in adolescent psychiatric inpatients was presented by Robbins and Alessi (1985). Sixty-four consecutively admitted adolescent psychiatric inpatients were interviewed with the Schedule for Affective Disorders and Schizophrenia (SADS). This standard research instrument, like the K-SADS, has four scales that measure aspects of suicidal behavior. The investigators evaluated the degree of correlation between each of these suicidal behavior scales and the relationship of the symptom items to depression. The results in this sample of adolescents, who had a heterogeneous array of psychiatric disorders, indicated that each scale for suicidal behavior was positively correlated with symptoms of depression. For example, the suicidal tendencies scale that measures severity of suicidal ideation and acts was highly correlated with depressed mood, negative self-evaluation, hopelessness, insomnia, poor concentration, and anhedonia. The number of suicidal gestures or attempts was associated with depressed mood, alcohol abuse, drug abuse, and negative self-evaluation. Seriousness of suicidal intent was associated with depression, negative self-evaluation, hopelessness, anxiety, indecisiveness, anhedonia, psychomotor agitation, insomnia, and alcohol abuse. Lethality of suicidal behavior was associated with depressed mood, negative self-evaluation, anhedonia, psychomotor agitation, and alcohol and drug abuse.

Another aspect of suicidal risk involves the relationship of depression and hopelessness to suicidal behavior. A number of studies in adults (Beck et al. 1985; Dyer and Kreitmen 1984; Wetzel et al. 1980) and in preschoolers (Kazdin et al. 1983) suggest that although depression and hopelessness are associated with suicidal behavior, hopelessness is a stronger predictor of suicidal behavior. One study (Rotheram-Borus and Trautman 1988) evaluates this association in suicidal adolescents. This study utilized 44 minority female suicide attempters. These adolescents reported high degrees of hopelessness and depression, but neither depression nor hopelessness predicted suicidal intent. Since this was a highly specific group of adolescents with certain demographic features, it is not clear whether these findings are generalizable to other groups of suicidal adolescents. Additional research is necessary to evaluate this issue.

The complexities of risk for nonfatal suicidal behavior in adolescent psychiatric inpatients were further elucidated in a record review of 200 consecutively admitted adolescent psychiatric inpatients. In this study, Pfeffer et al. (1988) evaluated correlates of suicidal behavior in male and female adolescents. The study suggested that there is an overlap in the types of factors associated with suicidal behavior in adolescent male and female psychiatric inpatients. This was illustrated by the fact that the history of suicidal behavior and the symptoms of depression were associated with suicidal behavior in males and females. Major depressive and alcohol abuse disorders were positively correlated with severity of suicidal behavior in males and females.

However, differences between suicidal adolescent males and females existed. For example, recent aggressive behaviors were associated with suicidal behavior in females. In females, borderline personality disorder was associated with suicidal behavior. Schizophrenia was negatively associated with suicidal behavior in males. Family factors that were associated with suicidal behavior in females were recent sexual abuse. Assaultive behavior of relatives and suicidal behavior of a sibling were associated with suicidal tendencies in males.

STUDIES OF DEPRESSED YOUNGSTERS WHO ARE SUICIDAL

Most reports compare depressed and nondepressed youngsters or compare suicidal and nonsuicidal youngsters. In fact, there are few systematic studies comparing depressed suicidal and depressed nonsuicidal youngsters. Studies of depressed youngsters suggest that not all depressed youngsters exhibit suicidal tendencies. This section highlights those factors in depressed youngsters that are associated with their propensity for suicidal tendencies.

Asarnow et al. (1987) studied 30 consecutively hospitalized depressed and nondepressed preadolescent psychiatric inpatients. Based on systematic assessments with standard research instruments, important findings emerged regarding differences between suicidal and nonsuicidal children and between depressed and nondepressed children. Compared with nondepressed children, depressed children had more hopelessness, lower self-esteem, and lower perceived cognitive competence. However, there were no associations between perceived competence and suicidal behavior. Furthermore, compared with nonsuicidal children, suicidal children perceived their families as having higher conflict, less cohesion, and less control over impulses. The investigators remarked that "the results of the study suggest that there are major differences in the correlates of depression and suicidal behavior" (p. 365). Depressed children have frequent negative cognitions, and suicidal children appear to have poor family social supports. This study, however, did not report on differences between depressed suicidal and depressed nonsuicidal children.

Another study whose main focus was to evaluate symptoms in depressed children and adolescents (Mitchell et al. 1988) offers information about developmental differences in the prevalence of suicidal behavior in depressed children, adolescents, and adults. However, this study also did not evaluate differences in symptoms of suicidal and nonsuicidal depressed individuals. This study of children and adolescents ages 7–17 years, who were evaluated in psychiatric inpatient and outpatient services, reported that among 45 depressed preadolescents, 67% had suicidal ideation and 39% attempted suicide. These percentages were similar to those observed in 50 depressed adolescents. However, when the preadolescent and adolescent samples were combined and compared with 100 depressed adults, the youths had a significantly higher rate of suicide attempts than the adults. Thirty-nine percent of the 95 depressed children and adolescents, compared to 15% of the 100 depressed adults, attempted suicide. However, the rates of suicidal ideation were similar in children, adolescents, and adults.

Kaplan et al. (1984) utilized the Beck Depression Inventory (Beck et al. 1961), a self-report measure of severity of depressive symptoms, and a Health Behavior Questionnaire to evaluate 447 high school students. The purpose of this study was to evaluate the relationships between suicidal behavior in depressed children and some factors that are involved with suicidal impulses. There were six behaviors on the Health Behavior Questionnaire found to be specifically associated with the "suicidal thoughts" item on the Beck Depression Inventory. These were cigarette smoking, beer drinking, liquor drinking, wine drinking, pot smoking, and use of other drugs. These adverse health behaviors involving substance abuse were associated with the total depression score on the Beck Depression Inventory. However, the "suicidal thoughts" item on the Beck Depression Inventory counted heavily in predicting these adverse health behaviors. This study pointed out that depressed youngsters often exhibit adverse health behavior specifically involving substance abuse. The fact that suicidal thoughts were associated with these adverse health behaviors suggests that clinical evaluation of suicidal risk should include evaluation of the level of depression and the history of substance abuse.

Types of depressive disorders were compared with conduct disorder and other psychiatric disorders in a study of 60 children and adolescents who were assessed in a psychiatric service (Fine et al. 1985). Suicidal ideation, as measured in clinical interviews, was more severe for the 13 youngsters with major depressive disorder than for youngsters with conduct disorder. Suicidal ideation was not more extensive for children with conduct disorders than for children with dysthymia, but it was more extensive for children with dysthymic disorder than for youngsters with nonmood disorders other than conduct disorders. This study pointed out that major depression, compared with other disorders, is associated with the highest intensity of suicidal ideation. However, it is not clear whether this association is based on the intensity of depression or on other factors associated with major depressive disorders.

One of the few studies (Friedman et al. 1983) to evaluate factors associated with suicidal behavior in depressed youngsters was conducted using 53 adolescents and young adults psychiatrically hospitalized for treatment of a mood disorder. These inpatients were studied by standard interview techniques. All patients had a mood disorder, and 78% met criteria for borderline personality disorder. Ninety-two percent of the patients with depression and a borderline personality disorder made at least one suicide attempt. This percentage was significantly higher than that for patients with depression and DSM-III Axis II disorders other than borderline personality disorder. Depressed patients with an Axis II personality disorder other than borderline personality disorder and depressed patients with no personality disorder had similar prevalences of suicidal attempts. The degree of lethality of suicidal attempts was greatest in patients with depression and borderline personality disorder. This study highlighted the important relationship between comorbid disorders and depressive disorders with respect to suicidal risk. It also highlighted the specificity of comorbidity of borderline personality disorder with mood disorders in increasing suicidal risk. (See Chapter 1.)

Strober and Carlson (1982) illustrated the importance of outcome studies in understanding the relationship between suicidal risk and mood disorders. Sixty consecutively hospitalized adolescents who were admitted for treatment of major depression were studied prospectively for 3–4 years. Each patient was evaluated systematically with standard research instruments initially and at follow-up. Mania developed in 20% of the patients during the follow-up period. These patients received a diagnosis at follow-up of bipolar disorder. The bipolar and nonbipolar patients were compared on many variables. With respect to suicidal behavior, the adolescents with nonbipolar disorders had more intense suicidal tendencies at the time of initial hospitalization. In addition, family histories of suicide were more common in patients with bipolar disorder at outcome, although the differences were not significant. This study suggests that factors that distinguish adolescents who have major depression with regard to the level of suicidal tendencies may be apparent or measurable at a later period of time. It may be that

vulnerability to certain disorders, such as bipolar disorder, is signaled by suicidal tendencies in a depressed youngster. (See Chapters 12 and 13.)

Other avenues of research that compare suicidal and nonsuicidal behavior in depressed individuals are those evaluating biological correlates of suicidal behavior. Essentially, this research involves neuroendocrine or
serotonergic neurotransmitter variables. These studies (Mann et al. 1989)
suggest relationships between neuroendocrine and serotonin metabolites
and suicidal behavior. However, no systematic studies to evaluate these biological correlates have been conducted in children and adolescents. This is
an important area requiring research attention.

CONCLUSION

This chapter outlines the important relationships among depressive symptoms, mood disorders, and suicidal behavior in children and adolescents.
One of the most consistent findings is a positive association between suicidal
tendencies and symptoms of depressive disorders. Populations studied had
a wide range of psychopathology and were studied in a variety of clinical
and nonclinical settings. These studies involved individuals who committed
suicide and those who exhibited nonfatal suicidal behavior.

Studies emphasize that suicidal behavior is a heterogeneous symptom
complex. Nondepressed youngsters also demonstrate suicidal ideation and
acts. In addition, some depressed children and adolescents do not exhibit
suicidal tendencies. What differentiates the suicidal depressed youngster
from the nonsuicidal depressed youngster is an issue requiring more extensive research.

Additional research is needed regarding the relationships among mood
disorders, suicidal behavior, family variables, and biological correlates. As
illustrated by one follow-up study, a prospective investigation of suicidal
youngsters would be important to evaluate continuities and discontinuities
of symptomatology. Certainly data already collected in existing studies
should be analyzed with regard to differences between suicidal and nonsuicidal youngsters both over time and in relation to their types of psychopathology.

From a clinical perspective, all depressed youngsters should be compre-
hensively evaluated for suicidal tendencies. Such youngsters require close
follow-up assessments. Any sign of increase in depressive symptomatology
should serve as a warning of a potentially increasing suicidal risk. Finally,
interventions that decrease depressive disorders, enhance social supports,
and strengthen adequate coping mechanisms should be aggressively used.
Each individual presents unique clinical issues that require closely watched
and carefully administered interventions. (See Chapters 7, 9, 10, and 11.)

REFERENCES

American Psychiatric Association: Diagnostic and Statistical Manual of Mental Disorders, 3rd Edition. Washington, DC, American Psychiatric Association, 1980

American Psychiatric Association: Diagnostic and Statistical Manual of Mental Disorders, 3rd Edition, Revised. Washington, DC, American Psychiatric Association, 1987

Apter A, Bleich A, Plutchik R, et al: Suicidal behavior, depression, and conduct disorder in hospitalized adolescents. J Am Acad Child Adolesc Psychiatry 27:696–699, 1988

Asarnow JR, Carlson GA, Guthrie D: Coping strategies, self-perceptions, hopelessness, and perceived family environments in depressed and suicidal children. J Consult Clin Psychol 55:361–366, 1987

Beck AT, Ward CM, Mendelson M, et al: An inventory for measuring depression. Arch Gen Psychiatry 4:561–571, 1961

Beck AT, Steer RA, Kovacs M, et al: Hopelessness and eventual suicide: a 10-year prospective study of patients hospitalized with suicidal ideation. Am J Psychiatry 142:559–563, 1985

Brent DS, Kalas R, Edelbrock C, et al: Psychopathology and its relationship to suicidal ideation in childhood and adolescence. J Am Acad Child Psychiatry 25:666–673, 1986

Brent DA, Perper JA, Goldstein CE, et al: Risk factors for adolescent suicide: a comparison of adolescent suicide victims with suicidal inpatients. Arch Gen Psychiatry 45:581–588, 1988

Costello AJ, Dulcan MK: DISC: Diagnostic Interview for Children. Unpublished manuscript, 1985

Dyer JAT, Kreitmen N: Hopelessness, depression, and suicidal intent in parasuicide. Br J Psychiatry 144:127–133, 1984

Fine S, Moretti M, Haley G, et al: Affective disorders in children and adolescents: the dysthymic disorder dilemma. Can J Psychiatry 30:173–177, 1985

Fowler RC, Rich CL, Young D: San Diego Suicide Study, II: substance abuse in young cases. Arch Gen Psychiatry 43:962–965, 1986

Friedman RC, Aronoff MS, Clarkin JF, et al: History of suicidal behavior in depressed borderline inpatients. Am J Psychiatry 140:1023–1026, 1983

Garfinkel BD, Froese A, Hood J: Suicide attempts in children and adolescents. Am J Psychiatry 139:1257–1261, 1982

Hoberman HM, Garfinkel BD: Completed suicide in youth, in Suicide Among Youth: Perspectives on Risk and Prevention. Edited by Pfeffer CR. Washington, DC, American Psychiatric Press, 1989, pp 21–40

Kaplan SL, Landa B, Weinhold C, et al: Adverse health behaviors and depressive symptomatology in adolescents. J Am Acad Child Psychiatry 23:595–601, 1984

Kazdin A, French N, Unis A, et al: Hopelessness, depression, and suicidal intent among psychiatrically depressed inpatient children. J Consult Clin Psychol 51:504–510, 1983

Khan AV: Heterogeneity of suicidal adolescents. J Am Acad Child Adolesc Psychiatry 26:92–96, 1987

Mann JJ, DeMeo MD, Keilp JG, et al: Biological correlates of suicidal behavior in youth, in Suicide Among Youth: Perspectives on Risk and Prevention. Edited by Pfeffer CR. Washington, DC, American Psychiatric Press, 1989, pp 185–202

Mitchell J, McCauley E, Burke P, et al: Phenomenology of depression in children and adolescents. J Am Acad Child Adolesc Psychiatry 27:12–20, 1988

Pfeffer CR: The Suicidal Child. New York, Guilford, 1986

Pfeffer CR, Newcorn J, Kaplan G, et al: Suicidal behavior in adolescent psychiatric inpatients. J Am Acad Child Adolesc Psychiatry 27:357–361, 1988

Rich CL, Young D, Fowler RC: San Diego Suicide Study, I: young versus old subjects. Arch Gen Psychiatry 43:577–582, 1986

Robbins DR, Alessi NE: Depressive symptoms and suicidal behavior in adolescents. Am J Psychiatry 142:588–592, 1985

Rotheram-Borus MJ, Trautman PD: Hopelessness, depression, and suicidal intent among adolescent suicide attempters. J Am Acad Child Adolesc Psychiatry 27:700–704, 1988

Shaffer D: Suicide in childhood and early adolescence. J Child Psychol Psychiatry 15:275–291, 1974

Shaffer D: The epidemiology of teen suicide: an examination of risk factors. J Clin Psychol 49:36–41, 1988

Shafii M: Completed suicide in children and adolescents: methods of psychological autopsy, in Suicide Among Youth: Perspectives on Risk and Prevention. Edited by Pfeffer CR. Washington, DC, American Psychiatric Press, 1989, pp 1–19

Shafii M, Whittinghill JR, Dolen DC, et al: Psychological reconstruction of completed suicide in childhood and adolescence, in Suicide in the Young. Edited by Sudak H, Ford AB, Rushforth NB. Boston, MA, John Wright PSG, 1984, pp 271–294

Shafii M, Carrigan S, Whittinghill JR, et al: Psychological autopsy of completed suicide in children and adolescents. Am J Psychiatry 142:1061–1064, 1985

Shafii M, Steltz-Lenarsky J, Derrick AM, et al: Comorbidity of mental disorders in the postmortem diagnosis of completed suicide in children and adolescents. J Affective Disord 15:227–233, 1988

Spitz RA: Anaclitic depression. Psychoanal Study Child 2:313–342, 1946

Strober M, Carlson G: Bipolar illness in adolescents with major depression. Arch Gen Psychiatry 39:549–555, 1982

Wetzel RD, Margulies T, Davis R: Hopelessness, depression, and suicide intent. J Clin Psychol 41:159–160, 1980

PART II

DIAGNOSTIC ASSESSMENT AND TREATMENT OF DEPRESSIVE DISORDERS IN CHILDREN AND ADOLESCENTS

Sadness is but a wall
between two gardens.

Kahlil Gibran

CHAPTER 6

Standardized Approaches to Clinical Assessment of Depression

Hartmut B. Mokros, Ph.D.
Elva O. Poznanski, M.D.

The traditional clinical approach to assessment of children and adolescents has been the unstructured interview. This approach stemmed from the conviction that the child or adolescent was not behaviorally or cognitively amenable to the demands of a direct interview. The parents were regarded as the primary and most reliable source of information; hence, the perceived need for direct interview of the youngster was negligible. However, recent research has indicated that children and adolescents may be directly and reliably interviewed, thus questioning the primacy of unstructured or play interviewing techniques for assessing child and adolescent psychopathology (Puig-Antich and Gittelman 1982).

Obviously, the unstructured interview has the advantage of testing a number of ongoing hypotheses about the youngster's difficulties. However, a clinician who relies exclusively on the unstructured interview runs the risk of neglecting certain symptomatology or focusing on his or her predisposed orientations. The lack of certainty about whether the systematicness of an unstructured assessment represented a critical obstacle to research and led to the development of standardized assessment techniques in child psychiatry.

The development of standardized assessment instruments represents important progress in child psychiatry for both clinical practice and research purposes. Standardized assessment instruments potentially serve four useful functions in clinical practice, although all four of these functions are rarely provided by any single instrument. First, they represent an economical screening device in the general evaluation of the patient population. Second, they contribute to diagnostic decision making by evaluating a specific disorder when this disorder is suspected or when the clinician wishes to rule out the disorder. Third, they provide an index of the severity of the disorder, thereby contributing to the evaluation of the severity of the episode, and may also be used as a follow-up measure during the course of treatment to monitor treatment response. Finally, and very importantly, these instruments provide a check on the clinician's systematicness of evaluation, as well as a framework for conducting the evaluation and keeping track of the current working assumption of what constitutes the disorder.

In this chapter we will first introduce some conceptual distinctions useful in distinguishing existing approaches to the evaluation of depression in youth. We will then describe and discuss the most prominent standardized approaches currently in use, followed by a brief review of psychometric considerations. Finally, we conclude with a summary and recommendations for the choice of instruments in clinical practice.

CONCEPTUAL DISTINCTIONS

Discussions of approaches to assessment commonly draw a distinction between self-report and interview measures (Kazdin and Petti 1982). The distinction between self-report and interview measures does not represent the actual practice in the use of these instruments. Although measures may be conceived of and referred to as self-reports, these types of measures are commonly administered in a quasi-interview fashion, with the interviewer reading items to the child and possibly recording the child's responses. Thus, the boundaries between self-report and interview instruments as used with children are often blurred.

A more useful distinction results by conceptualizing assessment procedures along two dimensions: the specificity of the instrument and the extent of structuring of the instrument. In the case of specificity, the key distinction is whether the instrument only evaluates depression or whether it evaluates depression within a broader diagnostic context. In the case of the structuring dimension, we may identify a distinction between instruments that are said to be structured and those that are semistructured.

The structured interview minimizes clinical judgment and the "creative" involvement of the clinician in the course of the interview by specifically defining the prompts of probes, the ordering or sequencing of these prompts and probe questions, and specifying explicit criteria for the interpretation or rating of the informant's responses to these probes. Structured evaluations may consist of scores obtained from ratings made by the clinicians, scores resulting from the child's self-report, or scores resulting from the reports about the child made by the child's significant others such as parents, siblings, attending nurses, or teachers.

In contrast, semistructured instruments are always administered by the clinician and thereby obtain ratings exclusively from the clinician about the child. Although reports of significant others are also obtained through semistructured evaluation, the important distinction is that scores generated in a semistructured context are always an interactive product, incorporating both the information provided by the informant and the evaluation of that information via clinical judgment by the clinician.

Besides actively capitalizing on the experience and knowledge of the clinician, the semistructured instrument provides the clinician with greater flexibility. Although probes or prompts are suggested, these are in fact modifiable in actual use, given specific pragmatic demands or constraints. Likewise, the ordering of items need not be absolute; the clinician has the opportunity to skip back and forth in any given case as the patient becomes more or less resistant toward the symptomatology being probed. However, this greater flexibility and greater involvement of the clinician in the structuring of the evaluation also potentially have a cost in that the clinician's involvement is now more actively represented in the ratings being made. The specific questioning frames the clinician invents online affect rater agreement; even the way he or she jumps around among questions may contribute to lower levels of rater agreement than when a structured approach is employed.

Likewise, the greater involvement of the clinician means that he or she must take greater caution in the rating of the symptom because of the possibility that the value placed on the symptom is not so much the "true" state of affairs but is a product of the way the question was asked and what the clinician believes constitutes supporting evidence. It is therefore exceedingly important with these types of instruments to provide documentation as to why a symptom was judged to be present—not merely to record the presence of a sleep disturbance, for example, but additionally provide the evidence that led to this judgment. Although the semistructured format certainly requires expert handling, its greater flexibility and reliance on established clinical expertise make it the optimal course of evaluation for diagnostic purposes.

Across both dimensions an additional distinction may be made between instruments that provide a categorical measure of disorder (presence versus absence) as opposed to those that measure the severity of a disorder. This distinction is embedded within the specificity distinction, where the aim of depression instruments is usually to provide a measure of severity, whereas the diagnostic instruments' aim is to provide a categorical decision. Nevertheless, the employment of cutoff scores in the case of depression instruments indicates that it is common practice to use these as preliminary diagnostic screening devices; however, such a practice should be discouraged.

Thus, although it is common in the literature to distinguish between self-report and interview-based assessment instruments, we suggest that this distinction in fact obscures two more fundamental distinctions: the distinctions of specificity and structuring. Nevertheless, the distinction between self-report and interview measures does offer an additional dimension, namely, the source of evaluations or ratings of the child. The most common rating sources consist of the child, the child's significant other (particularly parents), and the clinician. It should be noted that the type of rater who provides information about the child is not independent of the structuring dimension. That is, structured instruments designed to generate both diagnostic information about or severity measures of depression may theoretically be completed by any of the three rating sources. In contrast, semistructured instruments are always completed by the clinician on the basis of an interview. However, unlike clinician ratings based on structured instruments, semistructured instruments incorporate the involvement of the clinician. As such, these types of ratings reflect something of the clinician as well as the interviewee and therefore must be viewed as interactional products.

The two central distinctions, specificity and structuring, introduced in this section will serve as the basis of organization for the following discussion of the more prominent instruments currently used to evaluate childhood and adolescent depression. We will first describe and discuss key structured and semistructured instruments that provide diagnostic assessments and then describe and discuss key structured and semistructured instruments that provide depression severity assessments.

DIAGNOSTIC ASSESSMENTS

The first type of instrument we will consider provides the basis for a diagnostic evaluation of depression and affective disturbance. However, the key to these instruments is not that they merely evaluate depressive symptoms that are relevant to some diagnostic system; it is their emphasis on the evaluation of depressive symptoms within the context of a comprehensive evaluation of psychiatric symptomatology.

Structured Diagnostic Instruments

Structured instruments minimize the role of clinical inference and decision making in obtaining symptom information. Symptom data are usually scored categorically (e.g., as either present or absent), and diagnoses may then be reviewed in a checklist-like fashion against some set of criteria to determine the presence of any disorders.

The two most familiar structured diagnostic interview instruments are the Diagnostic Interview for Children and Adolescents (DICA), developed by Herjanic and Reich (1982), and the Diagnostic Interview Schedule for Children (DISC), developed by Costello et al. (1984). Separate formats for interviewing the parent and child are available for both of these instruments. In addition to these two interview instruments, the Child Behavior Checklist (CBCL; Achenbach and Edelbrock 1982), a paper-and-pencil measure, is a widely used diagnostic screen available in parent and teacher versions that may also be viewed as an example of a structured diagnostic assessment instrument.

Child Behavior Checklist. The CBCL is a widely used measure of childhood psychopathology completed by parents and appropriate for the evaluation of children between the ages of 4 and 16 years. The instrument assesses two areas: social competence (referred to as adaptive functioning in the teacher version) and behavior problems. The discussion below will focus on the portion of the instrument that assesses behavior problems. Both the parent and teacher versions of the "behavior problems" section consist of a set of 112 statements (although statements do differ between these two versions) describing behavior (e.g., "feels he or she has to be perfect") that the informant rates on a 3-point scale (0 = not true, 1 = somewhat or sometimes true, and 2 = very true or often true). In addition, a final item (#113) allows informants to enter problems not included in the inventory.

Informants are instructed to provide ratings for each behavioral statement to the extent that it describes the child "now or within the past 6 months" in the case of the parent version and "now or within the past 2 months" for the teacher version. The instrument is easily administered, takes no more than 15 or 20 minutes to complete, and may be scored by hand using scoring templates or by a computer program available from the developers of the instrument. The philosophy and theory behind the development of the CBCL differ sharply from those used in the development of all other instruments reviewed in this chapter. To accurately appreciate what the CBCL provides the clinician, it is necessary to first examine the theoretical orientation from which this instrument emerged.

Rather than approaching diagnosis from the perspective of rationally derived systems, Achenbach and Edelbrock (1984) argue for the development of an empirically derived approach to taxonomic classification. The point of view is that nosology of childhood pathology should be developed from data rather than fit to existing models. Hence, this orientation is also referred to as the statistical approach to classification. For example, they suggest that psychiatric disorders of children are better thought of in terms of "broad-band" disorders rather than "narrow-band" disorders like depression. This suggests that psychiatric disorders in children are less likely to be definable according to the specific diagnostic categories used in adults; rather, children will display a more diffused pattern of disturbance. Moreover, they additionally suggest that where there is a crystallization or clustering of specific problems, the manifestation may be developmentally unique, fluctuate in the course of developmental maturation, and potentially show differing manifestations in relation to various sociodemographic features, particularly gender.

Based on data obtained from large-sample, community-based and clinical studies of the instrument, Achenbach and Edelbrock have identified six unique factor structures (i.e., behavior problem groupings) according to the age and gender of the child. Thus, any given parental report on the CBCL is scored according to one of six distinct algorithms, three each for boys and girls depending on age, with the three age breaks being 4- to 5-year-olds, 6- to 11-year-olds, and 12- to 16-year-olds. For example, the factors for 6- to 11-year-old girls include depressed, social-withdrawal, somatic complaints, schizoid-obsessive, hyperactive, sex problems, delinquent, aggressive, and cruel, whereas the factors for 12- to 16-year-old boys include somatic complaints, schizoid, uncommunicative, immature, obsessive-compulsive, hostile-withdrawn, delinquent, aggressive, and hyperactive. These factors should not be confused with traditional diagnostic categories. Instead, they are labels assigned by Achenbach and Edelbrock to describe the commonalities among correlated subsets of items (i.e., factors) included in the checklist that have been statistically identified through factor analysis.

A second-order factor analysis (a factor analysis of the factors) identified two broad-band disorders referred to as "externalizing" and "internalizing" disorders. Again, as with the first-order factors, these broad-band factors are specific to the age and gender of the child. In the case of the 6- to 11-year-old girls, the internalizing factor groups the depressed, social-withdrawal, somatic complaints, and schizoid-obsessive first-order factors together, while the externalizing factor groups the hyperactive, sex problems, delinquent, aggressive, and cruel first-order factors together.

When a clinician scores a parental checklist, he or she obtains a series of summary scores that include scores for the first-order factors, the internalizing and externalizing factors, a total of the items endorsed, and the sum of these items. These scores are all also expressed as T-scores (which standardizes raw scores to a mean of 50 and a standard deviation of 10), which allows the clinician to compare the specific parental report of the child with normative data. That is, the clinician can assign a percentile rank of a problem area and, in the case of the first-order factors, a clinician T-score that provides a standardized comparison of a specific checklist with normative data from clinical samples. Additionally, the profile of a child's scores across all first-order factors is compared with clinical and profile types so that the clinician not only can compare the relative standing of a child with normative data from community and clinical samples, but also can determine in correlational terms how similar this child is to clinically developed profiles.

Clearly, the CBCL provides the clinician with a variety of indices of the child's behavior functioning for a fairly limited investment of time by the informant or the clinician in scoring the instrument. Additionally, the instrument has been widely used, thus making it possible to interpret data for a given child against both nonclinical and clinical norms. However, the interpretation of the profiles provided by the CBCL is by no means straightforward. First, the profile is based on parental (or teacher) perceptions. Although the checklist asks parents to make objective statements about the child's behavior, these statements are not free of parental interpretation and evaluation. The degree of parental involvement with the child, the ability or skill of the parent to provide accurate observational data, and the psychosocial state and characteristics of the parent are potential factors that may contribute to distortion in the parental report of the "true" behavioral problems of the child. Second, the labels of the factors evaluated by the CBCL do not directly translate into diagnostic categories familiar to the psychiatrist. The meaning of the factors needs to be considered in terms of the theory underlying the CBCL and should not be interpreted as equivalent to more familiar systems of classification.

Diagnostic Interview for Children and Adolescents. The DICA is a widely used instrument developed at Washington University over a period of 20 years (Welner et al. 1987). The most recent version was refined in the early 1980s by Herjanic and Reich (1982) and Reich et al. (1982). Available in both child and parent versions and also for use through face-to-face interview and through computer administration, the DICA is designed to evaluate children between the ages of 6 and 16 years.

The DICA is a structured evaluation that assesses the major diagnostic categories relevant to children and adolescents in DSM-III (American Psychiatric Association 1980) and DSM-III-R (American Psychiatric Association 1987) in its most recent updates. In addition to evaluating psychiatric symptom areas, the DICA also assesses various domains of social function. The results of the interview may be translated into DSM-III-R diagnoses.

The version of the DICA discussed by Herjanic and Reich (1982) consisted of a series of 168 questions. The following areas are covered by the interview (the number of questions included in each area is listed in parentheses): relationships at home (15), relationships with peers (10), homicidal thoughts (3), adjustment at school (19), social adjustment (10), medical history (5), phobias (4), obsessions (6), compulsions (4), depression (9), suicidal thoughts (5), somatic concerns (7), anxiety symptoms (6), "unusual" symptoms (e.g., couldn't move part of body) (5), nervous system (11), gastrointestinal system (7), encopresis (1), enuresis (2), genitourinary system (4), menstruation (3), sexual experience (7), self-concept (7), ideas of reference (3), depersonalization (2), derealization (2), passivity and control (4), hallucinations (5), and delusions (2).

The interview has since been both streamlined and expanded so that it is now structured in consort with DSM-III-R, consisting of 18 diagnostic subareas. Questions about psychiatric symptomatology are preceded by a series of 19 demographic questions designed to be administered jointly to both child and parent. Specific questions are provided for evaluating each symptom within a diagnostic area, with several questions included for many symptoms. Criteria for evaluating symptom presence (and past symptom presence for many items) are included, as are the DSM-III-R criteria for evaluating each diagnostic category.

The following diagnostic and thematic categories are evaluated in the child interview: attention-deficit disorder, oppositional disorder, socialization, conduct disorder, alcohol use, cigarette smoking, drug use, mood disorders (including depression and mania sections), separation anxiety disorder, overanxious disorder, simple phobia, obsessive-compulsive disorder, compulsions, anorexia nervosa, bulimia, somatization disorder, enuresis, encopresis, menstruation, gender identity disorder, sexual experience, psychotic symptoms including hallucinations and delusions, and psychosocial stressors. In the child interview, these areas are covered through the course of 246 questions with many embedded questions included when responses are positive. The interviewer is also asked to complete a series of additional questions that ask the clinician to evaluate general appearance, affect, motor behavior, speech, attention, flow of thought, general response to interview, and subjective clinical impressions of the interview.

Items to evaluate developmental history and medical history may either be addressed through joint interview or may be included only in the parent interview. Additionally, in the computer version of the instrument, certain symptom areas are only evaluated in the parent version. The computer version of the instrument allows the clinician to streamline the interview—to select only those symptom areas deemed of interest—rather than needing to go through the entire interview.

Diagnostic Interview Schedule for Children. The most recent version of the DISC, consisting of both a child and parent version, was developed by Costello and Dulcan (1985) under contract to the National Institute for Mental Health by Costello and others. Developed for epidemiological study, the DISC tends to emphasize sensitivity over specificity. Questions are worded to be understandable to the average 6- to 7-year-old, with alternative wordings of the same question available in cases where a child has difficulty understanding what is asked. These interview schedules are fully structured to ensure consistency among interviewers in administration. As such, the criteria for who may administer the DISC are relaxed compared with those for semistructured instruments. Indeed, Costello and Dulcan suggest that interviewers with no clinical experience achieve results comparable to those achieved by interviewers possessing clinical skills. The interviews are constructed such that responses may be easily transferred into computer files and then scored by computer programs.

The DISC-P has more questions and covers more topics than the DISC and therefore takes more time to administer. Although both interviews take more time as more pathology is indicated, the DISC may be completed in 45 minutes to 1 hour, whereas the DISC-P requires 1–1½ hours.

Questions in the DISC are organized to maximize naturalness. Rather than being organized around syndromes, the questions are organized around topics like home and school, beginning with a consideration of basic demographic information. Most questions are coded on a 3-point scale—No, Sometimes/Maybe, and Yes—although some provide only a binary choice of No or Yes and others request verbatim responses, such as for duration of symptoms. Interviewers are expected not to merely record Yes/No codings, but also to record as near verbatim as possible the basis of those codings. The interview is written in skip-forward structure. Thus, if a general query item is responded to as No, the interview skips forward past more specific prompts of that general query, which serves to greatly reduce the length of the interview. The DISC-P, for example, consists of 994 questions and 4 additional questions directed to the interviewer. In addition, interviewers are asked to supply their impression about the reliability of the information.

A training manual is available for use of the DISC and DISC-P (Dulcan et al. 1985). Additionally, computer programs have been developed both for interactive interviewing (direct input of data into the computer) and for scoring the protocol and determining diagnostic profiles (A.J. Costello, Instructions for DISC programs, unpublished manuscript, 1987).

In addition to major affective disorder, the DISC covers the following diagnoses: attention-deficit disorder, conduct disorder, separation anxiety, avoidant disorder, anorexia nervosa, bulimia, functional enuresis, functional encopresis, alcohol abuse/dependence, cannabis abuse/dependence, tobacco dependence, schizophrenia, cyclothymic disorder, agoraphobia, social phobia, simple phobia, panic disorder, obsessive-compulsive disorder, and substance abuse. The parent version also covers infantile autism, elective mutism, psychogenic fugue, hypochondriasis, Tourette's syndrome, pervasive developmental disorder, psychogenic amnesia, conversion disorder, and tic disorder.

Conclusion. These instruments, as a group, have some clear advantages and disadvantages relative to other modes of assessment that merit consideration. The primary advantage of these structured instruments is that they minimize the introduction of unsystematic practice by defining all the contingencies of the interview, the wording of questions, the sequencing of the questions, and the criteria for identifying evidence of disorder. A secondary advantage is that the level of training required of the person administering the interview is vastly reduced to the extent that researchers have developed variants of two of these instruments that eliminate the need for an intermediary altogether by allowing direct input of responses to computer screen prompts.

The advantages of these instruments in terms of systematicness and economy are clear. However, they also have significant limitations. First, these highly structured diagnostic interviews differ greatly from the typical clinical evaluation. This raises questions as to whether and to what extent information obtained in this fashion differs from the typical clinical assessment. The lack of clinical evaluation of a subject's responses, in particular, is certainly grounds for questioning the quality of the obtained data. For example, it may be unclear whether the subject truly understands the question posed, whether the symptoms reported co-occurred within a similar time frame, or whether the symptom definitions of the patient are consistent with those of the clinician. Moreover, establishing which disorder is primary in cases where multiple disorders are reported is difficult within a highly structured format. These difficulties are not necessarily inherent to the instruments themselves since there is, of course, no reason why structured instruments cannot be utilized in a semistructured fashion. However, they must be seriously considered when the instruments are applied in a highly structured format.

Semistructured Diagnostic Instruments

Whereas structured instruments minimize the role of clinical inference and decision making in obtaining symptom information, semistructured instruments maximize such involvement in both the process of evaluation and in the formulation of the diagnosis.

Two instruments of this type will be discussed. The first is the Child Assessment Schedule (CAS) (Hodges et al. 1982a, 1982b), which contains both structured and semistructured sections. The second are the two variants of the adult Schedule for Affective Disorders and Schizophrenia (SADS): the Schedule for Affective Disorders and Schizophrenia—Children's Version for the evaluation of current state or present episode (K-SADS-P; Puig-Antich et al. 1983) and a modification of this instrument intended for epidemiological study and referred to as the K-SADS-E (Orvaschel and Puig-Antich 1986). The K-SADS is the most comprehensive and commonly used semistructured instrument currently available.

The CAS and K-SADS were chosen for discussion because they provide somewhat differing approaches to evaluation and diagnosis within a semistructured orientation. An additional semistructured instrument that has been used extensively in the study of childhood depression is the Interview Schedule for Children (ISC) developed by Kovacs (1985a). This instrument will not be discussed since its format is essentially comparable to, but less elaborate than, the K-SADS.

Child Assessment Schedule. The CAS is a standardized diagnostic interview developed by Hodges et al. (1982a, 1982b). They emphasize that their aim in constructing the interview was to provide a developmentally sensitive diagnostic tool appropriate for use with children, one that was not overly lengthy, included interview prompts that could easily be understood by children, minimized the complexity of judgments children are asked to make about their symptomatology, and did not make unrealistic assumptions about the child's capability of understanding time-based concepts. Although the CAS is structured, the authors report that, when conducted by an experienced clinician, the interview is constructed so as to give the impression of an open-ended discussion of the child's life.

The CAS interview consists of two parts: 1) direct interview of the child about various experiential content and symptom areas, which may be administered in 45 minutes to 1 hour, and 2) the clinician's evaluation of the affective, verbal, nonverbal, and interactional style, and the child's performance in the course of the interview. The direct-interview component consists of 75 questions with responses to each question indicated in one of five categories: no, yes, ambiguous, no response, and not applicable. Although the intent of the instrument is to serve as a qualitative clinical tool that allows the clinician to gain an appreciation of dysfunctions in specific content as well as to develop and confirm diagnostic impressions, responses may also be more formally summarized for research purposes or systematic documentation. Ratings of 75 interview items and the results of the clinician's evaluation may be translated into a summary index of dysfunction, 11 content areas, and 9 symptom complexes. The content areas include school, friends, activities, family, fears, worries, self-image, mood, somatic concerns, expression of anger, and observational judgments by the interviewer. Symptom complexes include attention-deficit disorder (with and without hyperactivity), aggressive and nonaggressive variants of undersocialized conduct disorder and socialized conduct disorder, separation anxiety, overanxious disorder, oppositional disorder, and depression. Thought disorder symptomatology is also evaluated but not expressed as a summary scale.

Schedule for Affective Disorders and Schizophrenia—Children's Version (K-SADS). The K-SADS, developed by Puig-Antich et al. (1983), is the most widely and commonly used instrument for research of mood disorders in children and adolescents. It is a semistructured diagnostic interview designed for use with school-age children between ages 6 and 18 years, modeled after the adult SADS (Spitzer and Endicott 1978). Two versions of the K-SADS have been developed: the K-SADS-P, for the evaluation of current state or present episode, and the K-SADS-E, for the evaluation of both past and current episodes, designed for epidemiological study and lifetime history of a disorder. A major difference between these two instruments is in terms of the scoring or rating of symptomatology. Whereas the K-SADS-E requires only judgments about the presence or absence of a symptom, the K-SADS-P involves making judgments as to symptom severity. This means that the K-SADS-P is preferred when the clinician wishes to monitor change during the course of an episode, particularly when estimates of treatment response are of concern. Orvaschel and Puig-Antich (1986) suggested the joint use of the K-SADS-P and K-SADS-E for intake evaluations, with the K-SADS-P administered first to identify the presence of current episodes of the disorder and the K-SADS-E used to identify past episodes of this disorder and psychiatric disorders not currently manifested.

The typical procedure employed with the K-SADS is for the same clinician to first interview the parent and then the child. It is commonly assumed that children are better reporters of subjective symptoms and parents are better at reporting behavioral symptoms and the temporal parameters of prior episodes of disorder. Nevertheless, for certain types of behavioral symptomatology (such as conduct disorder and substance use), the child may provide a more reliable account. The authors of the K-SADS suggest that the clinician confront the child with any discrepancies between the child's and parents' reports to resolve discrepancies. This practice is certainly open to both ethical and empirical objections (Mokros et al. 1987). Once both the parent and child interviews have been completed, the clinician uses clinical judgment to combine this information with any other information about the child to achieve a summary rating for each symptom evaluated.

Before proceeding with the K-SADS interview, the clinician is expected to begin with an unstructured interview in which he or she explains the purpose and nature of the interview and in general attempts to establish rapport and relax the interviewee. This initial unstructured phase of the interview should also be used by the clinician to obtain a sense of the child's social environment and social functioning, such as family composition and relations, friendship patterns and peer relations, favorite activities, and attitudes and orientation at school. Since this initial unstructured phase of the interview overlaps with obtaining the sociodemographic and past and current treatment history information necessary to complete the interview, it provides the clinician with the opportunity to soften the transition from the unstructured to the structured phase of the interview and thereby serves to preserve a sense of rapport and naturalness.

It should be noted that any symptom information reported in this portion of the interview should be noted for reference in the course of formal symptom evaluation, particularly with regard to events and activities in the child's life. Discussion of autobiographical information provides the clinician with an initial sense of how reliably the child is able to report about onset and offset of symptoms. Since the goal of the clinician is to establish onset and offset of prior episodes of disorder and the onset of the current episode, it is critical both to establish the child's capacity to provide such information and to facilitate the child's ability to reconstruct from memory the time frames of his or her symptomatology. Thus, it is helpful if the clinician begins to develop in his or her notes a time line of autobiographical events discussed in the unstructured interview on which to anchor information introduced in the subsequent evaluation of symptom data.

Development of the K-SADS was strongly influenced by the Research Diagnostic Criteria (RDC). This fact is reflected in the types of items included in the evaluation of affective disorder in particular. The disorders evaluated by the K-SADS include, among other disorders, major depressive disorder, dysthymia, adjustment disorder with depressed mood, minor depression, manic disorder, cyclothymia, hypomania, and schizoaffective disorder—depressed and manic types. In addition, the K-SADS evaluates various anxiety disorders such as separation anxiety; panic disorder; phobic disorders; overanxious disorder; thought disorders including schizophrenia, schizophreniform disorder, and psychotic disorders; obsessive-compulsive disorder; eating disorders, namely anorexia nervosa and bulimia; various behavioral disorders of childhood such as attention-deficit disorder, conduct disorder, and oppositional disorder; and substance abuse and dependency. The K-SADS also evaluates suicidal behavior. Pervasive developmental disorder and autism are not evaluated by the K-SADS. Additionally, attention-deficit disorder and alcohol and substance use disorders are only evaluated in the K-SADS-E.

The K-SADS provides the clinician with a brief description of each disorder prior to the list of symptoms that need to be evaluated in order to determine whether there was an episode of the disorder. A series of interview prompts or questions are presented to facilitate the evaluation of each symptom, and criteria are presented for scoring the presence and severity of each symptom. The questions provided have been constructed such that the wording may be comprehended by even young prepubertal children. Since the K-SADS is a semistructured instrument intended for use by clinicians experienced in working with children and adolescents to assist them in making clinical judgments, the questions included are not intended to be adhered to religiously but to serve as a guide to the clinician. Thus, the clinician is free (and encouraged) to reformulate questions to meet immediate contingencies and to introduce additional questions when necessary.

In the process of evaluating symptomatology associated with a specific disorder, the K-SADS is structured so that the "essential symptoms" (Poznanski et al. 1985a) of a disorder are first evaluated to establish whether there is evidence for the presence of an episode of illness prior to the evaluation of additional "qualifying symptoms." Thus, the initial symptoms evaluated are screening items for the disorder in question. If there is no evidence for these symptoms, the K-SADS is structured so that the clinician then skips forward to the next diagnostic category. In the evaluation of depression, for example, the clinician first evaluates evidence of depressed mood and anhedonia and establishes the duration, frequency, and severity of these symptoms. If this evaluation fails to provide evidence of a depressive episode, additional symptoms associated with depressive episodes (e.g., appetite shifts, sleep disturbance, psychomotor retardation) are not evaluated. In those cases where the screening items do provide evidence of a disorder, the additional symptoms are evaluated and the results of this evaluation are then summarized to indicate whether or not diagnostic criteria for depression have been met. If diagnostic criteria have been met, the duration and period of worse functioning of the episode are defined. In this way, the clinician is actively developing a diagnostic profile of the child in the course of the interview, rather than waiting until the end of the interview to summarize the data obtained.

The K-SADS represents the most sophisticated approach to diagnostic evaluation in children and adolescents currently in use. This sophistication is expressed in the comprehensiveness and detail of the evaluation and thereby in the heavy demands on or expectations of the clinical sophistication of the interviewer. Additionally, if the K-SADS is indeed used as it is intended, particularly if both the K-SADS-E and K-SADS-P are administered to both the child and the parent, the administration can become quite time consuming, especially if multiple disorders are identified. Moreover, even the sophisticated clinician who is unfamiliar with the logic of the SADS approach will need to invest considerable time before he or she feels familiar and "fluent" in the administration of the K-SADS. As a result, use of the K-SADS is expensive; this must be considered prior to its adoption. Nevertheless, the centrality and highly successful use of this instrument in the most influential research on childhood mood disorders to date strongly suggest consideration of the instrument for clinical practice.

Conclusion. The semistructured interview bears a much closer resemblance to clinical practice than does the highly structured interview; in fact, it provides an optimal approach to symptom assessment. However, there are also disadvantages to the use of semistructured instruments. Most apparently, the use of these instruments assumes a high level of prior clinical sophistication, which thus makes their employment expensive. Because of the greater precision that a semistructured instrument is designed to establish, interview time will typically be longer than when a structured instrument is used. Of greater concern than the expense of using such instruments is the inevitable contribution of the interviewer to variation in ratings across probands and within probands over time. The highly active involvement of the interviewer in directing the course of the interview and in evaluating pro-band responses means that interrater variability will predictably increase over time. To guard against this inevitability, periodic reliability checks and retraining sessions are vital when semistructured instruments are used.

DEPRESSION RATING INSTRUMENTS

The second type of assessment instrument confines itself specifically to the measurement of depression. Although these instruments are inadequate for establishing diagnosis since they assess only depressive symptomatology, they are useful for both screening purposes and for documenting change in clinical status over time.

Structured Depression Rating Assessments

Structured depression measures include a wide range of instruments. These include the familiar self-report instrument, as well as such novel approaches as peer ratings of depression (e.g., Peer Nomination Inventory for Depression; Lefkowitz and Tesiny 1980), which, although useful for research purposes, have less utility in clinical practice. We will confine ourselves to discussing three instruments that are particularly appropriate to and commonly used in clinical practice: the Children's Depression Inventory (CDI), the Children's Depression Scale (CDS), and the Depression Self-rating Scale (DSRS).

Children's Depression Inventory. The CDI, developed by Kovacs (1985b), is one of the earliest developed and most commonly used self-report measures of depressive severity in children. The CDI, which consists of 27 items, was derived from the 21-item Beck Depression Inventory (Beck 1967), with all items reworked to make them age appropriate and with the 6 additional items specifically focused on such age-appropriate symptom areas as schoolwork. Whereas the CDI has been modified specifically for use in child populations as young as age 6 years, several versions of the adult Beck Depression Inventory have been applied in research on depression in adolescence with minor modification of content (Albert and Beck 1975; Kaplan et al. 1984; Reynolds 1983; Teri 1982).

The CDI covers a broad range of symptoms from multiple perspectives. Included are items evaluating dysphoria, pessimism, self-esteem, anhedonia, morbid concerns, suicidality, self-deprecation, social withdrawal, tendencies to ruminate, school performance, social conduct, and vegetative symptoms such as appetite and sleep disturbances, tiredness, and somatic complaints. Each of these items is rated along a 3-point scale from 0 (no problem) to 2 (severe problem), with the ordering of statements that reflect extreme scores randomized. That is, each item presents three statements or sentences; children are instructed to mark an X before the sentence that best describes them over the past 2 weeks. Kazdin and Petti (1982) report that these statements have readability at the first-grade level. However, one difficulty with this format, as Asarnow and Carlson (1985) suggest, is that asking children to make comparisons among three statements strains the attention span of child psychiatric inpatients and may in general exceed the attentional and cognitive capacities of younger children.

The CDI produces a single summary score ranging between 0 and 54, with no factor scores developed to date. A score of 19 or above has been reported to provide a useful cutoff for considering depressive disorder, with 90% of children in a normative sample scoring below this cutoff. The scale may be rapidly completed and may be read aloud to the child, as well as completed through self-report. The CDI with appropriate rewording of the items has been used to obtain parent ratings of the child.

Children's Depression Scale.   Rotundo and Hensley (1985) assert that the CDS, along with the CDI, are the two self-report measures most commonly used for the quantification of childhood depression. The CDS, developed by Lang and Tisher (1978; Tisher and Lang 1983), was initially developed as a Q sort of technique (Stephenson 1953). This technique involves having individuals sort through a deck of cards containing a set of statements that the individuals either judge as descriptive of themselves or not. The task may, but need not, involve a rank ordering of these descriptive statements. In the case of the CDS, 66 such cards were constructed; 48 of these cards provided depressive statements and 18 provided pleasurable or positive statements. The 48 depressive statements were divided among five factors associated with depression: affective responses (8 items), social problems (8 items), self-esteem (8 items), preoccupation with illness and death (7 items), and guilt (8 items). The cards are sorted into one of six boxes according to how closely the statement describes the child. The boxes are labeled "very wrong," "wrong," "don't know," "not sure," "right," and "very right." The scale is said to be appropriate for use with children and adolescents between ages 9 and 16 years; a parent-report version is also available. Reworded decks of cards have been developed for use with parents and significant others (e.g., siblings and teachers). The task is amenable to paper-and-pencil self-report, as illustrated by Rotundo and Hensley (1985).

Depression Self-rating Scale.   The DSRS, patterned after the Zung Depression Scale for adults (Zung 1965), was developed by Birleson (1981) as a screening instrument and severity measure of depression in children. The scale consists of 18 items that assess the range of symptoms associated with depression in children. Unlike the CDI, which presents children with three statements for each item scored, among which they are to choose the one that best describes them, the DSRS presents only a single statement for each item. Children are then asked to indicate whether they felt that way most of the time, sometimes, or never during the past week. To guard against response set bias, statements are constructed such that eight are problem oriented (e.g., "I think life isn't worth living," "I feel so sad I can hardly stand it") and the rest are statements of healthy functioning (e.g., "I look forward to things as much as I used to," "I like to go out to play"). Problem-oriented and healthy functioning statements are randomized in order of presentation, with responses indicating problems scored as 2, some degree of concern as 1, and no problem as 0.

The scale thus results in a summary score that may range between 0 and 36. Birleson (1981) reported mean scores for four groups of children including normal controls, maladjusted children in a residential school, a clinic control, and a depressed group, although sample sizes for each group were small. On the basis of analysis of these samples, he identified a cutoff score of 14 for identifying potentially depressed children. Although few studies of the DSRS have been published, the scale has attracted notable enthusiasm among several clinicians and researchers who find that its elegance and brevity make it an appealing alternative to the CDI.

Asarnow and Carlson (1985) developed a modified version of the DSRS, adding three additional depression items to more adequately cover DSM-III criteria. They also added three hopelessness items and two items assessing the child's capacity for empathy but retained these as separate factors.

Conclusion.   Instruments of this type are useful when the clinician is interested in rapidly screening for depression or when a severity measure of depression is needed to document change in the temporal course of a depressive episode. Additionally, responses to the instrument could serve as the basis for an interview evaluation of the child. Ratings are rapidly and economically obtained and scored even if, as is often done, an "interviewer" reads the instrument to the child as the child completes the ratings. Although the cost of generating information through such instruments is minimal, this information is only useful in combination with other measures. Reliance on self-report assumes that the child both is sufficiently motivated and possesses the cognitive ability to accurately describe his or her psychological states. On the basis of the results from such an evaluation alone, there is no easy way to determine whether the child was able to keep the called-for time frames in perspective when describing his or her symptoms, how the child interpreted each question, and whether that interpretation was consistent with the clinician's desired interpretation.

Semistructured Depression Instruments

Fewer semistructured than structured depression instruments have been developed. Below we will discuss two such instruments, the Bellevue Index of

Depression (BID) and the Children's Depression Rating Scale—Revised (CDRS-R).

Bellevue Index of Depression. The BID, developed by Petti (1978), consists in its most recent version (Petti 1985) of 40 items rated by clinicians on the basis of a semistructured interview. The BID represents a modified version of the evaluation instrument originally described by Weinberg et al. (1973). Fifty-two sample questions are provided for administering the scale and evaluating the 40 symptoms included. For example, for the evaluation of dysphoria, the following prompt is suggested: "How often do you look sad, lonely, or unhappy? Is this a problem?"

The 40 scaled items are organized according to 10 factors roughly associated with common symptoms of depression and manifestations specific to childhood (e.g., school performance and attitude issues). The 10 specific factors are as follows (the number of items involved in the evaluation of each factor is provided in parentheses): dysphoric mood (5), self-deprecatory ideation (5), aggressive behavior (5), sleep disturbance (4), change in school performance (7), diminished socialization (4), change in attitude toward school (2), somatic complaints (4), loss of energy (1), and unusual change in appetite and/or weight (2).

The evaluation procedure is to ask the child whether each item is perceived as a problem for the child or for others. If the child indicates that the item does represent a problem, the clinician further explores the extent of the problem by asking, "Is it a little problem, a big problem, a medium-sized problem, or not a problem?" (Petti 1985, p. 959). The child's response to this question is then translated into a rating along a 4-point scale, from absent to severe: 0 = not at all a problem, 1 = a little problem, 2 = quite a bit of a problem, 3 = very much of a problem.

Once an item has been described as problematic, the clinician then asks the child how long the problematic state has persisted. Here, Petti suggests four categories for the classification of the problem's duration: 1) less than 1 month, 2) 1–6 months, 3) 6 months to 2 years, and 4) always. Because of the difficulties many children (as well as adults) have in providing accurate temporal estimates of problem states, it is good practice, as Petti suggests, to provide anchors in terms of major cyclical and life events, such as birthdays, holidays, and deaths in the family, to facilitate an estimation of the symptom's time dimensions. For a symptom to merit clinical concern, the informant or child must view the symptom as a source of concern, with the symptom representing a notable change for the child and having a duration of at least 1 month. The clinician is expected to base his or her ratings of symptomatology on what is said, not on the clinical impression.

The scale has been recommended for use with children and parents, as well as significant others familiar with the child. A self-rated version of the scale has been developed for use with parents and significant others, although the interview format is also appropriate. The self-report format involves the rating of 52 items that correspond with the suggested queries posed to the child along the same two dimensions described for the interview format: degree of problem and length of problem. A total score is computed by adding the highest scores obtained from any source (e.g., child and parent) regarding all 40 symptoms. If the first factors on the scale—namely, dysphoric mood and self-deprecatory ideation—are both present (reflecting the Weinberg criteria for depression) and the total score across all 40 items is greater than 20, the child is considered "to have depressive features" (Petti 1985, p. 967). However, if only one of the first two factors is present or the total score is less than 20, depressive features are not indicated.

Children's Depression Rating Scale—Revised. The CDRS was developed by Poznanski in the late 1970s (Poznanski et al. 1979) and has since been revised (Poznanski et al. 1985b). The interview requires roughly 20–30 minutes to administer and score. It is useful both as an initial screen when depression is suspected or needs to be ruled out and for follow-up evaluation when a sensitive measure of change in depression status is called for. The CDRS-R is a semistructured, clinician-rated instrument designed for use with children between the ages of 6 and 12 years, although it has also been used effectively with adolescents.

The CDRS-R consists of 17 ordinally scaled items that evaluate the presence and severity of symptoms commonly associated with depression in childhood during the past month. The instrument may be used for direct interview of the child and/or the child's parents. Fourteen of these 17 items are rated by the clinician on the basis of the verbal responses of the informant. These include schoolwork, capacity to have fun, social withdrawal, appetite or eating patterns, excessive fatigue, physical complaints, irritability, guilt, self-esteem, depressed feelings, morbid ideation, suicidal ideation, and weeping. The remaining three items provide nonverbal indices of depressive features rated by the clinician on the basis of the child's appearance and demeanor during the course of the interview and are not used with informants other than the child. These include ratings of depressed affect, tempo of speech, and hypoactivity.

All items, with the exception of sleep disturbance, appetite or eating patterns, and tempo of speech, are rated on a 1- to 7-point scale with 1 indicating no evidence of problem or impairment and 7 indicating severe difficulties. The three remaining items are scaled from 1 to 5, with 1 again indicating no problem and 7 indicating severe difficulties. In addition, for two of these three items, an additional rating is made. In the case of the sleep item, if a sleep disturbance is reported, the clinician also indicates whether this difficulty occurs during the initial or middle stages of sleep or is manifested in early morning awakening. For the appetite pattern, the clinician indicates whether there has been an increase or decrease in appetite. Across all items, a rating of 3 indicates symptom presence at a level of clinical concern. Verbal descriptions of criteria are provided for the odd rating anchors (i.e., 1, 3, 5, 7) of each scale to assist the clinician in making rating decisions. The even anchors have been purposely left undefined to alleviate the inevitable difficulty presented when an informant's response is judged to fall between two descriptions. In their guide to the CDRS-R, Poznanski et al. (1985a, 1985b) provide examples of actual informant responses judged to match specific anchors for each item.

Besides identifying symptom presence, the CDRS-R may be used to obtain a severity index of depression by summing the scores across all 17 items, with possible scores ranging between 17 and 113. Poznanski et al. (1985a, 1985b) have reported that a summary score of 40 or above provides a useful index in clinical practice of a suspected major depressive disorder. Although a score of 40 or higher has been found to be a reliable indicator of depression, the summary score should not provide the basis for a diagnosis. Rather, it should serve as a heuristic and should be followed with a more comprehensive diagnostic evaluation.

The CDRS-R contains suggested prompts for each item evaluated. Since some children are developmentally unable to interpret questions about abstract concepts such as guilt, irritability, or suicide, the suggested prompts contain alternative ways of eliciting such information through wording specifically designed to be sensitive to the cognitive capacities of the child.

Additionally, the interview items are arranged so as to initially assess less threatening areas and gradually move toward more emotionally charged areas. However, since it is not uncommon for an informant to voluntarily introduce material that may appear as an area later in the questionnaire, it is important that the clinician capitalize on and thoroughly explore such revelations as they occur. Likewise, since it is also common to have informants who initially do not reveal or who deny the symptoms being assessed but who at some point begin to address such topics, the clinician necessarily must return to the earlier portions of the assessment and reconsider ratings that might have been previously made.

Thus, although a sequential format is suggested for the presentation of areas to be addressed, the intent of the CDRS-R is to serve as a guide for clinicians across the relevant terrain while establishing rapport and a sense of naturalness in the interview. This guide should be applied flexibly, with sensitivity to the course by which the informant chooses to traverse the terrain of interest. This intentional flexibility, which maximizes the analytic involvement of the clinician in the interview process, marks an important distinction between semistructured and structured approaches to evaluation.

Conclusion. Whereas structured measures of depression offer economy at the cost of uncertainty as to the quality of the data, the opposite is the case with semistructured depression evaluations. As with semistructured diagnostic instruments, use of these instruments necessitates clinical experience in the evaluation of childhood disorders. Because ratings obtained with these instruments are based on interviews, semistructured instruments cost much more to use than structured instruments. Additionally, as was discussed for semistructured diagnostic evaluations, it must be kept in mind that the clinician will always contribute to the ratings of the child. However, the data obtained through the semistructured evaluation are much less ambiguous than those obtained through structured evaluations in identifying whether a child has the cognitive capacity to understand the questions asked, whether mechanisms of distortion and denial were in evidence, and whether the child was motivated to respond and elaborate.

PSYCHOMETRIC ISSUES

Studies of the psychometric properties of most assessment instruments used in the evaluation of depression in childhood have been scant. This is true more for interview-based than for self-report instruments. Although common issues of reliability and validity have to some extent been explored for all of the instruments reviewed above, many important psychometric issues have been largely ignored. For example, although internal consistency has been investigated for several instruments, more sophisticated evaluations of the items included in instruments through factor analysis (e.g., CDI; Helsel and Matson 1984) and item-response theory are rare to nonexistent. Multitrait, multimethod approaches to evaluation of validity (Campbell and Fiske 1959) have only been applied to a few self-report measures (e.g., CDI and BID; Kazdin et al. 1983). Additionally, the effects of such sociodemographic variables as age, sex, and race have been highly underexplored, with the CBCL being a notable exception.

Semistructured and diagnostic instruments in particular (with the exception of the CBCL) have had insufficient psychometric evaluation, although some preliminary data have been reported for the DICA (Welner et al. 1987), the CAS (Hodges et al. 1982a, 1982b), the K-SADS-P (Chambers et al. 1985), the K-SADS-E (Orvaschel et al. 1982), the BID (Petti 1983), and the CDRS-R (Poznanski et al. 1984). This is in part due to the difficulty and expense involved in conducting large-sample, controlled studies when a high level of professional expertise is required to administer these instruments in order for the results to be reliable. Additionally, traditional ways of thinking about issues of reliability may prove overly dogmatic in the context of evaluating semistructured instruments precisely because use of these instruments relies on the active participation of the clinician.

The CDI has undergone the most extensive psychometric investigation. Normative data have been published for both normal children (Finch et al. 1985) and psychiatrically hospitalized children (Nelson et al. 1987). Reliability statistics for the CDI have, in general, been acceptable. Kovacs (1985b) reported high internal consistency and acceptable test-retest reliability. Saylor et al. (1984a) also reported high internal consistency, but found that test-retest reliability differed between depressed and normal children, with a high reliability coefficient for depressed children and a low coefficient for normal children. Finally, in a study of the reliability of the CDI over three repeat assessments during a 6-week period, Finch et al. (1987) found that CDI scores decreased significantly over time. The results of this last study have important implications for the use of the CDI as a treatment outcome measure.

Support for the validity of the CDI appears much more problematic (Costello and Angold 1988). Although Strauss et al. (1984) reported that children in the community who had high scores (above 19) on the CDI showed characteristics similar to those of clinically depressed children, data to indicate that the instrument distinguishes depressed from nondepressed children have been mixed. Thus, although Kovacs (1985b) reported that the CDI differentiated children who had major depression from both children who had adjustment disorder with depressed mood and children who had conduct/oppositional disorder, Saylor et al. (1984a) reported contradictory results. They found that the CDI discriminated children with emotional problems from normal controls but did not discriminate depressed from nondepressed children.

This failure to discriminate depressed children from a more general population of emotionally disturbed children may, in fact, result from the considerable overlap of the CDI with anxiety symptomatology (Wolfe et al. 1987). However, the finding of another study that the CDI fails to discriminate mood from conduct disorder diagnoses is still more problematic (Nelson et al. 1987). Indeed, when self-, peer, and teacher reports of depression (as well as of other traits) have been compared, little evidence for the convergent and discriminant validity of the CDI has been found (Saylor et al. 1984b). These data all suggest that the diagnostic sensitivity and specificity of the CDI are clearly limited. Supporting this conclusion, Kazdin et al. (1986) found that a CDI cutoff score of 19 resulted in a sensitivity of about 28.2% and a specificity of 75.3% based on child report and a sensitivity of 61.3% and specificity of 55.3% based on parent report.

In our opinion, this literature raises some serious concerns as to the validity of the CDI, in its current form, as a measure of depression for either clinical or nonclinical assessment. It is, of course, possible that similar conclusions apply to other instruments. The problem is that insufficient research has been carried out with other instruments to fairly evaluate them. Further consideration of the adequacy of available assessment procedures is certainly warranted (Costello and Angold 1988; Kazdin 1981; Kazdin and Petti 1982).

Additionally, further concern needs to be directed to the identification of strategies or decision rules for integrating information from multiple sources, including both differing types of instruments and particularly differing informants in the diagnostic process. It is, after all, common and appropriate practice to gather information from multiple perspectives for the purpose of formulating a diagnosis. As research on the relationship between child and parent accounts of the child's depression indicates, disagreements as to symptom reports are common and yet they are also not random (e.g., Mokros et al. 1987). How clinicians go about resolving discrepancies has a bearing on the diagnosis given and thereby merits the thoughtful consideration of both clinician and researcher.

CONCLUSION

Development of standardized instruments for the purpose of assessment was one of the earliest initiatives among researchers of childhood depression. This initiative was motivated by the recognition that variance in information was a key obstacle to acquiring knowledge through research. Although many instruments have been developed, the quality of these instruments, together with the meaning and significance of their information, merits continued scrutiny.

In discussion of prominent instruments used for the assessment of depression in childhood, we distinguished instruments along two dimensions. The first dimension drew a distinction between instruments that evaluated depression within a broader diagnostic context and those that specifically evaluated depression. We argued against the use of cutoff scores from depression measures to draw diagnostic conclusions. The second dimension suggested that instruments (or their use) may be described as either structured or semistructured. Conceptually, the differences between structured and semistructured instruments are in the assumptions made about the relationship between data and clinical judgment.

In the case of structured instruments, symptom ratings are based exclusively on the informant's responses to explicitly defined questions. The rating obtained with a structured instrument may (i.e., structured interview) or may not (e.g., self-report) involve an interviewer. If it does involve an interviewer, then the role played by the interviewer in making symptom ratings is intentionally minimized. Thus, the uninterpreted responses or data provided by the informant are the sole basis for all symptom ratings made.

In contrast, semistructured instruments always involve an interviewer (or interpreter) and require that this interviewer play an active role in the establishment of symptom ratings. Although questions and probes are provided in the semistructured instrument, the interviewer may expand these probes when further elaborations are judged necessary. This active participation of the interviewer is mostly directly expressed in the symptom rating process, where clinical judgment about the patient's responses, rather than the responses themselves, is the source of the ratings that are made. It is the central reliance on clinical experience, judgment, and knowledge that conceptually distinguishes semistructured from structured instruments. We believe that the assumptions underlying these conceptual distinctions are important considerations for the clinician who employs standardized instruments in the evaluation of depression in childhood and adolescence.

Thus, in this review we have examined four classes of instruments, with 10 measures described overall. Although no single instrument predominates, Petti (1985) notes a trend toward the use of three instruments in psychopharmacological research. These are the K-SADS-P, the CDRS-R, and the CDI. The K-SADS-P provides an interview format for comprehensive diagnostic evaluation of both affective and nonaffective psychiatric diagnoses, whereas the CDRS-R and the CDI provide severity measures of depression from the perspective of the clinician and the self-report of the child, respectively. Given the available psychometric literature, we advise caution in the use of the CDI and suggest the use of the DSRS in its stead when a quick self-report from the child is desired. Although we strongly endorse the use of the K-SADS, this instrument may not prove to be a manageable approach to diagnostic evaluation for many clinicians. As an alternative, we have found that the DICA in a semistructured context provides a useful basis for diagnostic evaluation.

Finally, interpretation of the results provided by any of these instruments for any given case requires that the clinician possess familiarity with the normative developmental course, know the cultural value systems of the child, have the ability to disambiguate what in the child's performance is a product of situational demands from what truly reflects the state of the child relative to the diagnosis of depression, and be able to estimate the contribution of the psychopathology (if any) of others, such as parents, to the reports they provide on the child. These considerations for interpretation should again underscore the fact that although standardized assessments provide a tool for the clinician, they are only a tool—nothing more.

REFERENCES

Achenbach TM, Edelbrock C: Manual for the Child Behavioral Checklist and Revised Child Behavior Profile. Burlington, University of Vermont, 1982

Achenbach TM, Edelbrock CS: Psychopathology of childhood. Annu Rev Psychol 35:227–256, 1984

Albert N, Beck AT: Incidence of depression in early adolescents: a preliminary study. Journal of Youth and Adolescence 4:301–307, 1975

American Psychiatric Association: Diagnostic and Statistical Manual of Mental Disorders, 3rd Edition. Washington, DC, American Psychiatric Association, 1980

American Psychiatric Association: Diagnostic and Statistical Manual of Mental Disorders, 3rd Edition, Revised. Washington, DC, American Psychiatric Association, 1987

Asarnow JR, Carlson GA: Depression self-rating scale: utility with child psychiatric inpatients. J Consult Clin Psychol 53:491–499, 1985

Beck AT: Depression: Clinical, Experimental, and Theoretical Aspects. New York, Harper & Row, 1967

Birleson P: The validity of depressive disorder in childhood and the development of a self-rating scale: a research report. J Child Psychol Psychiatry 22:73–88, 1981

Campbell DT, Fiske DW: Convergent and discriminant validation by the multitrait-multimethod matrix. Psychol Bull 56:81–105, 1959

Chambers WJ, Puig-Antich J, Hirsch M, et al: The assessment of affective disorders in children and adolescents: test-retest reliability of the Schedule for Affective Disorders and Schizophrenia for School-Age Children, Present Episode Version. Arch Gen Psychiatry 42:696–702, 1985

Costello AJ, Angold A: Scales to assess child and adolescent depression: checklists, screens and nets. J Am Acad Child Adolesc Psychiatry 27:726–737, 1988

Costello AJ, Dulcan MK: DISC: Diagnostic Interview for Children. Unpublished manuscript, 1985

Costello AJ, Edelbrock CS, Dulcan MK, et al: Report on the NIMH Diagnostic Interview for Children. Unpublished manuscript, 1984

Dulcan MK, Costello AJ, Kallas R: Training Manual for the Diagnostic Interview Schedule for Children. Unpublished manuscript, 1985

Finch AJ, Saylor CF, Edwards GL: Children's depression inventory: sex and grade norms for normal children. J Consult Clin Psychol 53:424–425, 1985

Finch AJ, Saylor CF, Edwards GL, et al: Children's Depression Inventory: reliability over repeated administrations. Journal of Clinical Child Psychology 16:339–341, 1987

Helsel WJ, Matson JL: The assessment of depression in children: the internal structure of the Child Depression Inventory (CDI). Behav Res Ther 22:289–298, 1984

Herjanic B, Reich W: Development of a structured psychiatric interview for children: agreement between child and parent on individual symptoms. J Abnorm Child Psychol 10:307–324, 1982

Hodges K, Kline J, Stern L, et al: The development of a child assessment interview for research and clinical use. J Abnorm Child Psychol 10:173–189, 1982a

Hodges K, McKnew D, Cytryn L, et al: The child assessment schedule (CAS) diagnostic interview: a report on reliability and validity. J Am Acad Child Psychiatry 21:468–473, 1982b

Kaplan SL, Hong GK, Weinhold C: Epidemiology of depressive symptomatology in adolescents. J Am Acad Child Psychiatry 23:91–98, 1984

Kazdin AE: Assessment techniques for childhood depression. J Am Acad Child Psychiatry 20:358–375, 1981

Kazdin AE, Petti TA: Self-report and interview measures of childhood and adolescent depression. J Child Psychol Psychiatry 23:437–457, 1982

Kazdin AE, French NH, Unis AS: Child, mother, and father evaluations of depression in psychiatric inpatient children. J Abnorm Child Psychol 11:167–180, 1983

Kazdin AE, Colbus D, Rodgers A: Assessment of depression and diagnosis of depressive disorder among psychiatrically disturbed children. J Abnorm Child Psychol 14:499–515, 1986

Kovacs M: The Interview Schedule for Children (ISC). Psychopharmacol Bull 21:991–994, 1985a

Kovacs M: The Children's Depression Inventory (CDI). Psychopharmacol Bull 21:995–998, 1985b

Lang M, Tisher M: Children's Depression Scale. Melbourne, Australian Council for Educational Research, 1978

Lefkowitz MM, Tesiny EP: Assessment of childhood depression. J Consult Clin Psychol 48:43–50, 1980

Mokros HB, Poznanski E, Grossman JA, et al: A comparison of child and parent ratings of depression for normal and clinically referred children. J Child Psychol Psychiatry 28:613–627, 1987

Nelson WM, Politano PM, Finch AJ, et al: Children's depression inventory: normative data and utility with emotionally disturbed children. J Am Acad Child Adolesc Psychiatry 26:43–48, 1987

Orvaschel J, Puig-Antich J: Schedule for Affective Disorder and Schizophrenia for School-Age Children, Epidemiological Version, 4th Edition (unpublished manuscript). Pittsburgh, PA, Western Psychiatric Institute and Clinic, 1986

Orvaschel J, Puig-Antich J, Chambers W, et al: Retrospective assessment of prepubertal major depression with the Kiddie-SADS-E. J Am Acad Child Psychiatry 21:392–397, 1982

Petti TA: Depression in hospitalized child psychiatry patients. J Am Acad Child Psychiatry 17:49–59, 1978

Petti TA: Childhood Depression. New York, Haworth Press, 1983

Petti TA: Scales of potential use in the psychopharmacological treatment of depressed children and adolescents. Psychopharmacol Bull 21:951–955, 1985

Poznanski EO, Cook SC, Carroll BJ: A depression rating scale for children. Pediatrics 64:442–450, 1979

Poznanski EO, Grossman JA, Buchsbaum Y, et al: Preliminary studies of the reliability of the Children's Depression Rating Scale. J Am Acad Child Adolesc Psychiatry 23:191–197, 1984

Poznanski EO, Mokros HB, Grossman J, et al: Diagnostic criteria in childhood depression. Am J Psychiatry 142:1168–1173, 1985a

Poznanski EO, Freeman LN, Mokros HB: Children's depression rating scale—revisited. Psychopharmacol Bull 21:979–989, 1985b

Puig-Antich J, Gittelman R: Depression in childhood and adolescence, in Handbook of Affective Disorders. Edited by Paykel ES. New York, Guilford, 1982, pp 379–392

Puig-Antich J, Chambers WJ, Tabrizi M: The clinical assessment of current depressive episodes in children and adolescents: interviews with parents and children, in Affective Disorders in Childhood and Adolescence: An Update. Edited by Cantwell DP, Carlson GA. New York, Spectrum, 1983, pp 157–179

Reich W, Herjanic B, Welner Z, et al: Development of a structured psychiatric interview for children: agreement on diagnosis comparing child and parent interviews. J Abnorm Child Psychol 10:325–336, 1982

Reynolds WM: Depression in adolescents: measurement, epidemiology, and correlates. Paper presented at the annual meeting of the National Association of School Psychologists, Detroit, MI, 1983

Rotundo N, Hensley VR: The Children's Depression Scale: a study of its validity. J Child Psychol Psychiatry 26:917–927, 1985

Saylor CF, Finch AJ, Spirito A, et al: The children's depression inventory: a systematic evaluation of psychometric properties. J Consult Clin Psychol 52:955–967, 1984a

Saylor CF, Finch AJ, Baskin CH, et al: Construct validity for measures of childhood depression: application of multitrait-multimethod methodology. J Consult Clin Psychol 52:977–985, 1984b

Spitzer RL, Endicott J: Schedule for Affective Disorders and Schizophrenia. NIMH Clinical Research Branch, Collaborative Program on the Psychology of Depression, 3rd Edition. Washington, DC, U.S. Government Printing Office, 1978

Stephenson W: The Study of Behavior. Chicago, IL, University of Chicago, 1953

Strauss CC, Forehand R, Frame C, et al: Characteristics of children with extreme scores on the children's depression inventory. Journal of Clinical Child Psychology 13:227–231, 1984

Teri L: The use of the Beck Depression Inventory with adolescents. J Abnorm Child Psychol 10:277–284, 1982

Tisher M, Lang M: The Children's Depression Scale: review and further developments, in Affective Disorders in Childhood and Adolescence: An Update. Edited by Cantwell DP, Carlson GA. New York, Spectrum, 1983, pp 181–203

Weinberg WA, Rutman J, Sullivan J, et al: Depression in children referred to an educational diagnostic center: diagnosis and treatment. Behavioral Pediatrics 83:1065–1072, 1973

Welner Z, Reich W, Herjanic B, et al: Reliability, validity, and parent-child agreement studies of the Diagnostic Interview for Children and Adolescents (DICA). J Am Acad Child Adolesc Psychiatry 26:649–653, 1987

Wolfe VV, Finch AJ, Saylor AJ, et al: Negative affectivity in children: a multitrait-multimethod investigation. J Consult Clin Psychol 55:245–250, 1987

Zung WWK: A self-rating depression scale. Arch Gen Psychiatry 12:63–70, 1965

CHAPTER 7

Dynamic Psychotherapy of Depression

Mohammad Shafii, M.D.
Sharon Lee Shafii, R.N., B.S.N.

The term *psychotherapy* is used loosely for many types of interactions. Defining psychotherapy is difficult. However, we have found that Jerome Frank's (1963) description of psychotherapy from a historical and transcultural perspective is comprehensive and yet specific:

> Attempts to enhance a person's feeling of well-being are usually labeled treatment, and every society trains some of its members to apply this form of influence. Treatment always involves a personal relationship between healer and sufferer. Certain types of therapy rely primarily on the healer's ability to mobilize healing forces in the sufferer by psychological means. These forms of treatment may be generically termed psychotherapy. (p. 1)

There are many kinds of psychotherapy. In this chapter, we will examine dynamic psychotherapy based on psychoanalytic and ego-psychological principles in the form of play therapy, talk therapy, and supportive-exploratory psychotherapy.

HISTORICAL PERSPECTIVE

The beginning of child psychotherapy is attributed to Freud (1909) with the publication of the classical case of the treatment of childhood phobia known as "Little Hans." Little Hans developed a severe phobia toward horses between the ages of 4 and 5 years. This phobia intensified after a tonsillectomy at age 5 years. Hans became so panic stricken that he could not leave his house because of a fear of horse-drawn carriages, a common mode of transportation in Vienna at the time. Freud did not treat Little Hans directly, but rather regularly met with Hans's father. Hans's father would report his son's worries, fears, and fantasies to Freud. Freud would suggest to the father how to treat Hans's phobia based on psychoanalytic principles. According to Freud's formulation, Hans's phobia was a displacement of his fear of his father to horses—a manifestation of underlying castration anxiety. Castration anxiety was the projection of Little Hans's phallic-oedipal aggressive and destructive wishes toward his father.

In searching the literature, one finds a precedence for adolescent psychotherapy approximately 1,000 years ago. Shafii (1972) reported on a case of a young prince, most probably in adolescence, who had the symptoms of severe weight loss, refusal to eat, and the delusion of being a cow who wanted to be slaughtered for making meat stew. Avicenna (d. 1037 A.D.), a Persian physician and philosopher, diagnosed this patient as having melancholia. He accepted the patient's delusion and communicated with the patient as if he were a "sick cow." Avicenna pretended to be a butcher who was preparing to slaughter this cow. He told the patient that he needed to be fattened before he could be slaughtered. Avicenna advised the patient's primary physicians and relatives not to challenge the patient's delusion, but to communicate with him as though he were a sick cow. They were to encourage him to take his food and medication so that he could be fattened for slaughter. Through this approach, the patient recovered a month later.

From a psychodynamic perspective, by accepting—not confronting or challenging—the patient's delusional system, Avicenna was able to establish rapport, basic trust, and therapeutic alliance. This approach resembles the psychoanalytic and psychodynamic method described by Ekstein (1966) of "communication within the delusional system" or "communication within the metaphor."

PRINCIPLES OF DYNAMIC PSYCHOTHERAPY

Psychotherapy based on psychoanalytic principles goes under various names: dynamic, exploratory, expressive, psychoanalytically oriented, uncovering, intensive, and insight-oriented psychotherapy (Gabbard 1990, p. 71). Psychoanalytic and ego-psychological principles are based on the unconscious, preconscious, and conscious aspects of the mind. According to psychoanalytic and psychodynamic concepts, mental contents, wishes, and drives ". . . which are unacceptable, threatening, or abhorrent to the moral, ethical and intellectual standards of the individual are repressed in the unconscious" (Moore and Fine 1968, p. 94). Repressed fantasies and wishes are the source of intrapsychic conflicts. Internal conflicts are the outcome of the intrapsychic struggle between the sexual and aggressive impulses of the id on the one hand and the sugerego prohibitions and external reality on the other hand. The ego (I, self) reacts to these internal conflicts through defense mechanisms. Defense mechanisms, then, are part of ego function. They are primarily unconscious and help an individual adapt to daily life (A. Freud 1936).

Defense Mechanisms

Meissner et al. (1975, pp. 535–536) classified defense mechanisms in the following way:

1. Narcissistic defenses—projection and denial
2. Immature defenses—introjection-identification, regression, acting out, and splitting
3. Neurotic defenses—repression, rationalization, displacement, intellectualization, reaction formation, and isolation
4. Mature defenses—altruism, anticipation, asceticism, humor, sublimation, and suppression

According to psychodynamic theory, some early childhood traumatic experiences such as separation from mother, parental deprivation, physical trauma, sexual overstimulation, overprotection, death of a loved one, chronic physical illness, bodily insult, parental disharmony, natural calamity, war, and disasters create overwhelming anxiety, particularly in infancy, childhood, and adolescence.

These overwhelming anxieties bring about a feeling of panic and helplessness. Also, for the most part through the defense mechanisms of the ego, these anxieties are repressed in the unconscious in the form of psychic trauma. When the individual reexperiences similar traumas or other overwhelming anxieties, the overwrought defense mechanism of repression fails to function effectively and various psychopathological symptoms and disorders may appear, such as depressive disorders.

The Dynamic Psychotherapeutic Process

In dynamic psychotherapy the patient is encouraged to express thoughts, feelings, sensations, wishes, ideas, and fantasies without any hesitation or censoring. The therapist, by an accepting, nonintrusive, and nonjudgmental attitude, encourages the patient to express conscious, preconscious, and unconscious thoughts and feelings openly.

In dynamic psychotherapy through free association, the patient is encouraged to remember, express, and reexperience earlier psychic traumas. The premise is that the patient gains insight into symptomatic behavior by becoming more aware of past experiences and by modifying repressed wishes, fears, and defensive postures. Understanding and insight help the patient to neutralize and master intrapsychic conflicts, leading to healthier adaptation.

According to Bibring (1954), five basic principles and techniques are used in psychoanalysis and dynamic psychotherapy: suggestions, abreaction (catharsis), manipulation, clarification, and interpretation. These same methods are employed in the dynamic psychotherapy of children and adolescents with depressive disorders.

Transference

The accepting, nonjudgmental position of the psychotherapist helps the patient to regress in the psychotherapeutic situation. Through this regression, the patient transfers unconscious feelings, wishes, desires, and expectations from meaningful persons of the past, particularly parental figures, to the therapist.

The discovery of the transference phenomenon and its effective use in psychoanalysis and dynamic psychotherapy was one of the most significant developments in understanding the psychology of the human mind in the twentieth century. Regarding the transference phenomenon, Greenson (1967) stated:

> The development of the technique of psychoanalysis has been determined essentially by the evolution of our knowledge of the nature of transference. The greatest advances in psychoanalytic technique were derived from Freud's (1905) major discoveries about the twofold power of transference; it is an instrument of irreplaceable value and it is the source of the greatest dangers. Transference reactions offer the analyst an invaluable opportunity to explore the inaccessible past and the unconscious (Freud 1919, p. 108). Transference also stirs up resistances that become the most serious obstacle to our work. . . . (p. 151)

The patient usually has ambivalent feelings toward the therapist. Based on this ambivalence, transference can be positive or negative. In positive transference, the patient has ". . . intense, positive, affectionate love and even sexual fantasies toward the therapist" (Shafii 1985, p. 79). In negative transference, the patient has ". . . unrealistic anger, hostility, and aggressive and destructive feelings. . . . " (Shafii 1985, p. 79).

In the past, there was considerable debate in the child and adolescent psychiatric literature on whether the transference phenomenon occurred in psychotherapy because parents still play an active role in the child's life. Now, it is generally accepted that the transference phenomenon in varying forms and intensities does occur in psychotherapy with children and adolescents (Chethik 1989, pp. 45, 122).

Resistance

Another important phenomenon that occurs in psychoanalysis and dynamic psychotherapy is resistance. The patient, whether child or adult, is ambivalent about change. A part of the patient wants to free the self from troublesome symptoms, and another part wishes to keep the status quo and resists and opposes change. Freud (1912) wrote that ". . . resistance accompanies the treatment step by step. Every single association, every act of the person and the treatment must reckon with the resistance and represents a compromise between the forces striving for recovery and the opposing ones" (p. 103).

Children and adolescents show more conscious and unconscious resistance toward psychotherapy because they usually do not want to come to therapy in the first place and feel forced by their parents to do so. Resistance is even more intense in the case of adolescents who also feel that the therapist as an adult is in "cahoots" with the parents.

Countertransference

The countertransference phenomenon is the unconscious or partly conscious attitude and feeling of the psychotherapist or psychoanalyst toward the patient. "In countertransference, the analyst [the psychotherapist] has displaced on to the patient attitudes and feelings derived from earlier situations in his own life" (Moore and Fine 1968, p. 29).

The therapist's awareness of countertransference feelings, such as irrationally liking or disliking the child, overprotecting the child, rejecting the child, overindulging the child, or competing with the parents, should be observed, examined, and worked through. Acting out countertransference feelings in the therapeutic setting exploits the patient, hampers the patient's progress, and may result in therapeutic failure. Also, the therapist's ". . . continuing scrutiny of his own countertransference feelings frequently provides correct clues to the meaning of the patient's behavior, feelings, and thoughts, and may facilitate more prompt *perception* of the patient's *unconscious*" (Moore and Fine 1968, p. 29).

DYNAMIC PSYCHOTHERAPY OF DEPRESSION IN THE INFANT FROM BIRTH THROUGH AGE 2 YEARS

Infants usually do not come to the attention of child psychiatrists or mental health professionals. Most often, they are referred by pediatricians, family physicians, or others because of suspicion of physical or sexual abuse, parental neglect, parental alcohol or drug abuse, or failure to thrive. (See Chapter 1.) In our experience, depression in infancy most frequently represents family dysfunction and parental psychopathology. After careful initial assessment depending on the severity and intensity of the infant's depression, parental psychopathology, and the availability of support systems, a decision can be made whether to treat the infant on an inpatient or outpatient basis.

Dolen (1982) stresses that although the infant is the perceived patient, actually the family as a whole needs the treatment. Fraiberg et al. (1980, p. 60) described three modes of psychotherapeutic intervention in infants.

1. *Brief crisis intervention.* This is indicated when an infant's depression is a reaction to a specific event such as the birth of a new baby, mother's hospitalization for physical illness, death in the family, or father's temporary absence. The parents need to be relatively healthy and able to benefit from brief psychological intervention.
2. *Developmental guidance—supportive therapy.* In this situation, parents generally have good parenting skills but, due to various reasons, they are under extreme distress. This approach can also be used when both child and the parents have severe emotional problems and "limited capacity" for psychological mindedness and ability to explore and work through unconscious conflicts. According to Fraiberg et al. (1980), ". . . our objective is to provide emotional support and to strengthen parenting capacities, while simultaneously providing developmental guidance in the form of information and discussion about the baby's needs" (pp. 60–61).
3. *Infant-parent psychotherapy.* This mode of treatment is indicated "when the parents have integrated the infant symbolically into their own neurosis so that the child represents a part of the 'parental past' or 'an aspect of the parental self that is repudiated or negated'" (Dolen 1982, p. 256).

In each of these modes of therapy, the infant and parent(s) or primary caregiver(s) should be seen together. Although the focus of therapy is the infant, parents are encouraged to share with the therapist their own backgrounds, marital relationship, childhood experiences, and relationships with their parents and significant others.

The therapist plays an active role in the therapeutic situation. In addition to being an attentive listener, he or she provides the parents with support, guidance, and education concerning child rearing and child development. The therapist also functions, at times, as a social intervener to help the family deal with outside social or health agencies if indicated. If the parents are suffering from severe forms of psychopathology, such as major depression, alcohol or drug abuse, psychosis, or acute or chronic physical illness, the therapist makes appropriate referrals.

In psychotherapy with depressed infants, home visits are essential. Fraiberg et al. (1980) suggest that psychotherapeutic interventions should occur at the infant's home. We suggest that, because of time and economic factors, psychotherapy or intervention could occur in a clinic or therapist's office, but occasional home visits significantly enhance the therapist's relationship with the family and therapeutic effectiveness.

In some cases, because of the limited ability of the parent(s) to cope with the infant on a 24-hour basis, we recommend the assistance of a nonthreatening and supportive homemaker on a regular basis, involvement of visiting nurses, early intervention programs, and/or day care placement. In severe cases of child abuse and neglect, the therapist may recommend placement of the child outside of the home.

In most cases of psychotherapy of depressed infants, the outcome is rewarding. Significant improvement occurs when the parents' attitude and interaction with the infant change and they provide a healthy, stimulating environment. Fraiberg et al. (1980) wrote, "Undo the impediments to forward movement and the baby lifts off! It's a little bit like having God on your side" (p. 53).

DYNAMIC PSYCHOTHERAPY OF DEPRESSION IN THE PRESCHOOL CHILD AGES 3–6 YEARS

Play is the language of the preschool-age child. Through play, the child enhances sensory motor functions, increases symbolic thought processes, imitates grown-ups, creates a world of make-believe, and expresses and acts out wishes and fantasies. Also, the child acts out prohibitions against wishes and fantasies. Through play, the child creates new situations, problems, and obstacles and makes every effort to overcome them. The child repeats past experiences, particularly traumatic experiences, through play. Through compulsion to repeat (Freud 1920), identification with the aggressor, and identification with the victim, the child attempts to cope with or master the past and deal with the present.

According to Schiller, "Man is perfectly human only when he plays" (Erikson 1950, p. 212). During this century with the works of Jean Piaget, Melanie Klein, Anna Freud, Virginia Axline, Erik Erikson, and others, we have become aware of the significance of play not only in child development but as an effective method of communicating with and treating children. Play therapy now has an important role in the assessment and treatment of preschool-age and school-age children.

Guidelines for Play Therapy

We have found Axline's (1947, pp. 93–94) guidelines for play therapy helpful in treating children with emotional disorders, including depressed children:

1. The therapist must develop a warm, friendly relationship with the child, in which good rapport is established as soon as possible.
2. The therapist accepts the child exactly as he is.
3. The therapist establishes a feeling of permissiveness in the relationship so that the child feels free to express his feelings completely.
4. The therapist is alert to recognize the feelings the child is expressing and reflects those feelings back to him in such a manner that he gains insight into his behavior.

5. The therapist maintains a deep respect for the child's ability to solve his own problems if given an opportunity to do so. The responsibility to make choices and to institute changes is the child's.
6. The therapist does not attempt to direct the child's actions or conversation in any manner. The child leads the way; the therapist follows.
7. The therapist does not attempt to hurry the therapy along. It is a gradual process and is recognized as such by the therapist.
8. The therapist establishes only those limitations that are necessary to anchor the therapy to the world of reality and to make the child aware of his responsibility in the relationship.

Individual play therapy of the preschool-age child should be accompanied by working closely with the parents in the form of parental psychotherapy, marital therapy, and parental education in child rearing. Preschool children with mild to moderate depression are usually seen for play therapy once to twice a week for 30–45 minutes. Parents are seen on a weekly basis for about 45 minutes. Generally, once or twice a month the parents and child are seen together for family therapy.

From a psychodynamic perspective, depressed preschool children usually have underlying concerns and worries about the consistency and quality of parental nurturance. Frequently, these children are inhibited. The defense mechanisms of suppression, repression, introjection, and reaction formation are overutilized.

Through play therapy, the child is encouraged to do or say anything as long as it will not hurt him or her, the therapist, or the "things around." The child is reassured that what is said or done is between the child and the therapist unless the child's life or someone else's life is in danger. If the therapist needs to share some information with the parents, the child should be told in advance. In this situation, when they meet together, the therapist shares the information with the parents and also encourages the child to express feelings and concerns. In psychotherapy with children and adolescents, it is important to let the patient know by word and deed that, for the most part, the therapist is on the youngster's side rather than on the parents' side. But this does not mean that the therapist will always agree with him or her. Openness, honesty, and consistency are the essences of psychotherapeutic work with children, adolescents, and their families.

Play therapy gradually helps the depressed child play out internal thoughts, worries, and concerns, especially through the defense mechanism of displacement. Children, particularly inhibited children, are reluctant to tell the therapist, especially in the early phase of treatment, how they feel or what is happening in their home. Doll houses and dolls dressed as children, grown-ups, doctors, nurses, teachers, policemen, and others become vehicles for the patient to assign the role of parents, siblings, teachers, friends, peers, and others. Puppets, clay, paper and crayons, blocks, tinker toys, and other creative toys also become vehicles for the child's expression and play. The therapist's "experiencing ego" regresses to the child's level and becomes the child's playmate. At the same time, the therapist's "observing ego" functions as a relatively objective observer to help the child master internal conflicts and improve behavior and attitude. The therapist follows the child's lead and encourages the child's involvement in fantasy play. This helps the child to decrease inhibitory tendencies such as suppression, repression, and introjection.

Through the process of suggestion, abreaction, and clarification, the child and parents become more familiar with their strengths and shortcomings and find ways to develop healthier relationships. An appropriate and timely confrontation and interpretation can decrease child and parental resistance and help them further along the path of exploration, self-discovery, and healing.

DYNAMIC PSYCHOTHERAPY OF DEPRESSION IN THE SCHOOL-AGE CHILD AGES 7–12 YEARS

The psychodynamic and psychotherapeutic principles discussed earlier in this chapter also apply to the depressed school-age child. Age-specific symptoms of depression that occur in this age group are intensification of suicidal behavior; verbalization of suicidal intent; development of a suicide plan; significant decline in school performance; withdrawal from peers and parents; and overwhelming feelings of guilt, self-blame, and worthlessness. (See Chapter 1.)

One of the developmental tasks of this age group is the toning down of oedipal, sexual, and aggressive wishes and fantasies toward parents through the intensification of the defense mechanisms of repression, suppression, and denial. The depressed school-age child's underlying anger and feelings of isolation and alienation from the parents are displaced to the therapist, making the task of psychotherapy more difficult. Also, at this age the defense mechanisms of isolation of affect and rationalization emerge. The depressed school-age child does not share thoughts, feelings, fantasies, and wishes with the therapist as readily as the preschooler does.

Differentiating the healthy and developmentally appropriate defense mechanisms of suppression, repression, denial, rationalization, and isolation of affect from the exaggerated and overwrought use of these same defenses in the depressed child is a difficult task. In a healthy individual, defense mechanisms are integrated into the personality and function smoothly; the defense mechanisms do not stand out. In an emotionally troubled individual, one or more of the defenses are noticeable; the defense mechanisms do stand out. The therapist's task is to help the patient become aware of the overuse of or rigid adherence to a particular defense mechanism(s). The therapist should encourage the patient to become more flexible in the choice and use of defense mechanisms through concrete examples based on the patient's behavior, attitudes, thoughts, and modes of problem solving.

Sometimes in psychotherapy, the depressed school-age child may immediately connect with the therapist and see the therapist as an ally. In this case, the child becomes involved in therapy readily, talking and initiating structured and unstructured games, play, and activities. The child uses the therapeutic situation to share thoughts, ideas, occasionally feelings, and to a lesser extent fantasies. Because a relative trust is established between the child and the therapist, the child is usually receptive to the therapist's suggestions, clarifications, gentle confrontations, and occasional interpretations.

However, at other times, the depressed school-age child may be uncooperative, extremely resistant, and defiant. In this situation the introduction of nonthreatening structured games such as checkers, cards, tic-tac-toe, hangman, and others are helpful, especially in the initial phase of therapy. Also, nonthreatening motor activity games such as baseball, basketball, and football using a Nerf ball even in the small space of an office are useful. Games help the patient become motorically expressive. Playing structured, nonthreatening games gradually helps the child verbalize thoughts and feelings initially about the games and, hopefully, later about school, peers, the family, and occasionally the self. After playing structured or motoric games, some of these depressed children move toward less-structured activities such as the use of modeling clay, drawing, and painting. Frequently children go back and forth between games and activities.

As the individual therapy progresses, the child becomes more expressive in family therapy and relies on the therapist for support and confirmation. When parents are confronted with their behavior or an issue by the therapist, the child often enjoys this confrontation and agrees enthusiastically with the therapist. The therapist needs to be sensitive to the child's feelings. But, at the same time, the therapist should handle the situation so that, even though the parents "feel the heat," they are not threatened so much so that they sabotage the child's treatment or terminate the child's therapy.

The emergence of the cognitive functions of serializing and separating objects into various groups, along with emergence of the defense mechanisms of isolation of affect and rationalization, can be used by the therapist to help the child separate and isolate personal problems from those of the parents, peers, or others. At this age the child is still at the concrete stage or preoperational stage of intelligence, meaning that "seeing is believing," and therefore relies on concrete sensory-motor and personal experiences to draw a conclusion. The child has not reached the stage of abstract thinking or formal operation of intelligence and thus does not have the ability to reason based on hypotheses or propositions or the ability to understand proverbs or metaphors. Abstract thinking does not usually occur until age 12 years or older. Because of this, the therapist needs to focus more on the here and now situations rather than on what will happen in the future.

The therapist not only functions as a primary therapist for the patient but also initiates and maintains contact with the school system, social agencies, and other settings if indicated. Home and school visits with the permission of the child and the family can be quite helpful.

When the inhibited and depressed school-age child begins to show aggressive behavior at home or at school or verbalize aggressive thoughts in the therapeutic session, the child is on the road to recovery. Parents, teachers, and the child should be informed about the possibility of this development and not be alarmed by it when it occurs.

In most cases, psychiatric hospitalization of a suicidal child or adolescent is strongly indicated. Hospitalization provides a physical environment that is relatively safe to protect the child from acting out suicidal impulses. Hospitalization underlines the seriousness of suicidal behavior and allows time for a more thorough assessment of patient and family psychopathology. (See Chapters 5 and 11.) After the child is discharged from the hospital, the therapist needs to be available to the patient and the family on a 24-hour basis. Also, it would be helpful to have a therapeutic contract with the patient: the patient promises the therapist not to do anything to hurt herself or himself or anyone else until talking it over with the therapist. If the patient feels or acts suicidal, the patient or the family should call the therapist, whether day or night.

Often, the therapist sees a patient who is depressed but at the same time manifests other psychiatric disorders (depression with comorbidity) such as oppositional disorder, conduct disorder, attention-deficit hyperactivity disorder, or others. (See Chapter 1.) In these situations, the therapist wants to encourage the patient not only to express hostile and aggressive feelings appropriately but also to modify troublesome behavior such as oppositional tendencies or the symptoms of conduct disorder. Teaching the patient through role-playing to express thoughts and feelings constructively and appropriately without "turning people off" or making them angry can be helpful. Also, the therapist can use role reversal to help the patient become more observant of behavior and attitudes to make appropriate changes.

Videotaping part or all of the session, whether individual or family therapy, and then playing it back immediately or at the next session can be an eye-opener. In reviewing the videotape, the therapist, the patient, and the family should feel free to stop at any moment to make comments on what has occurred. Some school-age children really enjoy "videotherapy" and learn from it. At midterm or the termination phase of therapy, the therapist, patient, and the family can review earlier tapes and see the changes that have occurred.

Psychotherapy of the depressed school-age child is rewarding. Through empathic identification the therapist feels and experiences the patient's sadness and unhappiness. Through months and months of the ups and downs and trials and tribulations of working together, the patient becomes more expressive and begins to work through internal and interactional conflicts. When the therapist sees a smile on the patient's face, notices that the patient is having fun even temporarily, or observes that the patient is free of suicidal thoughts and morbid wishes, it is indeed worth all the trouble.

DYNAMIC PSYCHOTHERAPY OF DEPRESSION IN THE ADOLESCENT AGES 13–18 YEARS

Psychotherapy of adolescents, including depressed adolescents, is challenging and tasks the ability, wit, and emotional strength of the therapist. Due to volatile mood, hormonal and emotional turmoil, struggle between dependence and independence, concern about physical changes and appearance, and acute sensitivity to peers' opinions and acceptance, adolescents are significantly more prone to depressive disorders than preschool-age or school-age children.

The prevalence of depressive disorders in the general population of adolescents is estimated to be 4.7%—close to the 5.7% prevalence observed in adults. This figure contrasts with a prevalence of 1.9% in school-age children. (See Chapter 2.) Adolescents have more proclivity toward depression, perhaps because of rapid hormonal and psychological changes. Emotional volatility, narcissistic preoccupation, disillusionment with parents and society, loneliness, isolation, overexpectation, and overachievement or underachievement all contribute to depression in adolescents.

Depressed adolescents are at high risk for suicidal preoccupation, suicide attempts, and actual suicide. Every year in the United States, close to 1,500 children and adolescents commit suicide. This is a threefold increase compared with the number of child and adolescent suicides in the 1960s and early 1970s. (See Chapters 1 and 5.)

In the psychological autopsy of completed suicide in children and adolescents in Louisville, Kentucky, we found that 95% of the suicide victims compared to 48% of the matched comparison group had at least one diagnosable psychiatric disorder. Major depressive disorder or major depression with comorbidity such as drug and alcohol abuse and conduct disorder was present in 76% of the cases. Unfortunately, only between 20% and 45% of the victims had at least one contact in their life with a mental health professional (Shafii and Shafii 1982; Shafii et al. 1985, 1988). Adolescents' behavioral and

emotional problems are frequently underrecognized or minimized, probably because of the adolescent's reluctance to communicate internal feelings
to adults and adults' difficulty in listening to adolescents in a nonjudgmental, empathic, and nonpatronizing manner.

In psychotherapy of depressed adolescents, the therapist needs to be
aware of countertransference feelings and observe and modify reactions accordingly. Remembering one's own adolescence, which is usually subject to
severe repression, is useful and helps the therapist avoid overidentification
or unhealthy emotional distance from the depressed adolescent. Even the
experienced psychotherapist might, at times, unconsciously assume the parental role, contributing to the adolescent's further rebellion, increased resistance, and possible disruption of the therapeutic relationship.

Most adolescents, including those who are depressed, are acutely aware
of the discrepancies or inconsistencies shown by therapists and by adults in
general, which they see as a sign of hypocrisy. They then use these discrepancies and inconsistencies to justify their lack of trust in the therapist and to
avoid commitment to the therapeutic process. Adolescents also can be mer-
ciless in pointing out the therapist's mistakes. Because of this, it is important
for therapists to be direct, frank, and honest and to get to the point immediately, rather than beating around the bush or couching their statements
in psychological or literary jargon. It is advisable for the therapist to use the
language of adolescents to communicate but at the same time be careful not
to overdo this and come across as "phony." The therapist needs to be aware
of the pitfalls of trying to become "one of the guys" in an attempt to win over
the adolescent. Usually this approach will backfire and may contribute to the
adolescent's acting-out behavior.

The most effective way of communicating with the depressed adolescent is to be straightforward and direct and to keep things aboveboard. This
approach helps to confront the adolescent's behavior and attitudes. Sharp-
ness in observation and immediacy in clarification and confrontation are important in the treatment of adolescents. One cannot wait for the next session.
If the therapist observes a particular attitude or behavior that is not healthy
or is destructive, it needs to be pointed out immediately. Psychotherapy with
depressed adolescents is like working in an emergency room. The therapist
needs to be alert and calm, but at the same time quick and decisive. At no
other age is the psychotherapeutic partnership more important than it is in
adolescence.

The psychodynamic and psychotherapeutic principles that were discussed earlier in this chapter, including the psychotherapy of both the depressed preschool-age child and the depressed school-age child, also apply
to the psychotherapy of the depressed adolescent.

Specific psychotherapeutic issues related to early adolescence (ages 12–

14 years) are the emergence of pubescence and the intensification of sexual and aggressive desires, wishes, and fantasies. Frequently the therapist sees the reemergence of phallic-oedipal conflicts that were relatively dormant between the ages of 7 and 12 years. Awareness of incestuous feelings and a guilty reaction to these feelings burden the depressed adolescent further.

With the emergence of abstract thinking or formal operation of cognitive functions, the adolescent is able to create hypothetical situations rather than merely relying on concrete thinking. At this age, the emergence of abstract thought and the defense of intellectualization move the psychotherapeutic transaction from play and games to verbal exchanges and talk therapy. In early adolescence, the patient at times may regress in the psychotherapeutic situation and use earlier modes of communication such as structured play and games and nonstructured creative activities.

In early adolescence, disorganization of thought processes, forgetfulness, and being "scatterbrained" occur frequently. In depressed adolescents, this thought disorganization and forgetfulness are intensified. At times, they are so severe that the patient appears to be "organic," although there is no evidence of gross organicity. Because of this developmental disorganization and depression, school performance may decline significantly in depressed adolescents. The therapist needs to be aware of these developmental changes and must separate normal developmental disorganization from cognitive dysfunction due to depression. The therapist should also help the patient, parents, and school authorities become aware of these developmental issues.

The defense mechanisms of projection, denial, isolation, and introjection are intensified in depressed adolescents. At one moment the adolescent blames parents, teachers, the therapist, and others for problems, and at the next moment, exaggerated self-doubt, self-criticism, and self-blame prevail.

In middle adolescence (ages 14–16 years) and late adolescence (ages 16–18 years), sexual and personal identity is established and consolidated. The depressed adolescent, on the other hand, begins to doubt identity and competency. Relationships with peers of the opposite sex become problematic. Depressed adolescents may avoid interacting with the opposite sex or may plunge into promiscuous sexual activities as a way of dealing with feelings of loneliness, isolation, and low self-esteem.

Antisocial and acting-out behaviors become prominent. Because of the tendency toward "acting out, "being "secretive," and "not leveling" with grown-ups (including the therapist), the therapist needs to be alert and look for various verbal and nonverbal cues in order to explore the adolescent's inner and interactional struggles. As soon as there is evidence or suspicion of a troublesome behavior or attitude, the therapist should explore it and gently but firmly confront the patient. The therapist's passivity, quiescence, or lack of active involvement is perceived by the adolescent as a sign of not caring, stupidity, collusion, or naïveté. Failure to immediately deal with relevant issues may contribute to the adolescent's further acting-out or self-destructive behavior.

Suicidal thoughts, attempts, and actual suicide are a major danger in depressed adolescents. In a review of 60 cases of children and adolescents ages 10–19 years who committed suicide in Jefferson County, Kentucky, we found that nearly half of all these suicides occurred at ages 17 (22%) and 18 (27%) years (Shafii and Shafii 1982). Late adolescence is the highest risk period for suicide in children and adolescents.

A recent survey of 5,500 freshman and senior high school students in Kentucky using the 70-item Youth Risk Survey developed by the Centers for Disease Control, Atlanta, Georgia, reveals alarming data concerning the physical and mental health of our youth (Table 7–1).

From the data shown in Table 7–1, it is clear that adolescents are at a high risk for suicidal behavior, alcohol and drug abuse, and sexual and aggressive behavior. Depressed adolescents frequently use alcohol and drugs for self-medication, as a way of dealing with their feelings of loneliness and isolation, and for gaining acceptance by peers. Therapists' awareness of and sensitivity toward these issues in treating depressed adolescents are important.

In late adolescence social consciousness, idealistic longings, and concern about the future emerge. In some depressed adolescents these issues become intensified and exaggerated. Some depressed adolescents become much more preoccupied and worried about the future, religious beliefs, and political, ecological, and racial issues. Guilt about one's own economic, social, and family status adds to the identity crisis of the depressed adolescent. The therapist's empathic identification with the patient helps the adolescent share these thoughts, feelings, and ideals—resulting in both a broader and deeper understanding of the issues.

The adolescent is hypersensitive concerning issues related to the self because of the reemergence of primary and secondary narcissistic tendencies. The therapist's clarifications and interpretations should be couched in such a way that the adolescent is not threatened by them and perceives them as his or her own (Kohut 1971, 1977). Supporting and underlining the attempts of the adolescent toward introspection, self-examination, and self-discovery help to enhance the therapeutic alliance. Confrontation is a double-edged sword. On the one hand, an adolescent who shows self-destructive or dangerous behavior needs to be confronted directly and immediately, but, on the other hand, the therapist needs to help the adolescent enhance self- observation and expand the observing ego. The aim of psychotherapy with the depressed adolescent is to help the adolescent become his or her own psychotherapist. This goal is accomplished by helping the adolescent become aware

Table 7–1. Survey of 5,500 freshman and senior high school students in Kentucky using the 70-item Youth Risk Survey

Behavior	Percent positive responses
1. Seriously thought about attempting suicide in the past 12 months	30
2. Specific plan for committing suicide	19
3. Suicide attempt	11
4. Have drunk alcohol	83
5. Drank alcohol during the last month	51
6. Had sexual intercourse	55
7. Sexual intercourse with more than one partner	32
8. Intercourse before age 14 years	17
9. Ninth-graders having had intercourse	41
10. Twelfth-graders having had intercourse	71
11. Pregnant or making someone pregnant (of those who had had intercourse)	8
12. Sexually transmitted disease (of those who had had intercourse)	4
13. Have tried cigarettes	75
14. Cigarette smoking during the past month	36
15. Carrying weapon (gun, knife, club)	21
16. Watching TV or playing video games on school days—3 or more hours	37
17. Never used marijuana	66
18. Never used illegal drugs	85
19. Never used cocaine	90

Source. Modified from Jennings 1990, pp. 1, 10.

of and work through the following tendencies: denying or minimizing troublesome or pathological behavior, deluding the self, avoiding examination of the consequences of one's behavior, projecting one's problems to others, and introjecting unnecessary and unrealistic self-blame.

DURATION OF PSYCHOTHERAPY

The length of psychotherapy for depressed children and adolescents depends on the severity and chronicity of the patient's depression, parental psychopathology, motivation for change, and the commitment and response to therapeutic intervention. After a few sessions, a number of mild to moderately depressed patients may feel better temporarily. This temporary improvement may lead the patient and the parents to want to stop the treatment. This phenomenon is referred to as "flight to health" and needs to be discussed with the patient and the family in advance and reexamined as it occurs. On the other hand, the patient and/or the family might feel worse after a few sessions, and this too should be discussed in advance and be reexamined as it occurs throughout therapy.

On the average, for short-term, goal-oriented dynamic psychotherapy, the frequency of the therapeutic sessions is one to three times weekly for 15–20 weeks with regular monthly or bimonthly follow-up. For more exploratory psychotherapy, intermediate or relatively long-term psychotherapy is in order with the same frequency of therapeutic sessions. Because most depressive disorders in children and adolescents are chronic disorders with a cycle of exacerbations, 1–2 years of outpatient psychotherapy are recommended. Parents are initially seen for a few months on a weekly basis with and without the child. If there is no evidence of moderate to severe psychopathology or marital disharmony in the parents, then the parents are seen as needed on a monthly or less-frequent basis. In the case of parental psychopathology or marital disharmony, the parents need to be assessed carefully and appropriate treatment recommended.

Although in the past, parents were seen by a different therapist than the child or adolescent's therapist, in recent years many therapists see both the child and the parents. Actually, we have found that this is a very effective way of being aware of the family milieu and that it helps in dealing with internal and intrafamilial conflicts.

With the limitations of third-party payments and managed care, the duration of psychotherapy with children, adolescents, and their families has been shortened. Unfortunately, however, there are no shortcuts. When depressed children and adolescents do not receive timely and appropriate care, their symptoms intensify. Eventually a number of them might undertake more drastic measures, such as suicidal ideation, threats, or attempts; drug and alcohol abuse; antisocial behavior; promiscuity; or homicidal behavior. Then inpatient hospitalization is required at a much higher cost.

Outpatient psychotherapy of depressed children and adolescents and long-term follow-up not only have a therapeutic indication, but are also needed for preventive purposes. We see long-term outpatient psychotherapy and follow-up as similar to the patient's treatment and follow-up by the pediatrician, family physician, or dentist. After termination of regular outpatient psychotherapy on a weekly basis, we like to see our patients and their families on an outpatient basis monthly or bimonthly for 2–3 years. After that, we encourage them to get in touch with us every 6 months to 1 year until they reach adulthood. A continuous relationship helps the patient and the family remain sensitive to the cyclic episodes of depression and encourages them to seek treatment immediately during a crisis or in anticipation of a crisis.

The essence of psychotherapy with depressed children and adolescents is providing consistent and caring human contact. No matter what type of therapy one uses or what type of orientation one has, providing caring human contact (such as spending time with and really listening to the troubled patient) has a profound healing effect beyond our present understanding and knowledge.

REFERENCES

Axline V: The eight basic principles, in Child Psychotherapy. Edited by Haworth M. New York, Basic Books, 1964, pp 93–94

Bibring E: Psychoanalysis and dynamic psychotherapies. J Am Psychoanal Assoc 2:745–770, 1954

Chethik M: Techniques of Child Therapy: Psychodynamic Strategies. New York, Guilford, 1989

Dolen D: Psychotherapy in childhood and adolescence, in Pathways of Human Development. Edited by Shafii M, Shafii SL. New York, Thieme-Stratton, 1982, pp 255–269

Ekstein R: Observations of the psychology of borderline and psychotic children, in Children of Time and Space, of Action and Impulse. New York, Meredith, 1966, pp 91–113

Erikson E (1950): Childhood and Society, 2nd Edition. New York, Norton, 1963

Fraiberg S, Shapiro V, Cherniss DS: Treatment modalities, in Clinical Studies in Infant Mental Health: The First Year of Life. Edited by Fraiberg S. New York, Basic Books, 1980, pp 53–61

Frank J: Persuasion and Healing. New York, Schocken, 1963

Freud A: The Ego and the Mechanisms of Defense. New York, International Universities Press, 1936

Freud S: Three essays on the theory of sexuality (1905), in The Standard Edition of the Complete Psychological Works of Sigmund Freud, Vol 7. Translated and edited by Strachey J. London, Hogarth Press, 1968, pp 135–243

Freud S: Analysis of a phobia in a five-year-old boy (1909), in The Standard Edition of the Complete Psychological Works of Sigmund Freud, Vol 10. Translated and edited by Strachey J. London, Hogarth Press, 1968, pp 1–149

Freud S: The dynamics of transference (1912), in The Standard Edition of the Complete Psychological Works of Sigmund Freud, Vol 12. Translated and edited by Strachey J. London, Hogarth Press, 1968, pp 99–108

Freud S: Beyond the pleasure principle (1920), in The Standard Edition of the Complete Psychological Works of Sigmund Freud, Vol 18. Translated and edited by Strachey J. London, Hogarth Press, 1968, pp 1–64

Gabbard GO: Psychodynamic Psychiatry in Clinical Practice. Washington, DC, American Psychiatric Press, 1990

Greenson RR: The Technique and Practice of Psychoanalysis, Vol 1. New York, International Universities Press, 1967

Jennings M: Students' replies on sex, suicide, alcohol alarm education chief. Courier-Journal (Louisville, KY), Nov 13, 1990, pp 1, 10

Kohut H: The Analysis of Self: A Systematic Approach to the Psychoanalytic Treatment of Narcissistic Personality Disorders. New York, International Universities Press, 1971

Kohut H: The Restoration of the Self. New York, International Universities Press, 1977

Meissner WW, Mack JE, Semrad EV: Theories of personality and psychopathology, I: classical psychoanalysis, in Comprehensive Textbook of Psychiatry, 2nd Edition, Vol 1. Edited by Freedman AM, Kaplan HI, Sadock BJ. Baltimore, MD, Williams & Wilkins, 1975, pp 482–566

Moore BE, Fine BD (eds): A Glossary of Psychoanalytic Terms and Concepts, 2nd Edition. New York, American Psychoanalytic Association, 1968

Shafii M: A precedent for modern psychotherapeutic techniques: one thousand years ago. Am J Psychiatry 128:1581–1584, 1972

Shafii M: Freedom From the Self: Sufism, Meditation and Psychotherapy. New York, Human Sciences Press, 1985

Shafii M, Shafii SL: Self-destructive, suicidal behavior, and completed suicide, in Pathways of Human Development: Normal Growth and Emotional Disorders in Infancy, Childhood and Adolescence. Edited by Shafii M, Shafii SL. New York, Thieme-Stratton, 1982, pp 164–180

Shafii M, Carrigan SP, Whittinghill JR, et al: Psychological autopsy of completed suicide in children and adolescents. Am J Psychiatry 142:1061–1064, 1985

Shafii M, Steltz-Lenarsky J, Derrick AM, et al: Comorbidity of mental disorders in the postmortem diagnosis of completed suicide in children and adolescents. J Affective Disord 15:227–233, 1988

CHAPTER 8

Group Therapy of Depression

Robert F. Baxter, M.D.
James F. Kennedy, Ph.D.

Although earlier clinicians such as Moreno, Adler, and Aichhorn pioneered therapeutic work with emotionally troubled adolescents in group settings, Slavson is generally credited with originating group psychotherapy for children in 1934 (Rachman and Raubolt 1984). His approach, known as activity group therapy, was designed to provide youngsters with socialization experiences not available in individual therapy (Slavson 1943). Since that time, numerous alternative forms of group therapy have emerged for children and adolescents.

Such alternatives have developed at least partially in response to patients' differing ages and stages of cognitive development. Clinicians' varying theoretical orientations also have stimulated the introduction of a variety of group approaches to treatment. Likewise, the structure of therapeutic groups for children and adolescents has been influenced by the nature of the clinical setting, whether an acute inpatient unit, a residential treatment facility, an outpatient clinic, or a private practice office.

Despite this evolution of therapeutic approaches to groups and an ever-expanding body of literature on group psychotherapy for children and adolescents, group therapy is often underutilized, particularly in outpatient settings. However, if the current trend of declining health insurance benefits (particularly coverage for mental health care) continues, utilization of group therapy is likely to increase because it provides care at less cost per patient than individual psychotherapy (Kraft 1979). Depressed youngsters, consequently, may be treated increasingly in groups, either as their primary therapeutic experience or as an adjunct to individual therapy and/or psychopharmacotherapy.

RATIONALE FOR GROUP THERAPY

Although depressed children and adolescents may present with a variety of symptoms, they most often share common problems in the social sphere; their depression tends to alter their interactions with peers and significant adults alike. The hypersensitive, dysphoric child, for example, may be viewed by classmates as a "cry baby" since he or she tends to overreact to their typical teasing and bantering. He or she thus may establish himself or herself in social relationships that ultimately lead to taunting provocation and rejection by age-mates. This, in turn, may serve to diminish self-esteem and increase the child's sense of despair and hopelessness, thereby reinforcing the depressive feelings.

Similarly, the more agitated, perhaps aggressive, but nonetheless depressed young adolescent may come to be labeled a "bully" by peers and, minimally, a disrespectful, disruptive menace by teachers. Criticism and rejection by one or both groups may follow, further enhancing a sense of loneliness and supporting the adolescent's self-perception of inadequacy.

Thus, some depressive symptomatology may be maintained through the youngster's inadequate socialization skills and consequent relationships (or lack thereof) with parents, siblings, and peers and with adults outside the family. Psychopharmacological treatment with antidepressant medication cannot directly address this interactional aspect of depressive psychopathology, and various forms of individual psychotherapy may do so only partially. However, group psychotherapy offers an opportunity for depressed children and adolescents to more fully explore the social dimensions of their illness and to develop more functional, gratifying coping styles and modes of interaction. (See Chapters 7, 9, and 10.)

Case Example

Ten-year-old D. was evaluated following several weeks of angry, destructive behavior, refusal to obey or follow his mother's rules, and a long history of oppositional behavior. The mental status examination revealed an angry, sullen lad with little spontaneity who stared at the floor. His only comment was that his mother did not love him or want him and he was thinking about suicide. He was admitted to the inpatient service where he did relate to his peers but remained aloof from adults. Several antidepressant medications were prescribed at various times while he was in the hospital. The best results were obtained with imipramine, which was continued while he was an outpatient. D. was also referred for outpatient group psychotherapy. During the first several group sessions, D. had slow, lethargic movements. He sat at the table, looked sad and unhappy, and said nothing. This was a well-behaved group of 10- and 11-year-old males, several of whom were thoughtful and sensitive to each other. One in particular was very friendly to newcomers, asking about their problems and inviting them to participate in games such as basketball. The therapists used the introductions for D. to share the reasons for his hospitalization and to hear about the problems of the other patients. The supportive patient empathized with D.'s family problems and made it a point to select him on his team for kickball.

D.'s fourth and fifth sessions (which occurred just prior to Christmas) demonstrate the value of group psychotherapy for depressed children. While group members were excitedly anticipating the holiday and gift giving, D. remained depressed and unhappy. Therapists involved the group in trying to understand and support D., who explained that he did not want to stay with his mother during vacation because of her criticism, neglect, and rejection. During the fifth session, one patient brought a gift-wrapped can of mixed nuts for the therapists, who opened it and shared them with the group. All the patients eagerly ate the nuts except D., who declined, saying he did not like nuts but preferred grapes. He did not join in group games, but sat sadly at the table. He was later observed to eat some nuts, suggesting an effort to seek nurture in the group. While the others talked excitedly about Christmas and vacation, D. shook his head dejectedly and said he was not excited. The sensitive patient quickly recalled D.'s previous complaints about his angry, punitive mother and led the others in offering suggestions to D., one being to discharge his anger by hitting the punching bag. D. began to hit the bag and, with group support, his movements became more spirited and he cheered up a bit.

During the weeks following the vacation, D. received group support about his anger at his mother and encouragement to actively play group games. His sad, quiet times at the table gradually decreased, and his active physical involvement increased. When another new patient entered the group, D. asked if he had been on the inpatient unit. Then, he shared his own wish to stay there rather than go home to his angry mother.

D.'s mother began to cancel appointments, complaining about insurance problems. D. returned to the group after a 3-week absence, asked about several absent patients, and expressed his sadness that one patient had to leave the group because his family moved to another state. D. wrestled and was physically active with peers. Toward the end of that session, he asked if he could print his name on the wall near the names of the other group members, reflecting his identification with and feelings of acceptance in the group. As his depression lifted, more anger and oppositional behavior began to surface, particularly toward a patient who set himself up to be scapegoated.

Unfortunately, D. was abruptly withdrawn from group therapy by his mother because their health maintenance organization (HMO) decided not to further underwrite his case. The HMO said that it would not authorize further treatment because his depression had improved and the insurance did not cover oppositional disorder. This was an unfortunate, shortsighted, antitherapeutic decision because D. felt that he was part of the peer group and needed their continuing support to displace and sublimate his anger and to develop effective coping mechanisms to prevent further recurrences of depression.

A Sense of Universality

In part, group therapy may be an effective therapeutic intervention because it offers patients reassurance that others share similar feelings and, often-times, experiences. This sense of what Yalom (1975) referred to as "universality" can prove to be particularly supportive to depressed youngsters since they tend to view themselves as alienated and alone at the very time when age-mates all appear to be comfortably situated with their peer group. Furthermore, this perception of group supportiveness may make the child or adolescent feel safer in exploring his or her problems than he or she would have felt in the singular therapist-patient, adult-child relationship.

Case Example

R. was a 9-year-old female evaluated because of a sudden drop in school grades from As to Cs, with distractibility, daydreaming, and re-fusal to do schoolwork. Mental status examination revealed an articu-late, knowledgeable, pseudomature female with an IQ of 130. How-ever, she expressed that she felt unloved by her mother, who was too busy to understand or listen, and rejected by her stepfather, who fa-vored his two younger daughters. R.'s underlying depression was de-fended against by suppression of feelings as well as by verbosity.

R. was added to an ongoing group of 9- and 10-year-old females. She arrived late for her first session. She responded to the attention of the group by extending her introduction of herself and her problems to de-scribing how she felt unloved by her family, that everyone was too busy for her, and that she might as well be dead. The group became anxious but responsive and supportive. One patient supportively sub-grouped with her. The therapists responded on the group level, which allowed the members to say that they had experienced similar feelings.

In the next two sessions, R. ventilated anger at her stepfather and ambivalence about her mother's lack of emotional support. She also mentioned missing her natural father. R.'s expression of anger allowed other patients to acknowledge their own anger, aiding identification and cohesion in the group.

R. arrived late for her fourth group session. She was angry at her teacher for not allowing her to leave early for the session. The patients were talking about anger at mothers, and R. went to the punching bag and began hitting it, slamming it and scowling as her anger escalated. She withdrew to a closet and took the punching bag with her. She hit it and fell to the floor sobbing. The other group members offered support and comfort. Since the session was ending, a cotherapist remained with R. as she sobbed about her mother's aloofness, feeling exploited about housework, being prohibited from expressing her anger and com-plaints, and sharing her wish that her natural father and mother were still together.

This emotional outburst created anxiety for the group, but also pro-vided reassurance that the group therapists would respond appropriately and protectively and that the expression of such emotion was acceptable within the group. In subsequent sessions, R. felt the acceptance and safety of the group and was able to vent anger and share fantasies about her mother leaving the stepfather. The group offered support and advice on a cognitive level, as well as encouragement to discharge affect through games, play, and activity. R. and the group suggested that the therapists work with R.'s mother and gave them permission to do so. R.'s mother was also depressed and unhappy with her marital and family circumstances and agreeable to her own psychotherapy.

Expression of Feelings and Thoughts

At times, feelings and cognitions may be more fully expressed in group psychotherapy settings than in individual therapy. Depressed adolescents in particular are often more reticent and less than articulate in describing their internal experiences. The multiple relationships and interactions available in a group can foster such expression. In a therapeutic group, youngsters have the option of referencing others' statements, making comparisons, indicating differences, and responding to multiple questions. All of these assist in drawing a fuller picture of their emotional status and psychological dilemmas. In addition, the language of the group, consistent with that of the contemporary peer culture, helps in making self-expression easier than it would be in a dyadic relationship with an adult therapist.

Over time, the therapeutic group, regardless of its theoretical orientation, offers its members opportunities to reevaluate their self-perceptions (which are often considerably distorted) in the light of others' perceptions about them. Depressed youngsters frequently view themselves as inept, unworthy, and unlovable. This self-image is increasingly difficult to maintain in a setting where there is repeated feedback, either behavioral or verbal, to the contrary. This is especially true when such feedback comes from other group members, rather than the therapist.

Increased Awareness

Not only does group psychotherapy offer opportunities for depressed children and adolescents to modify their self-perceptions, it also provides a structured, protective situation in which they can develop an increased awareness of their own behavior and its impact on others. With the support of the therapist and other group members, these youngsters can then experiment with, and practice, new behaviors that might lead to better peer relationships and an improved self-image.

Case Example

The group consisted of teenagers who presented with problems of aggressive acting out, depression, and drug abuse. Most of them were

bright, attractive, and socially skilled. B., a 16-year-old male with severe congenital defects consisting of exstrophy of the bladder, incomplete external genitalia, clubfoot, and spina bifida, was added to the
group. Due to optic atrophy, he lived at the school for the blind and
began acting out by stealing and carrying pictures of nude females. He
was accepted into the group and took a quiet role, but vicariously identified with the behavior discussed by members of the group. Later, he
began to express his intense anger emanating from the unfairness of his
handicaps.

D., one of the group members, was a large, muscular, articulate boy
with an impulse control problem. He openly discussed his difficulty in
controlling his anger. D., despite a tough, macho exterior, could be
quite sensitive and perceptive to the needs of others. However, when
he became angry, some members felt anxious and threatened by his
temper, but he did comply with the group rule of no physical acting
out. Also, at other times, D. would become withdrawn or pouty. B. and
D. began to good-naturedly joke with each other and developed a
friendship in the group.

During a session in the spring of the year, a depressing theme
emerged about the futility of life, the prospects of nuclear war, and
teenage peers being killed in auto accidents. B. suddenly interrupted
and said that the school for the blind was having a sports banquet and
that he could invite two outside people as guests. They could be friends
or family, but he had no known relatives as he had lived in foster
homes since early childhood. He then turned to D., who represented
everything B. was not and could not be, and asked him if he would
attend the sports banquet. D. was quiet, and it was apparent that he
was struggling for a reply that would not hurt or reject B. Finally, D.
said he would like to attend but he would have to first talk with his
mother, who controlled his time and schedule.

B.'s physical appearance was in marked contrast to the other physically healthy group members. Despite his handicaps, B's optimism and
enthusiasm had a decided positive effect on the depression, gloom, and
negativism of the other teenagers in the group. Acceptance of B. into
the group not only increased B.'s self-esteem, but helped the physically
healthy teenagers to temper their own self-doubts by contrasting the
physical assets they took for granted with the obstacles B. had to cope
with.

Increased awareness, changes in self-perception, better peer relationships, and other socially acceptable behaviors can develop from observing
others. Group members, as well as the group therapist, may serve as role
models. It is not unusual for a depressed child or adolescent to observe another youngster in the group handling a problem that he or she has experienced and then to imitate that youngster's approach. This may occur either
spontaneously or, in some behaviorally oriented therapy groups, during
specifically planned role-playing exercises.

INDICATIONS AND CONTRAINDICATIONS FOR GROUP THERAPY

Group psychotherapy offers potential benefits to most depressed children and adolescents. However, except in hospital settings, group therapy is infrequently included in the initial treatment plan. Referrals to a therapeutic group are most often made as youngsters demonstrate progress in individual treatment. It should be noted, however, that decreases in insurance coverage are likely to stimulate more emphasis on group treatment as an economical primary therapeutic modality for depressed children and adolescents.

At the present time, many clinicians view group psychotherapy as a significant adjunctive intervention rather than as a primary treatment strategy. Perhaps this reflects their recognition that the depressed youngster's self-deprecatory hypersensitivity to others, anhedonia, and diminished socialization combine to make him or her a resistant candidate for group therapy during the early phase of treatment. These therapists tend to add group psychotherapy to the treatment regimen as the patient's depressive symptomatology begins to wane and he or she becomes more accessible to group influences.

Case Example

B. was initially evaluated at age 8 years because of preoccupation with his uncle's suicide, his denial of the suicide, and his hallucinatory reports that he had seen his uncle. Also, he worried about his parents' health and safety. B. had a long history of fighting with peers who teased him about being overweight. B. had evidenced poor self-esteem. He was diagnosed as having major depression and was seen for a year of individual outpatient psychotherapy with reduction of worries about his parents, death, and thoughts of his uncle. Because B.'s low self-esteem, doubts, and conflicts with schoolmates persisted, he was referred for group psychotherapy and joined a group of 9- and 10-year-old males. He seemed comfortable in the group, shared his problems, and entered into group activities.

He gradually began to show irritation with a patient who sought attention by loud yelling, sexual comments, teasing, and curiosity. B. subgrouped with two other patients against the loud patient and voiced his anger toward him. The therapists intervened individually and on the group level by discussing the need to be accepted and liked and the difficulty some children have in finding acceptable ways to gain attention. B. struggled to control his own anger and was active in planning with his subgroup how to talk with this patient about his unacceptable behavior. B. continued to complain about being teased by his schoolmates, which periodically precipitated suicidal thoughts and depressive feelings.

The group was encouraged by the therapists to suggest ways to help B. deal with the teasing. B. also acted out peer conflicts in the group, enabling group members and therapists to observe firsthand B.'s over-sensitivity to criticism, followed by anger and fighting. He participated in wrestling and football in activity group therapy. B.'s poor self-esteem and sensitivity became evident in his overreaction to rule viola-tions, complaints, and arguing. Therapists interpreted the meaning of these behaviors when they were acted out, as well as supported B. by pointing out similar problems in other group members.

Pfeifer and Spinner (1985) and Bromfield and Pfeifer (1988) have dis-cussed both the benefits and the potential risks of combining individual and group psychotherapy in children, especially with the same therapist. Others may introduce group therapy during the termination phase of a child or adolescent's individual treatment. In this situation, the group generally is viewed as a setting in which the youngster can solidify any further therapeu-tic gains and strengthen social skills in order to maintain improvement.

In the hospital setting, unlike the situation in the outpatient clinic or the private practice office, group psychotherapy is commonly utilized as part of the initial treatment strategy for depressed children and adolescents. In this situation, emphasis is usually placed on the "here-and-now" events of patients' lives on the inpatient unit and on problem-solving activities rele-vant to their current environment.

Indications for group psychotherapy of depression in children and ado-lescents far outweigh contraindications, of which there are a few. The occa-sional youngster who manifests extreme impulsivity and aggression as part of the total symptom complex, thereby potentially endangering other group members, should be excluded. Likewise, an occasional youngster may prove to be overly stimulated, disruptive, and unmanageable in a group setting, particularly if it is a relatively unstructured group. This patient might better be excluded from the group.

Traditionally, another reason for excluding a depressed child or adoles-cent from participation in a particular therapy group had to do with the so-called balance of the group—the mix of passive, assertive, provocative youngsters, etc. Too many depressed patients, for example, were thought to slow the pace of the group, tipping the balance toward passivity and a help-less, overly dependent group culture (Berkowitz 1972). However, recent re-ports on psychotherapy groups designed specifically for depressed children and adolescents (Fine et al. 1989; Schachter 1984) suggest that this conven-tional wisdom may not hold in appropriately structured groups, particularly in the case of behavioral group therapy.

GROUP THERAPY STRUCTURES

Group psychotherapy structure must take into account the members' psy-chosocial and cognitive development, as well as their phase-specific orientation to group interaction. Certainly therapeutic groups that consist of children and adolescents of mixed ages have been reported. But in such situations, the patient tends to identify primarily with other group members of a similar age, feels threatened by older members, and in turn looks down on and threatens younger participants (Kennedy 1982). Thus, most group therapists have found greater success, both in terms of management and of therapeutic efficacy, with groups of youngsters of similar age.

Elementary-School-Age Group

Regardless of the theoretical orientation of the group therapist, many therapy groups for elementary-school-age children utilize activity and play extensively. This was true of the psychoanalytically oriented activity group therapy introduced by Slavson (1943) and it remains true today, despite the development of numerous modifications, including behavioral group therapy. However, depending on the orientation of the therapist, the actual use of play activities may vary considerably from one therapy group to the next.

A modification of activity group therapy is activity-interview group therapy, described by Schiffer (1977). Activity-interview group therapy combines the child's need for activity as a means to discharge anxiety, relate to peers, and symbolically play out conflicts with problem-focused discussion periods within the session. Whereas group-level verbal interventions by the therapist will build cohesion and encourage the group process, individual interventions with group members are also appropriate for specific issues. Sugar (1974) discussed the use of interpretations in groups for children.

Psychodynamically oriented group therapy. In groups that are psychodynamically oriented, structure and limits tend to be kept to a minimum and the therapist's posture is relatively nondirective. Meeting in an appropriately equipped playroom, youngsters are encouraged to play out their fantasies and conflicts, giving expression to their underlying emotions. However, careful, thoughtful planning of the physical environment of the children's group therapy room is a very sensitive variable that has a decided effect on the behavior of the children and the development of group structure and intergroup controls. Schamess (1986) has dealt with the dynamic interplay between such environmental factors as size and design of the room, play materials and furnishings, the activity of the therapist, the phase-specific developmental needs of each child, the diagnosis, and the level of character pathology. Schamess captures the complexity of child group psychotherapy by considering levels of personality development, psychopathology, and group dynamic principles.

In such a group, the depressed child is likely to remain aloof, initially appearing sullen and withdrawn and relying on helplessness, which invites taunting from peers and elicits protective responses from the therapist.

These behaviors, if they continue, reinforce the child's self-image of inadequacy. However, the therapist's relative neutrality (accepting but not rescuing the patient) and gentle encouragement for other group members to attend to their own activities usually prove frustrating to the child, ultimately encouraging experimentation with other behaviors that may prove more acceptable and rewarding.

In groups of older elementary-school-age children, the therapist might well enhance the group experience with interpretations of the children's actions and statements, but with younger children, such interpretative interventions are rarely used. Rather, the focus remains on play and its pivotal role in children's development (Kraft 1979).

An example follows of a preschool-age group in which discussion of shared feelings and concerns about family and developmental issues was integrated with play.

Case Example

A. was 5 years old when he was referred for an evaluation because of the fear of leaving his mother when he had to have an examination at the health clinic. While separation anxiety and fear of strangers were the presenting symptoms, A. also manifested depressive symptoms of dysphoric mood, slow movements, lack of interest, and low energy. A. was assigned to a group of 5- and 6-year-old males and females.

A. sat quietly at the table while the other children talked about their fears, worry, anger, and rivalries. A.'s sad look and slow movements indicated depression, and he talked only when spoken to and then scarcely above a whisper. The group of six was a mixture of active, aggressive children and fearful, depressed children. A. repeated the comments of the others about feeling sad and worrying about his "mama." He did not attempt to reach out or subgroup with peers. The group therapists encouraged other children to help A. to participate in games and activities. But A. would sit quietly, staring blankly, and only gradually explored some of the toys. He would passively allow more aggressive children to grab toys out of his hands and take things from him. The group therapists also intervened on a group level to protect and support A. with comments dealing with the group rules, fairness, sharing, and rivalry.

A. gradually began to play but would withdraw if confronted by another child. He began to subgroup with less-aggressive children to wash and clean the windows, to serve make-believe food, and to build with blocks. With support, he gradually began to test himself with more aggressive children and became more assertive, defending himself in conflictual disputes. As this behavior became more frequent, his mood brightened, his active participation increased, and a spark of enthusiasm and spontaneity in play began to emerge.

Behavioral group therapy.   In contrast to psychodynamically oriented groups for elementary-school-age children, behavioral group therapy is conceptualized in terms of basic learning theory; the goal is behavior change rather than personality change. In this model, the therapist is active and directive in facilitating appropriate social behavior and utilizing multiple behavioral techniques such as reinforcement, modeling, behavioral contracting, and rehearsal (Rose 1972).

In a behavioral therapy group, the therapist might specifically structure the session, or part of the session, to increase socialization and cooperative play if one or more of the group members are depressed and withdrawn. A game or activity might be introduced, for example, that requires the children to work in teams. Successful completion of the game or activity might then be rewarded with tokens to support and reinforce cooperative interaction.

Because behavioral group therapy focuses specifically on inappropriate, maladaptive behaviors, youngsters who share similar problematic behaviors are often grouped together. Thus, a depressed child might find himself or herself in a group with others who appear timid, reluctant, and withdrawn. Their diagnoses might differ, but group activities are structured to benefit them all. Clearly, this orientation to symptomatic homogeneity differs from many other groups, where efforts are made to achieve a balanced distribution of symptoms and personality styles.

Regardless of orientation, however, it is preferable for elementary-school-age groups to consist of members of the same gender, reflecting their age-appropriate tendency to form isosexual play groups. However, since far fewer females in this age range are referred for treatment, it is often difficult to form female groups. In this case, females and males can be treated in the same group, but it is best to have equal numbers of each, since they tend to quickly form subgroups differentiated by gender.

The Pubescent and Early-Adolescent Group

Therapy groups for pubertal children and even young adolescents continue to be organized by gender, if possible, again following the "natural" preference of youngsters in this age range. It also is recommended that the therapist be of the same gender as the patients, thereby providing a role model for identification.

These groups, like those for younger children, continue for the most part to be activity oriented, since the group members still experience difficulty in conceptualizing. Early-adolescent groups may involve some amount of discussion, depending on the patients' cognitive skills, but the intense sexual curiosity and anxiety these youngsters experience can quickly lead to disruption of any protracted discussion.

Therapy groups involving pubertal children and young adolescents are usually conceptualized as peer groups rather than as substitute families, a common conceptualization of groups designed for younger children (Kraft 1979; Slavson 1943). The therapeutic focus is likely to be the socialization process itself; issues of identification, sexual curiosity, and competitive striving become important in the group culture.

In such groups, whether behaviorally or psychodynamically oriented, the therapist generally takes an active and sometimes directive role, maintaining a firm position around the structural boundaries of the group (e.g., time boundaries, space limitations) and rules of engagement (e.g., no fighting). Such a posture prevents the youngsters' intense anxiety and competitive provocativeness from overwhelming them and disrupting the group experience.

Initially, depressed group members are likely to find pubertal and early-adolescent therapy groups very stressful, just as they do peer groups at school or in the community.

Case Example

R. was a member of a 12- and 13-year-old males' group. He was short for his age, wore glasses, and became depressed because of his diabetes. Onset of juvenile diabetes occurred at age 5 years, and R. was hospitalized several times in acute distress because of noncompliance with medical management and refusal to take insulin. R. was a friendly, verbal person who gained peer attention through clowning and joking. At other times he would seriously share his fear of becoming blind and dying at a young age as his father had because of his diabetes. He was a popular member of the group and was missed when he was absent due to being hospitalized for depression and suicidal ideation. He returned to the outpatient group sessions while still in the hospital. Several of the group members expressed their concern for R. and their disappointment that he did not call them for help when thinking of suicide. They gave R. their telephone numbers and asked him to promise to call them when he was depressed in the future.

Youngsters in this age group tend to provoke, taunt, and scapegoat peers whom they perceive to be weak or otherwise vulnerable. Depressed children all but advertise their availability for the role of "target." Insecure in their own identity and convinced of their own inadequacy, they may have trouble joining the competitive norms of the group, either retreating totally or being unduly belligerent and hostile.

Case Example

J. was evaluated at age 8 years because of suicidal thoughts, self-critical comments, and complaining for several months that school peers did not like him. J. had had difficulty adapting to his parents' divorce a year ago in another city. Following the separation, J. and his mother moved to this city and his father stayed in another city 400 miles away. After evaluation, J. was admitted to the inpatient children's psychiatric unit.

Diagnostically, J. presented a mixed picture of depression, anxiety, and borderline traits. Following discharge, he was seen in outpatient individual psychotherapy and, after a year, was also included in a psychotherapy group because of the persistence of poor peer relationships.

J.'s hunger for peer acceptance was evident immediately from his monopolizing, attention-seeking behavior and bragging. He functioned best in structured, physically active games such as kickball and basketball, where his energy was focused and contained. He could talk about his problems with the group, describing how his hurt that others disliked him led to depressed and hopeless feelings. Unfortunately, his anxiety was manifested in provocative behavior toward others, resulting in anger and dislike by them. The therapists intervened individually and on a group level to prevent J. from putting himself in a scapegoat role. Interpretations regarding his self-defeating behavior were made to protect J. and to defuse the anger toward him. Both J. and the other group members discussed ways for J. to control his behavior and not overreact to criticism. J.'s behavior vacillated from conscious efforts to suppress anger and control provocative behavior to loss of control precipitated by a combination of events in his family and school life, as well as in the group.

The value of peer group psychotherapy for a youngster with poor self-esteem, depressive features, and the capacity to seek insight and self-understanding was evident in a recent session. J. had been scapegoated by another angry patient, leading to threats of physical attack. The therapists had the patients discuss the issues and conflict. During the discussion, J. described the dynamic of projective identification that occurs in scapegoating in groups. J. turned to the hostile antagonist and said that the qualities he did not like in J. were qualities he did not like in himself. J.'s ability to be aware of this identification aided him in feeling less self-critical and more reassured in terms of himself.

Over the course of time, the group offers opportunities for depressed patients to glimpse other members' own insecurities and vulnerabilities and, in response, to tentatively try out new behaviors, often emulating those of the therapist or other youngsters in the group. The ultimate goal is for the depressed youngster to become appropriately assertive on his or her own behalf and to develop social skills that will enhance self-esteem and increase comfort with peer-relatedness.

The Middle- to Late-Adolescent Group

Therapy groups organized for middle- and late-adolescent patients tend to differ from those for younger children in both format and composition. Increased cognitive skills, including development of the capacity for abstract reasoning and the diminution of anxiety, allow for a shift away from activities and toward discussion during group sessions. Thus, in this sense, psychotherapy groups for middle and late adolescents resemble those formed for adult patients. However, more emphasis needs to be placed on group rules regarding physical contact (either sexual or aggressive), confidentiality, and extra-group relationships between members, particularly in groups for mid-adolescent patients, than would be the case in adult groups (Kennedy 1982).

Unlike therapeutic groups for younger patients, most adolescent groups include both male and female patients unless the setting (e.g., a residential treatment facility for emotionally disturbed males) prevents this. By this age, sexual identity is generally more secure, and a gender-heterogeneous group more nearly approximates the adolescents' appropriate social milieu.

As with adult therapy groups, adolescent groups have developed from a variety of models that range from the psychoanalytic-interpretive to the cognitive-behavioral model. Therefore, some group therapists emphasize the development of insight and intrapsychic change, whereas others focus primarily on behavioral adaptation. Nonetheless, regardless of the therapist's orientation, there is significant overlap in these various groups: the development of self-understanding is valued, and positive emotional and behavioral changes are supported.

In any of these groups, the depressed, hopeless adolescent is likely to present initially as a reluctant, unenthusiastic participant. The depressed adolescent will typically devalue both the experience and the other group members, as well as the therapist, so that he or she once again establishes himself or herself in an isolated, alienated position. Therefore, the group's early work with this patient will focus on inclusion, assisting the patient in recognizing that he or she is not, in fact, alone with his or her struggles and that his or her contributions have meaning and value to the group.

Once the inclusion work has been accomplished, various groups, according to the preference and theoretical orientation of the therapist, will proceed in different ways with the depressed adolescent. Some may strive for the development of insight into the origins of his or her depression, while other groups will focus primarily on current, conscious dilemmas and interpersonal relationships, either in the group or outside of it. Some groups will provide information and deliberately teach socialization skills, either through discussion or practice using a variety of role-playing techniques. Still other groups will emphasize cognitive skills, teaching the depressed adolescent about faulty, distorted cognitions and offering corrective experiences. Here, again, approaches may vary considerably. However, all group psychotherapies for depressed adolescents are directed toward the goals of alleviating the burdensome depression and improving socialization.

It has been long accepted that adolescents identify with each other because of common concerns and quickly form cohesive groups. Quite often, depressive themes are clearly evident, such as anger at punitive parents, feeling rejected by peers, and disappointment and hopelessness about political and religious leaders, nuclear war, crime, etc. Identifying with peer anger is reassuring to adolescents and, in a balanced group with counterforces, can allow ventilation but also help the angry adolescents to develop more acceptable defensive and coping abilities. One such group consisted of 15- and 16-year-old males and females with male and female cotherapists.

Case Examples

U. was a 15-year-old female who had made a suicide attempt when feeling depressed and helpless after learning that she was pregnant. She was vocal in the group and talked easily about her feelings and at the same time was supportive of other members.

B. was a 16-year-old male whose grades deteriorated as a result of becoming depressed, withdrawn, and hopeless following the sudden and unexpected divorce of his parents. He was very open in describing his unhappiness and loneliness due to parental conflicts and his father's rigid strictness. B. took an active role in the group and, because he found it a safe and protective environment, he began to ventilate his extreme rage and anger about his situation. Initially, his anger was displaced onto the male therapist as a transference figure for his father. Other group members would object to his overt and loud anger toward the therapist. B. would stop and explain that he liked the therapist and that this was the only place in his life where he could vent his feelings. Through therapeutic interpretations, he became aware of his intense anger toward his father, whom he had feared all of his life. When he was young, his father had punished him for showing feelings and had taught him that it was a sign of weakness.

D. was a 16-year-old female living in a foster home because of neglect and abuse by her antisocial mother. Her depression was masked by anger, cynicism, and criticism of others. During the initial phases of group therapy, she subgrouped with B. in ventilating anger about parents, teachers, and society in general. The anger and hopelessness were most evident during the Christmas holiday season. Gradually D. began to subgroup with U. and some of the less angry members of the group. She was able to accept questions, criticism, and suggestions regarding her own impulsiveness and poor judgment.

J. was a 15-year-old male who was referred after expressing suicidal thoughts to his school counselor in reaction to his parents' stormy divorce. He initially took the role of superego in the group, objecting to or criticizing questionable behavior of others. He was a very sensitive and perceptive person who later became an indigenous therapist, making accurate observations and interpretative comments about the others. The group accepted him in this role and gave him recognition, which later enabled him to reveal his own feelings of loneliness, lack of confidence, and sensitivity to peer rejection. The group both identified with him and empathized with his feelings.

M. was a short 17-year-old female who entered the group after re-vealing her depression, loneliness, self-consciousness about her size, fear of peer rejection, and suicidal thoughts. She gradually became comfortable in the group and shared her concerns about peer accep-tance and her anger at her anxious parents. She was surprised and reas-sured to hear other more attractive group members say that they felt the same about peer rejection. M. gained peer support and with it self-confidence and became more active in discussions, identifying with J. and confronting others about questionable judgment, behavior, and values.

H. was a 17-year-old male who entered the group because of missing school, with underlying depressive feelings associated with frustration and failure due to learning deficiencies. He was a handsome, imposing, articulate young man looked up to by the others. Psychological evalua-tion revealed low-average intelligence, which he denied and found un-acceptable because of a family history of above-average functioning and success. He had unrealistically lofty ambitions. Understandably, it took H. a much longer time to begin to acknowledge some of his own self-doubt and discouragement, first to himself and then to the group.

In this cohesive group, these depressed adolescents experienced safety, protection, identification with each other and the therapist, and support. The repetitive themes of loneliness, despair, and anger that were shared pro-vided the unifying force for the development of cohesion. Common com-plaints about parents, teachers, and other adults solidified the mutual iden-tification and provided a framework within which they could confront and challenge each other. Also, they began to care for each other. They offered to help each other in times of crisis, such as when a group member felt like running away, was having recurring suicidal thoughts, or reported abuse. The realization that one is not all alone and that other teenagers have similar problems is a powerful dynamic force in reducing uncertainty, confusion, and self-doubt in depressed adolescents.

PHASES OF TREATMENT

Multiple schemata have been put forth to describe phases of group develop-ment. They focus on the group as a closed system with consistent member-ship and a specific time boundary. These schemata are, of course, of theoret-ical importance, but they do not necessarily reflect on the experience of the individual group members. Furthermore, many depressed children and ad-olescents who are treated in groups do not become members of consistent, time-limited groups, although some have been reported (Fine et al. 1989). More often, they are treated in ongoing therapeutic groups that add or termi-nate a member. Therefore, the phases of treatment for the individual child or adolescent in a group become more important than the phases of group development.

Introductory Phase

The introductory phase may extend over one or many sessions, depending on the individual's experience and availability for affiliative relationships. Such availability is generally low in depressed children and adolescents, so this phase can be protracted.

During the introductory phase, the patient usually participates reluctantly and sometimes negatively, if at all. Rather, the patient tends to be anxious and to remain quietly vigilant while studying the group to which he or she does not yet belong. This is the time during which the patient is learning about the group's norms and expectations; introductory explanations given by the therapist and other members of the group can facilitate the introductory phase.

Investment and Commitment Phase

The investment and commitment phase is initiated when the youngster begins to experience himself or herself as a member of the group and recognizes some loyalty to its members. A sense of affiliation, though still weak, emerges, and the patient begins to identify with the therapeutic goals of the group. Borrowing from the language of individual psychotherapy, this phase is characterized by a "therapeutic alliance" between the patient and the group, including the therapist.

During this middle phase, the depressed child or adolescent undergoes a major transition with the active support of the group. The specific nature of the therapeutic work varies, depending on the structure and orientation of the group, but the youngster's investment in, and commitment to, the group is the foundation upon which psychological improvement is built.

Separation and Termination Phase

Hopefully, the separation and termination phase follows a period of significant change and marks the patient's final involvement in the life of the group. Although patients, particularly adolescents, attempt to deny any problems concerning separation and termination, this phase is often difficult for the youngster who has found understanding, tolerance, support, and guidance in the group.

The child or adolescent usually handles this phase clumsily, at least initially. He or she either demonstrates regressive behavior, in a thinly disguised attempt to remain dependent on the group, or "leaps" into a differentiated, nonmember stance while attempting to avoid the pain inherent in the disruption of meaningful relationships. However, sensitive interpretation and adequate time devoted to the total group's experience of the pending separation can greatly assist the youngster's transition out of the group.

SPECIAL CONSIDERATIONS FOR THE GROUP THERAPIST

Depressed children and adolescents often present the group therapist with special problems due to their initial reluctance to join in group activities or discussion and their vulnerability to being victimized and scapegoated by other group members. Like other adults, the therapist may experience strong desires to make the youngster feel happier. Thus, the therapist becomes vulnerable to unconsciously colluding with the depressed patient's perceived helplessness, tending to overprotect the patient and rescue him or her from peers. This, however, does not bring positive results since it confirms and reinforces the youngster's feelings of inadequacy.

Collusion in another direction can be equally problematic. Depressed children and adolescents can prove to be exasperating over time since their progress may be very slow, particularly in the early stage of treatment. In such situations, other group members may criticize and verbally attack the patient out of their frustration with his or her isolated, poorly integrated stance. The therapist may share this frustration and impatience. There is the danger of inadvertently supporting scapegoating behavior toward the patient, thereby reinforcing the depressed youngster's low self-esteem.

The group therapist must continually guard against colluding with unhealthy aspects of the depressed youngster's personality. Fortunately, group members can help the therapist avoid this collusion. Among these children or adolescents, there are usually some who will comment on, inquire about, or directly confront the therapist's behavior, and the therapist would do well to listen.

SUMMARY

In this chapter, we have presented clinical examples to demonstrate the group psychotherapy process with depressed children and adolescents. Group therapy is particularly useful to improve social skills and strengthen self-images. Acceptance by and identification with same-age peers play a crucial part in reducing the isolation and aloneness experienced by depressed children and adolescents. Hearing from happier-appearing peers that they also experience hurt, sadness, hopelessness, and suicidal thoughts provides a sense of belonging and reassurance that "I'm not really the only one to feel this way." Systematic outcome research in the effectiveness of group psychotherapy is needed (Dies and Riester 1986).

REFERENCES

Berkowitz IH: On growing a group: some thoughts on structure, process and setting, in Adolescents Grow in Group: Experiences in Adolescent Group Therapy. Edited by Berkowitz IH. New York, Brunner/Mazel, 1972, pp 6–28

Bromfield R, Pfeifer G: Combining group and individual psychotherapy: impact on the individual treatment experience. J Am Acad Child Adolesc Psychiatry 27:220–225, 1988

Dies R, Riester A: Research on child group therapy, in Child Group Psychotherapy: Future Tense. Edited by Riester A, Kraft IA. Madison, CT, International Universities Press, 1986, pp 173–220

Fine S, Gilbert M, Schmidt L, et al: Short-term group therapy with depressed adolescent outpatients. Can J Psychiatry 34(2):97–102, 1989

Kennedy JF: Group psychotherapy: in childhood and adolescence, in Pathways of Human Development: Normal Growth and Emotional Disorders in Infancy, Childhood and Adolescents. Edited by Shafii M, Shafii SL. New York, Thieme-Stratton, 1982, pp 270–281

Kraft IA: Group therapy, in Basic Handbook of Child Psychiatry, Vol 3. Edited by Harrison SI. New York, Basic Books, 1979, pp 159–180

Pfeifer G, Spinner D: Combined individual and group psychotherapy with children: an ego developmental perspective. Int J Group Psychother 35:11–35, 1985

Rachman AW, Raubolt RR: The pioneers of adolescent group psychotherapy. Int J Group Psychother 34:387–413, 1984

Rose SD: Treating Children in Groups: A Behavioral Approach. San Francisco, CA, Jossey-Bass, 1972

Schachter RS: Kinetic psychotherapy in the treatment of depression in latency age children. Int J Group Psychother 34:83–91, 1984

Schamess G: Differential diagnosis and group structure in the outpatient treatment of latency age children, in Child Group Psychotherapy: Future Tense. Edited by Riester A, Kraft IA. Madison, CT, International Universities Press, 1986, pp 29–68

Schiffer M: Activity-interview group psychotherapy: theory, principles and practice. Int J Group Psychother 27:377–388, 1977

Slavson SR: An Introduction to Group Psychotherapy. New York, The Commonwealth Fund, 1943

Sugar M: Interpretive group psychotherapy with latency children. J Am Acad Child Psychiatry 13:648–666, 1974

Yalom ID: The Theory and Practice of Group Psychotherapy, 2nd Edition. New York, Basic Books, 1975

CHAPTER 9

Cognitive Therapy of Depression

G. Randolph Schrodt, Jr., M.D.

The development of cognitive therapy represents a major advance in the treatment of depressive disorders. The early theoretical and technical work of Albert Ellis (1962) and Aaron T. Beck (1967, 1976) initiated a generation of research on basic cognitive pathology, treatment methods, and clinical outcome. Cognitive psychotherapy has a short-term treatment format, formalized training manuals (Beck et al. 1979; Meichenbaum 1977), and reliable measures of therapist competency (Vallis et al. 1986), and it has lent itself to extensive empirical outcome research.

Hollon and Najavits (1988) reviewed the empirical literature evaluating the efficacy of cognitive therapy for depression in adults. They concluded that this approach is at least as effective as any other intervention for treatment of the acute episode and may be superior in preventing subsequent relapse. Dobson's (1989) meta-analysis of 28 studies of cognitive therapy concluded that it produced a greater improvement than that observed with waiting-list or no-treatment controls, pharmacotherapy, behavior therapy, or other psychotherapies. However, findings of the National Institute of Mental Health Treatment of Depression Collaborative Research Program (Elkin et al. 1989) do not support such a robust claim for cognitive therapy.

The efficacy of cognitive therapy for the treatment of adults with depression has encouraged research on other psychiatric conditions and special patient populations. This chapter will review the basic theoretical and technical aspects of cognitive therapy as they apply to depressed children and adolescents.

THEORETICAL ISSUES

Schemata and Information Processing

Cognitive therapy is based on the premise that an individual's self-knowledge and mode of processing information about the world are primary determinants of mood and behavior. Guidano and Liotti (1983) have synthesized a developmental model of cognitive processes that emphasizes that the growth and refinement of self-knowledge are a result of the complex interactions of the child with his or her environment and significant adults. This active, gradual developmental process leads to the establishment of relatively stable and enduring assumptions, attitudes, beliefs, and modes of information processing.

Schemata are the organizing principles that govern perceptions, predictions, and actions. They serve an important role in screening of sensory inputs and are the silent rules used to evaluate the significance of events. Although this active process of structuring and organizing phenomenological experience usually serves an adaptive function (e.g., "I am a competent person" or "I should try my best"), disturbances in early attachment experiences may lead to the development of depressogenic schemata.

Depressogenic schemata are frequently characterized by rigid, absolutistic standards of conduct and self-evaluation and typically refer to events and situations within one's "personal domain" (Kovacs and Beck 1978). When these latent cognitive constructs are activated by stress or biological events, the symptoms of depression are triggered and maintained (Kovacs and Beck 1978). Certain types of life events appear to be most commonly associated with initiation of depression, particularly those involving loss of or failure in a significant interpersonal relationship or an important personal goal. For people with schemata such as, "I must be loved to be happy" or "My life is meaningless if I am not a success," stressful events can assume catastrophic significance.

Depressed patients often employ a negative explanatory style for stressful life events, which leads to increased helplessness and decreased coping behavior (Abramson et al. 1978). When a negative life event occurs, it is attributed to internal, global, and invariant causes: "I lost the swim meet because I'm a terrible swimmer who will never be any good." In contrast, most nondepressed persons demonstrate an even-balanced or self-serving cognitive bias: "I lost the swim meet because I had bad luck (external), I wasn't really into training (specific), and anyway, I'll do better the next time (variable)."

Automatic Thoughts and Cognitive Errors

Children and adolescents commonly make statements such as, "I got an 'A' on my exam and I'm happy," "My boyfriend didn't call me and I'm sad," and "My father won't let me go out and I'm angry." Each statement describes the emotion as a result of the event. The cognitive model emphasizes that every "objective" event is in fact perceived and processed in very unique and, at times, idiosyncratic ways (Figure 9–1). The cognitive appraisal of events constitutes an individual's stream of consciousness, so-called automatic thoughts, or visual images. These conscious thoughts and images are termed *automatic* because they occur rapidly in response to situations and are often not subjected to systematic, logical analysis. Although a person may be unaware of the presence or significance of automatic thoughts, most individuals can be trained to recognize them. At first, the patient's appraisal of an event may appear to be a perfectly plausible and accurate representation of reality, but a sampling of the automatic thoughts of depressed patients usually reveals extensive negative distortions and logical errors.

Common cognitive distortions include personalization ("It's all my fault"), overgeneralization ("Nothing ever works out for me"), absolute categorization ("I'm worthless"), and invariant predictions ("I'll never have a satisfying relationship"). Depressed patients frequently draw arbitrary inferences ("He hasn't called yet—he's probably out with another girl") or selectively focus on aspects of their experience that are consistent with themes of personal inadequacy, helplessness, and hopelessness about the future. These conclusions are often reached even in the presence of contradictory details. Negative events are magnified in significance, and positive experiences are disqualified. These persistent negative and erroneous assessments lead to

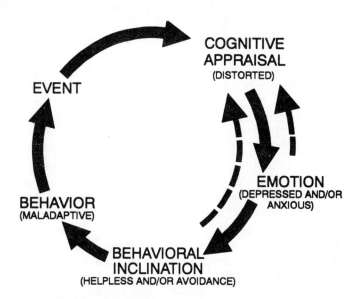

Figure 9–1. A cognitive model of depression. Reprinted from Wright JH: Cognitive therapy of depression, in American Psychiatric Press Review of Psychiatry, Vol 7. Edited by Frances AJ, Hales RE. Washington, DC, American Psychiatric Press, 1988. Reprinted with permission. Copyright 1988 American Psychiatric Press.

sad mood, lowered self-esteem, guilt, apathy, withdrawal, amotivation, and suicidal wishes.

Cognitive errors are not specific to depression and are frequently observed in patients with other psychiatric conditions, such as anxiety and eating disorders. Indeed, most people jump to inaccurate conclusions or misperceive events at some time. However, depressed patients demonstrate a pervasive ruminative stream of negative, distorted thoughts. Beck (1967) has defined the negative cognitive triad of depression: negative views of the self (worthlessness), the world (helplessness), and the future (hopelessness). The cognitive therapist teaches the patient to identify, test, and modify these negative automatic thoughts and associated depressogenic assumptions. Improvement of depressive symptoms is facilitated when a more accurate and adaptive cognitive style is maintained.

Cognitive Processes in Depressed Children and Adolescents

Application of the cognitive model to depressed children and adolescents has received substantial empirical support. Depressed children and adolescents demonstrate a distinct negative bias in their thinking and report more depressive, distorted thoughts than nondepressed control subjects (Haley et al. 1985; Leitenberg et al. 1986). Grade school children with high scores on self-measures of depression typically show low self-esteem, self-directed hostility, and shame (Blumberg and Izard 1985; Kaslow et al. 1984). Hospitalized depressed adolescents also have a broad range of self-image disturbances, including poor body image, low personal esteem and self-concept, and a low sense of self-efficacy (Koenig 1988; McCauley et al. 1988; Schrodt et al. 1989).

Depressed children and adolescents also have a negative outlook on their environment. Teri (1982) noted that high school students with depressive symptoms report negative family relations, poor impulse control, and low sense of mastery of the external world. These students were also more maladaptively assertive than their classmates who had low depression scores (Teri 1982). Hospitalized adolescents with a diagnosis of major depressive disorder expressed significantly more concern about peer relations, sexual acceptance, social tolerance, family rapport, and academic confidence (Schrodt et al. 1989).

In addition to their negative view of self and the current situation, depressed children and adolescents view the future in a pessimistic, hopeless fashion (Kazdin et al. 1983; McCauley et al. 1988; Rotheram-Borus and Trautman 1988; Schrodt et al. 1989). Children with repetitive suicidal thoughts or recent suicide attempts scored high on a measure of hopelessness, but the correlation between hopelessness and suicidal intent was not observed in depressed adolescents (Rotheram-Borus and Trautman 1988).

Depressed children and adolescents tend to perceive that they have little influence over their environment, are not responsible for negative life events, and do not have the capacity to deal with stress (Mullins et al. 1985; Schrodt et al. 1989). Hospitalized children and adolescents who showed elevated Children's Depression Inventory (Kovacs 1983) scores also showed a low rating of personal competence and sense of control (Weisz et al. 1989). Fourth- and fifth-graders with high scores for depressive symptoms performed significantly worse than children with fewer depressive symptoms on a measure of problem-solving ability that included considering alternatives and consequences, planning steps, and anticipating obstacles (Sacco and Graves 1984). Another study of 11-year-olds found that depressive symptomatology was associated more with negative self-appraisal of ability than actual decreased performance on measures of intelligence (McGee et al. 1986).

An attributional style characteristic of the reformulated learned helplessness model (Abramson et al. 1978) has been repeatedly observed in children with depressive symptoms. (See Chapter 2.) Grade school children who attribute bad events to internal, stable, and global causes are more likely to report depressive symptoms, low self-esteem, and poor academic achievement (Blumberg and Izard 1985; Fielstein et al. 1985; Kaslow et al. 1984; Nolen-Hoeksema et al. 1986; Seligman and Peterson 1986; Seligman et al. 1984). This maladaptive explanatory style also appears to be a risk factor for future depressive symptoms (Nolen-Hoeksema et al. 1986; Seligman and Peterson 1986; Seligman et al. 1984).

McCauley et al. (1988) found that clinically depressed children and adolescents showed an externalized locus of control and attributed positive events to external, unstable, and specific causes. However, their way of explaining failure was not significantly different from that of patients whose depression was in remission or of patients who had other nondepressive psychiatric disturbances. In a 36-month follow-up study of their original report, McCauley et al. (1989) found that depressed teenagers' cognitive response style (low self-concept, hopelessness, and negative attributions) normalized with resolution of depressive symptoms. However, their thinking again became "depressive" with recurrence of a depressive episode.

TECHNICAL ISSUES

The Therapeutic Relationship

Cognitive therapy is an active, goal-directed psychotherapy. In general, the focus is on current problems and issues. A short-term format of 16–20 sessions has been described for adults, although the optimum frequency and duration of therapy sessions have not been established for depressed children and adolescents. However, significant clinical improvement appears largely dependent on establishing a working therapeutic alliance. As with all effective psychotherapies, nonspecific therapist variables such as warmth, empathy, and rapport are important contributors to treatment outcome. Patience, tolerance, and a nonjudgmental attitude facilitate the development of a positive working alliance. However, there are a variety of intrinsic and extrinsic obstacles to the development of a collaborative relationship with children and adolescents.

Children and adolescents typically do not initiate requests for therapy. Parents, teachers, or social agencies often identify depressive behaviors such as social withdrawal, conflicts with family, school failure, substance abuse, or self-harm behaviors and refer the child or adolescent for treatment. Children, and especially adolescents, are extremely sensitive to criticism and the stigma of psychiatric care, which they believe means that they are "crazy." In response to this insult to their self-esteem, and in part due to cognitive limitations, children and adolescents commonly externalize the source of the problems and contend that they do not need therapy. An unwillingness to participate in therapy also frequently may reflect a general mistrust of adults and suspicions regarding the motives and intentions of the therapist. Issues of autonomy, control, and confidentiality are especially common with adolescents.

These negative thoughts can often be elicited by asking the child or adolescent about his or her reaction to being brought to a professional for treatment. At other times, negative reactions to therapy must be inferred from lack of clinical improvement or failure to complete self-help assignments. A psychoeducational approach regarding the goals and process of therapy enhances socialization to cognitive therapy. Distorted attitudes and beliefs about the therapeutic relationship can also be modified by standard cognitive techniques. Most importantly, the therapist emphasizes that the therapeutic relationship is explicitly for the benefit of the child or adolescent and acknowledges that his or her view of the current situation will be taken into account.

Another problem that complicates the establishment of an effective therapeutic alliance is cognitive immaturity. Most children, and many adolescents, do not have the capacity to "think about their thoughts," an abstract cognitive task. A second cognitive deficit involves the inability to consider alternatives. The egocentric, personalized, and occasionally illogical thinking processes of normal children and young adolescents have been described by Elkind (1967). The structured learning approach of cognitive therapy appears to modify some of these cognitive limitations. There is evidence that abstract, hypothetical reasoning skills can be learned through brief, formal training (Nisbett et al. 1987).

Agenda Setting and Structure of the Therapy Session

Cognitive therapy sessions begin with agenda setting, the specific listing of issues to be discussed during the available time. Agenda setting represents a significant theoretical and technical departure from traditional psychodynamic psychotherapy. Some modes of psychodynamic therapy emphasize silence and nondirectiveness on the part of the therapist, especially at the beginning of the therapy session. In contrast, the cognitive therapist assumes that depressed patients may interpret this lack of direction or feedback as evidence that their situation is hopeless and can actually lead to a worsening of depressive symptoms.

Agenda setting serves a variety of functions. It is a formal symbol of the collaborative nature of the therapeutic relationship and emphasizes the active participation of the child or adolescent. An agenda focuses on specific target symptoms for intervention and aids in judicious use of therapy time. This structured therapy approach also enhances a sense of accomplishment and promotes the use of logical problem-solving skills. Finally, the review of the agenda at the end of the session provides a context for mutual feedback and a reemphasis of important points of the session.

Effective agenda setting typically begins with a review of recent events, including delayed reactions from the last session. A brief clinical assessment or use of a short self-report instrument, such as the Children's Depression Inventory (Kovacs 1983), can assist in identifying any particular symptoms that need to be addressed, such as hopelessness or suicidal thoughts. (See Chapter 6.) A review of previous therapy homework assignments provides an opportunity to assess the child or adolescent's understanding and mastery of therapy concepts and reinforces the importance of self-help in clinical improvement. The agenda may also include "leftover" items from previous sessions. The therapist can suggest and give feedback about agenda items that are not raised by the child or adolescent but appear to be important. Finally, contact with parents, teachers, social workers, or others is discussed to generate additional topics for the agenda.

After listing the agenda, the therapist and patient collaborate in prioritizing the most important or troubling issues or symptoms. Decisions are made about what can be dealt with in the available time. Depressed children and teenagers often perceive problems as overwhelming and diffuse; mastery of this method of efficient time management and specific goal setting can have a positive influence on problem-solving abilities in general.

The therapist facilitates an agenda that is geared to the stage of the therapy and the clinical status of the patient. In early stages of therapy (sessions 1–3, and often longer), much of the agenda is directed toward enlisting the child or adolescent in a therapeutic alliance and identifying goals for change. Middle therapy sessions (sessions 3–12) often focus on specific events and the monitoring, identification, and modification of depressive automatic thoughts and behaviors. The agenda of later sessions (sessions 12–20) may include reality testing of underlying assumptions, refinement of new coping skills, or practice of relapse prevention techniques. Severely depressed children or adolescents require a more narrow, focused agenda, such as an activities schedule. As depression improves, more complex behavioral tasks or cognitive approaches are possible.

Despite the efforts of the therapist to engage the child or adolescent in this collaborative process, at times topics or issues are avoided or there is a "hidden agenda." Attention to nonverbal messages or mood changes may suggest important automatic thoughts that can be elicited directly in the therapy session. The failure to establish a working agenda can be an indication of therapeutic alliance problems. When the therapeutic alliance has been solidified, it typically only takes 5–10 minutes to set an effective agenda for the session.

A sensitive and empathic cognitive therapist will add, delete, or modify agenda items as the need arises. However, the therapist also assumes the responsibility to focus on the topics and goals identified at the outset. At the end of each session, the agenda is reviewed and note is made of items for the next session.

Eliciting and Testing Automatic Thoughts

In addition to the relief of specific target symptoms, cognitive therapy has several general goals and objectives:

1. Identify negative automatic thoughts and their relationship to dysphoric mood and maladaptive behavior.
2. Pinpoint cognitive errors.
3. Test distorted automatic thoughts and underlying assumptions.
4. Replace or modify self-defeating cognitive styles with a more realistic, adaptive perspective.
5. Improve sense of self-efficacy by developing social skills and problem-solving abilities.
6. Prevent relapse.

Most automatic thoughts can be elicited by a guided discovery approach that focuses on "What were you thinking that led you to feel that way?" as opposed to "How did it make you feel?" Younger patients can often relate to the analogy of a videotape machine: "When you feel sad or upset, stop the tape and rewind it a few feet, then play it back in slow motion so you can remember what you were thinking." Emotional shifts within the session often provide an excellent opportunity to practice this method of enhanced self-awareness. Visual imagery techniques can be used to re-create an event or a personal interaction that occurred outside the therapy setting. Depressive thinking processes can also be identified by review of journals, diaries, or more formal mood-thought records.

A 15-year-old male had difficulty during early cognitive therapy sessions in identifying the thoughts he had that led to his chronic, severe depression. He was encouraged to write in his therapy journal the thoughts he had when he felt depressed.

> There are many things that I hate about myself. I hate that I am shy, I can't go up to someone I am not familiar with and talk to them comfortably. I hate that I always do the wrong thing. I hate my hair. I hate my body. I hate my face. I hate that I have a hard time making myself do schoolwork. I hate that I have a hard time trying anything new. I hate that I have no self-confidence. I hate being quiet. I hate being lonely sometimes. I hate being afraid or worried that I'm not doing something right. I hate that I feel like I never fit in or am part of something. I hate being depressed.

Once automatic thoughts have been identified, the connection to a change in attitude, mood, and behavioral response is explored. The young man in the example was able to see that this negative, pessimistic, and helpless outlook on himself and the world led to his depressed, agitated mood, social withdrawal, and resistance to change.

The child or adolescent is encouraged to consider his or her thoughts as "hypotheses" (possible explanations of data) rather than absolute facts. However, many depressed children and adolescents are unable or reluctant to conceptualize or accept alternative points of view. They may also not be convinced that change is desirable. The therapist accepts that the patient's point of view may possibly be accurate, but encourages consideration of alternatives before coming to premature closure. A skillful, empathic cognitive therapist can usually engage a child or adolescent in the discussion and review of his or her thoughts without resorting to debate or argument. Rather, the therapist provides a role model for a more positive, less distorted way of dealing with life stresses and assists the patient in exploring these possibilities (Schrodt and Fitzgerald 1987).

The cognitive therapist can employ a variety of cognitive interventions to test automatic thoughts (Table 9–1). In many cases, simply focusing attention on automatic thinking leads to recognition of cognitive errors and their modification. A very useful cognitive technique is the five-column Realistic Thoughts Worksheet (Table 9–2). In the first column, a factual description of the event or situation that triggered a dysphoric mood is recorded. In the second column, the child or adolescent is encouraged to write down his or her automatic thoughts and to rate the degree of belief in that thought on a 1–100% scale, with 0% meaning "not at all" and 100% meaning "completely." In the third column, the associated mood is recorded. This task is

Table 9–1.   Cognitive techniques

Guided discovery
Visual imagery
Realistic Thoughts Worksheets
Identifying cognitive errors
Examining the evidence
Focus on language and use of labels
Considering alternatives
Reattribution
Reframing
Decatastrophizing
Weighing the advantages and disadvantages

Table 9–2.   Realistic Thoughts Worksheet

Situation	(1) Automatic thoughts (2) Degree of belief (0–100%)	(1) Mood (2) Strength of emotion (0–100%)	(1) Realistic response (2) Degree of belief (0–100%)	(1) Outcome (2) Strength of emotion (0–100%)
Lost baseball game	If I lose at something I'm a failure (95%)	Upset (100%)	Everybody loses sometime (100%) It doesn't matter if you win or lose (10%)	Upset (40%)
	I should have played better (100%)	Angry (98%)	I should practice more (80%)	Angry (10%)
	The team blames me (90%)	Sad (90%)	No one said anything, other people made mistakes (100%)	Sad (30%)
Overdue school assignment	The teacher thinks I'm a loser (100%)	Sad (100%)	If I talk to him maybe I can get an extension (80%)	Anxious (50%)
	I might as well give up; I'll never get it (95%)	Hopeless (100%)	I guess I have learned hard things before (90%) A tutor might help (90%)	Worried (50%)

often facilitated by having a list of adjectives that describe various mood states. The patient is instructed to rate the strength of the emotion on a 0–100% scale. The fourth column is used to formulate a "realistic response" or reevaluation of the original automatic thoughts. Children and teenagers can be taught to use a self-questioning approach to their own thinking, often guided by written questions provided by the therapist. The fifth column is used to rate the outcome or change in emotional tone as a result of the cognitive reappraisal.

The opportunity to look at one's written thoughts enhances the ability to observe, rather than react to, automatic thoughts. Guided by the therapist, older children and teenagers are encouraged to ask themselves a series of questions:

1. "What's the evidence?" The technique of examining the evidence is designed to identify exaggerated statements or conclusions reached without sufficient support. The first step involves the identification of cognitive errors: for instance, the use of absolutistic or categorical words such as "always," "never," "worthless," or "must." Positive events, experiences, or accomplishments that were previously excluded from consideration can be recognized. A review of the ratings given for belief in automatic thoughts and intensity of mood can be used to explore dichotomous thinking or a tendency to magnify or minimize.

2. "Are there alternative explanations?" This analysis may lead to reframing and reattribution of automatic thoughts. Reframing includes the redefinition of problems and modification of negative labels. For example, the statement, "I always screw up" can be more accurately reframed as, "I sometimes don't do as well as I'd like." Reattribution techniques can be used to modify cognitive errors such as personalization or taking excessive responsibility or blame for certain events.

3. "What's so awful or upsetting about this event?" Many negative automatic thoughts that lead to depressed or dysphoric mood are in fact not "distorted." Actual events such as failure in athletic competition represent real cause for distress. Nevertheless, depressed children and adolescents with a low sense of self-efficacy and poor problem-solving skills often catastrophize the significance of these events.

4. "What can I do about it?" This question encourages positive adaptive responses and a critical evaluation of personal strengths and abilities. The ability to consider options and alternative reactions often leads to a decrease in feelings of helplessness and hopelessness. The therapist and child or adolescent can then identify specific adaptive-skills deficits and formulate further goals for therapy. In some cases, depressive automatic thoughts are in response to something that might occur, rather than an event that has actually happened. The child or adolescent can be encour-

aged to imagine the worst possible scenario and then to develop coping strategies.

The young man in an earlier example who had written in his journal about the things he hated about himself showed improvement with pharmacotherapy and cognitive therapy. Four weeks later, he wrote the following entry:

> My doctor told me to write of my top 10 goals for the summer. One goal is for me to try to be less shy around people my own age that I am not familiar with. Another is for me to choose what school I will be going to. Also, I want to practice driving more since I haven't had my license too long. To fulfill more of an image I have of myself. To stick with lifting weights. To get a new girlfriend. To buy some stock in Textron. To spend most of my summer nights out with my friends. To give my parents a chance for me to see if they really are going to be able to change. Last, to take things less seriously so I will possibly be less stressed.

This entry represents a "realistic response" to the pervasively worthless, helpless, and hopeless thoughts that he had earlier described. It shows indications of motivation, initiative, and a commitment to making personal changes in thinking and life-style. However, simply understanding what needs to be done does not ensure that behavior will change and, in many respects, represents only a blueprint for further therapeutic intervention.

Behavioral Techniques and Homework

There are a number of reasons that behavioral techniques are useful in the treatment of depressed children and adolescents (Table 9–3). The behavioral manifestations of depression in children and adolescents have been well characterized and are now included as "age-specific features" of major depressive episodes. (See Chapter 1.) Prepubertal children frequently have somatic complaints, psychomotor agitation, phobias, and separation anxiety (Geller et al. 1985; Ryan et al. 1987). Adolescents commonly present with hypersomnia, weight change, use of alcohol and drugs, antisocial behavior, and suicide attempts (Geller et al. 1985; Ryan et al. 1987). There is also evidence that maladaptive behaviors associated with adolescent depression persist into young adulthood, as noted by increased rates of hospitalization,

Table 9–3. Behavioral techniques

Behavioral analysis	Graded task assignments
Activity schedules	Rehearsal
Social skills training	Role-playing
Problem solving	Homework

use of minor prescription tranquilizers among women, more deviant activities, and reduced ability to establish intimate heterosexual relations as young adults (Kandel and Davies 1986). The use of specific tactics to modify these behaviors may improve recovery from depression and may have an impact on long-term functioning.

Behavior modification appears to be an essential component of sustained cognitive modification. "Understanding" may lead to a change in mood, decreased helplessness, and increased engagement and participation in behavioral experiments. However, enduring change at the schemata level requires a change in behavior. Albert Bandura (1977) has described the development of self-efficacy expectations and established the relationship of the strength of these beliefs to the persistence of effort an individual displays when confronted with obstacles. Belief in self-efficacy has been shown to be a uniformly accurate predictor of performance on tasks varying in difficulty and presenting different degrees of personal threat. Although vicarious experience, verbal persuasion, and emotional arousal may have some impact on self-efficacy beliefs, successful task performance produces the most significant change.

The most common behavioral technique is behavioral analysis. The therapist works to define a stimulus-response pattern of dysfunctional thoughts and behaviors. Children and their parents can use this information to modify environmental events and contingencies and to promote more adaptive problem-solving responses. Boredom, inactivity, and poor time management are common problems in depressed children and adolescents. Lack of involvement in activities that provide a sense of enjoyment and mastery is commonly observed. An activity schedule can be used to monitor mood changes as well as encourage new behaviors. Many children and adolescents are unable to generate new ideas regarding activities or are convinced that "I can't do anything without money" or "There's nothing to do in this town." The use of a structured survey such as the Pleasant Events Schedule (Lewinsohn et al. 1986) can often identify activities that would promote a sense of enjoyment and mastery.

Many depressed children and adolescents have actual skills deficits in addition to a negative appraisal of their abilities. For example, impulsive children and adolescents typically do not stop to think before they act. Kendall and Braswell (1985) have described guidelines for teaching reflective thinking and self-control to impulsive children through the use of adaptive "self-statements." Social skills training teaches communication, including assertiveness, methods of negotiation and compromise, and accurate listening. The problem-solving method can be taught to depressed children and adolescents in a brief, didactic training session. First, attention is placed on identifying the specific problem. Second, a list of possible options or courses of action is generated. Third, the child or adolescent weighs the advantages and disadvantages of each alternative. Next, he or she is assisted in choosing one option and formulating a realistic plan. Finally, ways of evaluating outcome and responding to feedback are refined.

Complicated behavioral goals such as planning summer activities, getting a job or a driver's license, or talking with an estranged parent can often be fostered by use of a graded task assignment. With this method, a complex problem is broken down into more easily manageable steps. Mastery and refinement of the skills necessary to complete each step can be enhanced by use of behavioral rehearsal, including role-playing that allows a child or teenager to take an alternative point of view. Relaxation training can be a useful adjunct for children and adolescents who experience significant emotional or physiological arousal when confronting problems and obstacles.

Depressed children and adolescents will commonly ask, "How can talking about problems for an hour a week make any difference in my life?" This is an important and sensible question. Most people assume that homework or practice is an integral part of learning to play the piano, remembering the multiplication tables, or learning to shoot a basketball. However, many therapists overlook the importance of practicing the complex skills learned in psychotherapy. Not surprisingly, completion of homework assignments appears to be essential to good outcome of cognitive therapy (Person and Burns 1985; Person et al. 1989).

Children and adolescents are encouraged to take notes or, at times, make an audiotape of the therapy session. A therapy journal can be used to review the topics discussed in the session and to record homework assignments. A workbook or collection of reading assignments also facilitates the educational aspect of cognitive therapy (Burns 1981, 1989; Lewinsohn et al. 1986). Many depressed children and adolescents benefit from a psychoeducational approach that provides accurate information on topics such as sexual abuse, drug education, and contraceptive counseling.

The concept of homework is well understood by children and adolescents because they are accustomed to homework from school. Their reaction to psychotherapy homework frequently parallels their positive or negative reaction to school assignments. Homework assignments are most effective if they are clearly defined and relate to the material discussed in the therapy session. When children or adolescents perceive that an assignment is irrelevant or "busy work," they are significantly less likely to complete it. Assignments should have a reasonable expectation of success and can often be designed to provide useful information even if the specific goals are not accomplished. There are a number of common cognitive-behavioral homework assignments, including reading, keeping an activity schedule, or using the Realistic Thoughts Worksheet. The most effective homework assignments are customized to the child or adolescent's specific needs. Children and adolescents usually have an immediate reaction to a homework assignment and commonly report that they know whether they are going to complete it or not. Negative reactions such as, "It's impossible" or "That's a dumb idea" need to be checked out before the end of the session. Finally, the therapist reinforces the importance of self-help by regularly checking homework activities.

There are many reasons that children and adolescents fail to complete therapy homework assignments. In some cases, a homework assignment is perceived as a test of worth or skill and induces anxiety or feelings of helplessness. Feelings of hopelessness, lethargy, and impaired concentration are especially common in depressed children and adolescents. Competing priorities or a lack of planning can often undermine completion of self-help tasks.

Family Therapy

Family involvement is a critical variable in the treatment of depressed children and adolescents. Parents and other family members often have distorted perceptions and attitudes about the identified patient. Some parents have difficulty accepting the idea that their child or teenager is depressed, or that treatment is indicated. They may also reinforce negative or depressogenic attitudes ("You're hopeless"), self-statements ("You're worthless"), and behaviors ("You're lazy"). A number of researchers have found that the negative explanatory style of depressed children was also observed in their mothers (but not their fathers), suggesting a mutually learned or reinforced style (Nolen-Hoeksema et al. 1986; Seligman and Peterson 1986; Seligman et al. 1984).

Cognitive and behavioral techniques can be integrated into standard family therapy methods. More specific cognitive-behavioral approaches have been described for families of adolescents with disruptive behavior disturbances, a common feature of teenage depression (DiGiuseppe 1988).

In the early stages of family therapy, it is important to establish realistic treatment goals. Diagnosis, treatment options, and recommendations are thoroughly discussed. If medication is recommended, a formal psychoeducational approach and analysis of family attitudes can enhance acceptance of and compliance with pharmacotherapy (Wright and Schrodt 1989). An explanation of the basics of the cognitive therapy approach is enhanced with the use of reading materials geared toward the family (Beck 1988).

Problems and goals are defined in behavioral, operational terms: "He never does what he's supposed to" can be reframed as "The goal of our family sessions will be to clarify each person's responsibilities and to improve our cooperation in seeing that they are met." It may be necessary to specify that changes are often required from other family members for the depressed child or adolescent to improve. Silent expectations that the therapist "fix" or change the child or adolescent to conform to a preconceived norm need to be modified for treatment to be successful. When family members share goals and expectations for treatment, they are more willing to participate in family homework assignments such as scheduling family meals together or attempting to resolve conflicts without screaming or cursing.

OUTCOME RESEARCH AND DIRECTIONS FOR FUTURE DEVELOPMENT

Although adaptations of cognitive therapy to the treatment of depressed children and adolescents have been described (Bedrosian 1981; Bedrosian and Epstein 1984; DiGiuseppe 1981; Schrodt and Wright 1986; Schrodt and Fitzgerald 1987; Trautman and Rotheram-Borus 1988; Wilkes and Rush 1988), little empirical research exists to evaluate efficacy. Werry and Wollersheim (1989) have reviewed the literature on behavior therapy with children and adolescents and have concluded that behavioral approaches are useful with a number of specific problems commonly observed in child and adolescent depression, such as anxiety, disturbances of eating, and disruptive behaviors.

Reynolds and Coats (1986) described a study of cognitive therapy conducted within a high school setting. Subjects were recruited from a larger pool of students who were screened with self-report measures and a structured clinical interview scale. They were randomly assigned to a cognitive-behavioral group ($n = 9$), group relaxation training ($n = 11$), or a waiting list ($n = 10$). Cognitive-behavioral therapy emphasized training in self-control skills, including self-monitoring, problem solving, developing a self-change plan, and self-reinforcement. The second group was taught traditional progressive muscle relaxation techniques. All subjects who received relaxation training practiced at home and kept a log; both groups met for 10 sessions in 5 weeks. Treatment groups were led by the same therapist, and adherence to the protocol was monitored by random review of audiotaped therapy sessions. Dropout rates were low in both active treatment groups, and 67–68% of homework assignments were completed.

Adolescents in the cognitive-behavioral and relaxation therapy groups had lower posttreatment depression scores than the waiting-list controls. Seventy-five percent of the relaxation therapy subjects and 83% of the cognitive-behavioral subjects had posttreatment Beck Depression Inventory (BDI) (Beck et al. 1961) scores in the normal range, compared with none of the waiting-list subjects. These findings were observed both at posttreatment and at 5-week follow-up. Roughly equivalent results were noted in the two active treatment groups. No significant differences were noted on general self-concept measures. Both groups showed significant improvement in academic self-confidence, although relaxation training was slightly more effective in reducing state anxiety levels.

This study has several limitations, including small sample size and failure to use standard diagnostic criteria. As estimated from BDI scores, these students had moderate levels of depression and may not be representative of adolescents seen in clinical settings.

Lewinsohn et al. (1989) reported on a study designed to test the efficacy of group cognitive-behavioral therapy. In one treatment group, the adolescents alone received this therapy. In a second group, adolescents and their parents received this therapy separately. Adolescents placed on a waiting list served as controls. Forty-eight students ages 14–18 years completed a structured diagnostic interview and were found to meet criteria for major depressive and/or dysthymic disorder. Lewinsohn's "Coping With Depression" (1986) course was presented in a group format. Each session was 2 hours long, and the sessions were held twice a week for 8 weeks. The course focused on mood monitoring, social skills, increasing pleasant activities, controlling depressing thoughts, relaxation, and improving communication, negotiation, and problem-solving skills. The parents' group met weekly and included material about teenage depression, communication, negotiation, and solving family problems. Both active treatment groups improved significantly as measured by BDI scores. The subjects who improved showed a decrease in depressogenic cognitions and parent-adolescent conflicts and an increase in perceptions of social competence and parent problem-solving abilities. Adolescents whose parents also received cognitive therapy did not show significantly greater improvement in depression scores than did the adolescent group alone, but parents' perceptions of their teenager did improve. At 24-month follow-up, 85% of subjects had sustained remission.

These two studies offer support for further research on cognitive therapy with clinically depressed children and adolescents. Comparative studies with other treatments such as pharmacotherapy, family therapy, and interpersonal psychotherapy (Klerman et al. 1984) have not yet been undertaken in children and adolescents. Future studies should include evaluation of individual and family cognitive therapy approaches, as well as further research on group methods.

CONCLUSION

This chapter has reviewed the theoretical and technical aspects of cognitive therapy with depressed children and adolescents. The cognitive model offers a useful paradigm for the study of depression in this age group. The short-term, active, goal-oriented approach of cognitive therapy is well suited to children and teenagers. Minor modifications of standard adult techniques may be necessary for children with cognitive immaturity or skills deficits, and involvement of the family in treatment may be particularly critical. Early outcome studies are encouraging, although further research is needed to determine whether improvement of depression is specifically related to the cognitive and behavioral skills taught by this approach.

REFERENCES

Abramson LY, Seligman ME, Teasdale JD: Learned helplessness in humans: critique and reformulation. J Abnorm Psychol 87:49–74, 1978

Bandura A: Self-efficacy: toward a unifying theory of behavioral change. Psychol Rev 84:191–215, 1977

Beck AT: Depression: Causes and Treatment. Philadelphia, University of Pennsylvania Press, 1967

Beck AT: Cognitive Therapy and the Emotional Disorders. New York, International Universities Press, 1976

Beck AT: Love Is Never Enough. New York, Harper & Row, 1988

Beck AT, Ward CM, Mendelson M, et al: An inventory for measuring depression. Arch Gen Psychiatry 4:561–571, 1961

Beck AT, Rush AJ, Shaw BF, et al: Cognitive Therapy of Depression. New York, Guilford, 1979

Bedrosian RC: The application of cognitive therapy techniques with adolescents, in New Directions in Cognitive Therapy. Edited by Emery G, Hollon SD, Bedrosian RC. New York, Guilford, 1981, pp 68–83

Bedrosian RC, Epstein N: Cognitive therapy of depressed and suicidal adolescents, in Suicide in the Young. Edited by Sudak HS, Ford AB, Rushforth NB. Boston, MA, John Wright PSG, 1984, pp 345–366

Blumberg SH, Izard CE: Affective and cognitive characteristics of depression in 10- and 11-year-old children. J Pers Soc Psychol 49:194–202, 1985

Burns DD: Feeling Good: The New Mood Therapy. New York, New American Library, 1981

Burns DD: The Feeling Good Handbook. New York, Morrow, 1989

DiGiuseppe RA: Cognitive therapy with children, in New Directions in Cognitive Therapy. Edited by Emery G, Hollon SD, Bedrosian RC. New York, Guilford, 1981, pp 50–67

DiGiuseppe RA: A cognitive-behavioral approach to the treatment of conduct disorder children and adolescents, in Cognitive-Behavioral Therapy With Families. Edited by Epstein N, Schlesinger SE, Dryden W. New York, Brunner/Mazel, 1988, pp 183–214

Dobson KS: A meta-analysis of the efficacy of cognitive therapy for depression. J Consult Clin Psychol 57:414–419, 1989

Elkin I, Shea MT, Watkins JT, et al: National Institute of Mental Health Treatment of Depression Collaborative Research Program: general effectiveness of treatments. Arch Gen Psychiatry 46:971–982, 1989

Elkind D: Egocentrism in adolescence. Child Dev 38:1025–1034, 1967

Ellis A: Reason and Emotion in Psychotherapy. New York, Stuart, 1962

Fielstein E, Klein MS, Fischer M, et al: Self-esteem and causal attributions for success and failure in children. Cognitive Therapy and Research 9:381–398, 1985

Geller B, Chestnut EC, Miller MD, et al: Preliminary data on DSM-III associated features of major depressive disorder in children and adolescents. Am J Psychiatry 142:643–644, 1985

Guidano VF, Liotti G: Cognitive Processes and Emotional Disorders. New York, Guilford, 1983

Haley GMT, Fine S, Marriage K, et al: Cognitive bias and depression in psychiatrically disturbed children and adolescents. J Consult Clin Psychol 53:535–537, 1985

Hollon SD, Najavits L: Review of empirical studies on cognitive therapy, in the American Psychiatric Press Review of Psychiatry, Vol 7. Edited by Frances AJ, Hales RE. Washington, DC, American Psychiatric Press, 1988, pp 643–666

Kandel DB, Davies M: Adult sequelae of adolescent depressive symptoms. Arch Gen Psychiatry 43:255–262, 1986

Kaslow NJ, Rehn LP, Siegel AW: Social-cognitive and cognitive correlates of depression in children. J Abnorm Child Psychol 12:605–620, 1984

Kazdin AE, French NH, Unis AS, et al: Hopelessness, depression, and suicidal intent among psychiatrically disturbed inpatient children. J Consult Clin Psychol 51:504–510, 1983

Kendall PC, Braswell L: Cognitive-Behavioral Therapy for Impulsive Children. New York, Guilford, 1985

Klerman GL, Weissman MM, Rounsaville BJ, et al: Interpersonal Psychotherapy of Depression. New York, Basic Books, 1984

Koenig LJ: Self-image of emotionally disturbed adolescents. J Abnorm Child Psychol 16:111–126, 1988

Kovacs M: The Children's Depression Inventory: a self-rated depression scale for school-aged youngsters (unpublished manuscript). Pittsburgh, PA, University of Pittsburgh School of Medicine, April 1983

Kovacs M, Beck AT: Maladaptive cognitive structures in depression. Am J Psychiatry 135:525–533, 1978

Leitenberg H, Yost LW, Carroll-Wilson M: Negative cognitive errors in children: questionnaire development, normative data, and comparisons between children with and without self-reported symptoms of depression, low self-esteem, and evaluation anxiety. J Consult Clin Psychol 54:528–536, 1986

Lewinsohn PM, Muñoz RF, Youngren MA, et al: Control Your Depression. New York, Prentice-Hall, 1986

Lewinsohn PM, Clarke G, Rohde P: The Adolescent Coping With Depression Course. Paper presented at the annual meeting of the Association for the Advancement of Behavior Therapy, Washington, DC, November 1989

McCauley E, Mitchell JR, Burke P, et al: Cognitive attributes of depression in children and adolescents. J Consult Clin Psychol 56:903–908, 1988

McCauley E, Mitchell J, Calderon R: Cognitive attributes of depression in children and adolescents: changes with remission and recurrence of depression.

Paper presented at the World Congress of Cognitive Therapy, Oxford, England, June 1989

McGee R, Anderson J, Williams S, et al: Cognitive correlates of depressive symptoms in 11-year-old children. J Abnorm Child Psychol 14:517–524, 1986

Meichenbaum D: Cognitive-Behavior Modification: An Integrative Approach. New York, Plenum, 1977

Mullins LL, Siegel LJ, Hodges K: Cognitive problem-solving and life event correlates of depressive symptoms in children. J Abnorm Child Psychol 13:305–314, 1985

Nisbett RE, Fong GT, Lehman DR, et al: Teaching reasoning. Science 238:625–631, 1987

Nolen-Hoeksema S, Girgus JS, Seligman MEP: Learned helplessness in children: a longitudinal study of depression, achievement, and explanatory style. J Pers Soc Psychol 51:435–442, 1986

Person J, Burns DD: Mechanisms of action of cognitive therapy: the relative contribution of technical and interpersonal interventions. Cognitive Therapy and Research 9:539–551, 1985

Person J, Burns DD, Perloff JM: Predictors of dropout and outcome in cognitive therapy for depression in a private practice setting. Cognitive Therapy and Research 12:557–575, 1989

Reynolds WM, Coats KI: A comparison of cognitive-behavioral therapy and relaxation training for the treatment of depression in adolescents. J Consult Clin Psychol 54:653–660, 1986

Rotheram-Borus MJ, Trautman PD: Hopelessness, depression, and suicidal intent among adolescent suicide attempters. J Am Child Adolesc Psychiatry 27:700–704, 1988

Ryan ND, Puig-Antich J, Ambrosini P, et al: The clinical picture of major depression in children and adolescents. Arch Gen Psychiatry 44:854–861, 1987

Sacco WP, Graves DJ: Childhood depression, interpersonal problem-solving, and self-ratings of performance. Journal of Clinical Child Psychology 13:10–15, 1984

Schrodt GR Jr, Fitzgerald BA: Cognitive therapy with adolescents. Am J Psychother 41:402–408, 1987

Schrodt GR Jr, Wright JH: Inpatient treatment of adolescents, in Cognitive Therapy: Applications in Psychiatric and Medical Settings. Edited by Freeman A, Greenwood V. New York, Human Sciences Press, 1986, pp 69–82

Schrodt GR Jr, Fitzgerald BA, Wright JH, et al: The negative cognitive triad in depressed adolescents. Paper presented at the World Congress of Cognitive Therapy, Oxford, England, June 1989

Seligman MEP, Peterson C: A learned helplessness perspective on childhood depression: theory and research, in Depression in Young People: Developmental and Clinical Perspectives. Edited by Rutter M, Izard CE, Read PB. New York, Guilford, 1986, pp 223–249

Seligman ME, Peterson C, Kaslow NJ, et al: Attributional style and depressive symptoms among children. J Abnorm Psychol 93:235–238, 1984

Teri L: Depression in adolescence: its relationship to assertion and various aspects of self-image. Journal of Clinical Child Psychology 11:101–106, 1982

Trautman PD, Rotheram-Borus MJ: Cognitive behavior therapy with children and adolescents, in American Psychiatric Press Review of Psychiatry, Vol 7. Edited by Frances AJ, Hales RE. Washington, DC, American Psychiatric Press, 1988, pp 584–607

Vallis TM, Shaw BF, Dobson KS: The cognitive therapy scale: psychometric properties. J Consult Clin Psychol 54:381–385, 1986

Weisz JR, Stevens JS, Curry JF, et al: Control-related cognitions and depression among inpatient children and adolescents. J Am Acad Child Adolesc Psychiatry 28:358–363, 1989

Werry JS, Wollersheim JP: Behavior therapy with children and adolescents: a twenty-year overview. J Am Acad Child Adolesc Psychiatry 28:1–18, 1989

Wilkes TCR, Rush AJ: Adaptations of cognitive therapy for depressed adolescents. J Am Acad Child Adolesc Psychiatry 27:381–386, 1988

Wright JH, Schrodt GR Jr: Combined cognitive therapy and pharmacotherapy, in Handbook of Cognitive Therapy. Edited by Freeman A, Simon KM, Arkowitz H, et al. New York, Plenum, 1989, pp 267–282

CHAPTER 10

Pharmacological Treatment of Major Depression

Neal D. Ryan, M.D.

Multiple lines of evidence support strong similarities and relationships among the child, adolescent, and adult types of major depressive disorder. The clinical picture of depression during childhood and adolescence is stable and similar to that observed during adulthood (Ryan et al. 1987a). The duration and pattern of recurrence of depression in school-age children are also like those observed in adults (Kovacs et al. 1984a, 1984b). Studies of familial transmission of depression throughout the life span show that there is an increased rate of depression in adult family members of depressed children and adolescents. An increased rate of depression occurs in the child and adolescent offspring of depressed adults (Merikangas et al. 1985; J. Puig-Antich, unpublished data, 1986; Puig-Antich et al. 1989; Weissman et al. 1987). From school-age children through reproductive-age adults, the younger the age at onset of major depression, the more depression found in family members. Recent evidence suggests that increases in the rate of depression in children and adolescents parallel those found in adults (N.D. Ryan, unpublished data, 1989). Also, strong similarities exist between neuroendocrine changes in child and adolescent depression and those found in adult depression (Goetz et al. 1987; Puig-Antich et al. 1983, 1984a, 1984b, 1984c, 1984d; Ryan et al. 1988a). (See Chapters 1, 2, and 3.)

The biological and psychological factors, consequences, and correlates of depression are not constant throughout the life span. Biological developments that are probably central to the control of affect include the ongoing maturational development of noradrenergic central nervous system (CNS) pathways throughout the late teens and into the early twenties (Goldman-Rakic and Brown 1982) and the changing sex steroid milieu of the brain that occurs with adolescence. Evidence for a biological effect of maturation on control of affect is provided by the observation by Rapoport et al. (1978) that the stimulant amphetamine rarely, if ever, causes euphoria in prepubertal children, whereas that compound regularly produces euphoria in adolescents and adults.

In this chapter the pharmacokinetics, pharmacodynamics, indications, contraindications, and side effects of tricyclic antidepressants (TCAs) in the treatment of depressed children and adolescents are discussed. Brief reference is made to the use of nontricyclic antidepressants such as fluoxetine and monoamine oxidase inhibitors (MAOIs). Clomipramine, trazodone, carbamazepine, and valproic acid are sometimes used in treatment-resistant depression in adults. Their use in children and adolescents with depressive disorders is not a common practice and they will not be reviewed.

TRICYCLIC ANTIDEPRESSANTS

Given the experience with using tricyclics in prepubertal children for the treatment of enuresis and given the data reviewed above showing strong similarities among child, adolescent, and adult forms of depression, clinicians began openly treating both children and adolescents with tricyclic-type antidepressants. These early open treatment reports suggested efficacy of TCAs in this age group (Geller et al. 1983; Petti and Conners 1983). Before considering controlled clinical studies, we consider developmental effects on the pharmacokinetics and pharmacodynamics of these medications.

Pharmacokinetics and Pharmacodynamics of Tricyclic Antidepressants

As with the majority of medications, TCAs are metabolized most rapidly by children, somewhat less rapidly by adolescents, and even more slowly by adults. There is extensive first-pass metabolism of these compounds by the liver and extensive protein binding (70–95% in adults, somewhat less in younger people). Tricyclics are metabolized primarily in the liver by oxidation, aromatic hydroxylation, and demethylation. About 5% of the population are slow hydroxylators of these compounds, resulting in a much higher plasma level of the parent compound and a much longer half-life (Potter et al. 1982); this characteristic is genetically determined (Sjoqvist and Bertilsson 1984). Adults who receive similar doses show a more than 30-fold difference in plasma levels (Sjoqvist and Bertilsson 1984); the same wide variation occurs in children and adolescents (Preskorn et al. 1983; Ryan et al. 1987b).

The difference in the pharmacokinetics and pharmacodynamics of TCAs in children and adolescents compared with adults has several implications. Children and adolescents may require a relatively higher weight-adjusted dose to achieve the same plasma level as has been found therapeutic in adults with depression. Unfortunately less appreciated, children and adolescents are more vulnerable to the anticholinergic withdrawal effect because of the rapid metabolism and subsequent rapid clearance of these compounds from the blood. An example of the latter is the occasional adolescent on a once-a-day dose who is found to have nausea and myalgia shortly before the next medication dose is due. This effect could easily be confused with medication toxicity. The key here is if the side effects are seen shortly before rather than after the next medication dose, then the reaction is most probably related to withdrawal. Not unexpectedly, the author has seen this withdrawal reaction more frequently in younger children, in whom even a twice-daily dosage schedule will frequently be insufficient. As reviewed by Dilsaver and Greden (1984), the most common symptoms associated with stopping antidepressant medication, probably due to anticholinergic withdrawal effects, are somatic or gastrointestinal distress, anxiety, agitation, sleep disturbance characterized by excessive vivid dreaming, initial and middle insomnia, and psychic and behavioral activation.

Requirement for Frequent Electrocardiograms in Children and Adolescents Receiving Tricyclic Antidepressants

The juvenile cardiac system, both in humans and animals, is much more susceptible to the cardiotoxic effects of TCAs (Ryan et al. 1987b). For this reason, electrocardiograms (ECGs) should be obtained more frequently when treating a child or adolescent than when treating an adult patient. A baseline ECG should be obtained prior to starting therapy with tricyclics. ECGs are needed for two reasons: 1) to serve as a comparison for later ECGs and 2) to rule out the existence of an aberrant cardiac conduction system. For example, some children have a congenital anomaly of the electrical system of the heart (Wolff-Parkinson-White syndrome is the most significant of such congenital conduction anomalies) that provides a split pathway for conduction of the electrical signal. If the conduction times are delayed, which is an effect of tricyclic medications, a reentrant pathway can be established (i.e., a signal can go around and around in a circle), causing the heart to go into fibrillation and the patient to die. Thus, a baseline ECG is strongly recommended to rule out this unlikely but important possibility in an otherwise healthy child.

The ECG rhythm strips are recommended at intervals throughout the tricyclic titration period, not simply upon achieving a therapeutic dose. I recommend the following cardiac limitations to tricyclic titration: PR interval of no more than 0.21 second, QRS widening that represents no more than a 30% increase over the baseline QRS interval, heart rate of no more than 120 beats per minute, and blood pressure of no more than 135 mmHg systolic and 85 mmHg diastolic. Although hypotension is occasionally seen and is frequently dose limiting, vascular barometric changes are much more likely to be in the *hypertensive* direction in both children and adolescents; these are frequently dose limiting.

Other Side Effects

In children and adolescents, the other side effects of TCAs are virtually identical to those in adults. Most prominent are the anticholinergic side effects, including dry mouth, constipation, delayed micturition, etc. Usually these side effects are not dependent on dosage. Side effects should be handled in the same way as they are handled in adults. For dry mouth the clinician may suggest a sugar-free gum or sugar-free sour candy to avoid an increase in dental caries. For constipation a diet higher in fiber or Metamucil is recommended—not a laxative.

Mild confusional states have also been reported, especially with higher plasma levels (Preskorn et al. 1983), which may well necessitate dose reductions. Other clinically significant side effects seen throughout the age range include lowering the seizure threshold, enhancing CNS depressant effects of alcohol or other CNS active compounds, photosensitivity, induction of mania or psychosis, peripheral neurological symptoms, and gynecomastia in the male or breast enlargement and galactorrhea in the female.

The only other side effect that I have observed with surprising frequency is a rash that is generally not linked to the antidepressant compound itself but to the yellow dye, FD&C Yellow No. 5 (tartrazine), which is added to many but not all tricyclic formulations. In the event that the patient experiences a rash, the first thing to do is contact the pharmacy to find out whether the particular strength of the particular compound dispensed to that individual did indeed contain tartrazine.

Interaction of Tricyclic Antidepressants With Other Medications

The clinical significance of interactions of TCAs with other medications in children and adolescents includes potentiation of CNS depressants such as alcohol. When used concomitantly with barbiturates or with cigarette smoking, TCAs are metabolized at an increased rate, resulting in lowered plasma levels, possibly below the therapeutic range. When used concurrently with oral birth control pills and other estrogenic compounds, TCAs are metabolized at a decreased rate, possibly leading to toxicity. The use of marijuana with TCAs increases sinus tachycardia. Phenytoin toxicity increases with the use of TCAs (Rizack 1989).

Plasma Level Ranges Used in Clinical Treatment

In the absence of definitive controlled studies, TCAs are prescribed to children and adolescents in order to achieve therapeutic plasma levels similar to those in adults. With nortriptyline, a plasma level of 75–150 ng/ml is usually sought (Geller et al. 1983, 1985), and with imipramine or amitriptyline a total plasma level of parent compound plus demethylated metabolites of 200 ng/ml or slightly more is targeted (Preskorn et al. 1982; Strober 1989).

No definitive guideline can be given for the optimum length of treatment before declaring a patient unresponsive to TCAs. Studies with adults suggest that a 6- to 8-week trial, with plasma levels in the therapeutic range, should be completed before medication is discontinued.

If TCA therapy seems to produce substantial therapeutic improvement in a child or adolescent, no data exist to serve as a guide to the length of treatment. Therefore, the best advice is to continue the medication for 4–6 months, as in an adult. The astute clinician will taper the medication during the summer or during a school holiday. However, medication should not be tapered off before the adolescent takes the important college examinations such as the entrance examinations.

CONTROLLED STUDIES OF TRICYCLIC ANTIDEPRESSANTS IN CHILDREN AND ADOLESCENTS

Surprisingly, placebo-controlled studies have yet to clearly demonstrate the efficacy of TCAs for mood disorders in children and adolescents. In children, a major difficulty in demonstrating the efficacy of TCAs has been a relatively high placebo response rate over the short term for major depressive disorder. At present, no studies have been done to determine whether a high placebo response rate is seen over the long term.

If TCAs do prove to be effective for at least some adolescents with major depression, it is quite possible that the effect will not be as strong *on average* as it is in adults, for two reasons: 1) the improvement achieved by many adolescents who receive TCAs may be more modest than that achieved by adults, or 2) some adolescents may benefit as much as adults from TCAs, but at the present time, we cannot distinguish their group from nonresponders.

Two types of control studies have been done regarding the efficacy of TCAs in children and adolescents. The first type is an open-label, plasma level–response study. In this type of study, the research clinician knows which medication is being used. When patients are treated with a fixed (weight-adjusted) dosage of TCAs, a large variation in plasma levels occurs. The researcher looks for the relationship between the plasma level of TCAs and the clinical outcome.

In prepubertal children, open-label, plasma level–response studies have strongly indicated the efficacy of imipramine. Preskorn et al. (1982) suggest a therapeutic window of 125–225 ng/ml for imipramine, which is similar to the therapeutic window of nortriptyline in adults. Puig-Antich et al. (1987) report a threshold effect of imipramine with plasma levels over 150 ng/ml, but without an upper range in children and adolescents, typical of adult studies of imipramine plasma levels.

In adolescents, two studies using this design have been reported. In one, 34 outpatient adolescents were treated with imipramine titrated to 5 mg/kg/day as limited by side effects, achieving a mean dose of 4.5 mg/kg/day (Ryan et al. 1986). In this study, there was no evidence of a plasma level threshold or window within which imipramine was efficacious. In another study using a similar design, imipramine was given to inpatient adolescents. This study also did not find a statistically significant therapeutic threshold. However, there was an almost statistically significant trend for a better response to higher plasma levels (Strober 1989).

The second and more definitive type of control study is the medication/placebo type. In this type of study, subjects are randomized to receive either medication or placebo. Neither the patient, the family, nor the research clinician knows whether the child or adolescent is being treated with medication or placebo.

In prepubertal children, results of medication/placebo studies are mixed. One group reported very interesting data on a small sample, suggesting that medication is superior to placebo in dexamethasone-nonsuppressing prepubertal children (Preskorn et al. 1987). Two other studies, one of imipramine (Puig-Antich et al. 1987) and another of nortriptyline (Geller et al. 1989), found no differences between medication and placebo. A possible confounding variable is the high rate of response to placebo frequently seen in younger children.

In adolescents, two medication/placebo studies have been completed. The first used amitriptyline (Kramer and Feiguine 1981). Because of a small cell size (10 subjects each receiving medication or placebo), the negative finding of this study was not surprising—a larger sample was probably required to show a significant effect, if there were one. More recently, Geller (1989) reported negative findings when adolescents were treated with nortriptyline titrated to achieve a plasma level in the therapeutic range (plasma levels, in general, titrated to 75–100 ng/ml). This study gave absolutely no indication by any analysis that medication was superior to placebo.

Nevertheless, despite these mixed and somewhat negative early data, the returns are not in yet on the final efficacy of TCAs in treating adolescents with major depression. Very few studies have been reported. More importantly, the total number of adolescents entered in all medication/placebo studies to date combined is under 100. On the other hand, only 30 of the 50 well-controlled, double-blind studies of imipramine in adults have found that the active compound is superior to placebo. In addition, it must be emphasized that there are no other pharmacological or psychological treatments whose efficacy has been demonstrated by controlled studies in either children or adolescents with major depression.

It is possible that with more study tricyclics will eventually prove to be as effective in child and/or adolescent depression as they are in adult depression. Alternatively, tricyclics may prove to be quite effective in one subgroup of children or adolescents with major depression but not in others, or tricyclics in general may prove to be less effective or not superior to a placebo in this age group.

The possible reasons that TCAs are less effective include maturational changes in the brain that make the same disorder unresponsive to certain pharmacological interventions during childhood or adolescence but more responsive in adulthood; effects of the particularly high levels of sex steroid hormones found during adolescence on the central control of mood; the possibility that children or adolescents may require different plasma levels (either higher or lower) for optimal efficacy of TCAs (although this is somewhat unlikely); and the strong possibility that more children and adolescents who have major depression will turn out with time to have bipolar disorder, which may be relatively less responsive to TCAs. (See Chapters 12 and 13.)

Summary of Tricyclic Antidepressant Studies

Plasma level–response data from prepubertal children give significant evidence for tricyclic efficacy in this age group, but definitive data from medication/placebo studies do not as yet corroborate these findings. In adolescents, data from controlled studies are not available to demonstrate the specific efficacy of any pharmacological treatment. Without a doubt, all treatments have a considerable nonspecific effect, including both the placebo effect with medication and the general expectancy effects seen in virtually all studies of psychotherapy for all psychiatric disorders. Therefore, all of these treatments "work," but none is shown to work through specific mechanisms rather than simply the nonspecific effect of treatment expectation and seeing a therapist weekly.

NONTRICYCLIC ANTIDEPRESSANT TREATMENT

Although most studies on the use of nontricyclic antidepressants in depressed prepubertal children report a high overall response rate, the response rate appears to be lower in adolescents. In any group of adolescents treated with TCAs, many will have, at best, a partial response. Therefore, we need to look at the efficacy of other, nontricyclic antidepressants. Three will be reviewed: fluoxetine, a nontricyclic antidepressant that, like some tricyclics, blocks serotonin reuptake; lithium augmentation of TCAs; and MAOIs.

There are few data on the use of fluoxetine in children or adolescents with major depressive disorder, although several groups are now collecting open pilot data. Just as when this compound is used in adults, the clinician must remember its remarkably long half-life. This long half-life is most critical in the compound's interactions with MAOIs. Specifically, the clinician must wait the full 2 weeks after stopping MAOIs before starting fluoxetine. Fluoxetine and MAOIs should not be used in combination because, like other serotonergic reuptake blockers, fluoxetine is extremely dangerous when combined with MAOIs. However, unlike all other medications, *after stopping fluoxetine, a hiatus of 6 weeks or more is required before starting MAOIs.* This cannot be overemphasized.

Of two open clinical trial reports concerning the use of lithium augmentation in patients unresponsive to tricyclics, one was positive and one was negative. One report, on outpatients, suggested that about half of the adolescents unresponsive to tricyclics showed moderate or better improvement with the addition to their tricyclic therapy of lithium titrated to approximately 0.6 mEq/L (Ryan et al. 1988c). The other report, on inpatients, failed to suggest efficacy of lithium augmentation (Strober 1989). In the outpatient study, which did suggest efficacy, there continued to be improvement between weeks 3 and 6. There was no evidence of an improvement within a day or two of starting lithium, which had been suggested in the earliest reports about open lithium augmentation of a TCA response in adults. In adolescents, as in adults, this combination should be tried for a month to 6 weeks before deciding that it is not helpful.

There is only one report of open trial treatment with MAOIs in adolescents with major depression (Ryan et al. 1988b). In this study, about 50% of the adolescents had both significant clinical improvement and reliably followed the MAOI diet. Dietary noncompliance and potential interaction with other medication or street drugs are of paramount concern with MAOIs. Most of the necessary sacrifices required by the MAOI diet are not problematic for adolescents because, in general, they have less of a taste for fermented and aged foods. (The exceptions, however, may be pizza and beer.) Surprisingly, a portion of adolescents who achieved moderate or marked improvement while taking MAOIs nevertheless could or would not follow the diet and required discontinuation of MAOI therapy. MAOIs are not recommended for impulsive adolescents or those with unreliable families, even while the adolescent is hospitalized, because an improvement during the hospitalization does not seem to be helpful in encouraging the adolescent to reliably follow the MAOI diet after discharge.

PHARMACOLOGICAL FLOW SHEET

Table 10–1 presents a suggested flow sheet for the pharmacological treatment of children and adolescents with major depressive disorder.

Table 10–1. Flow sheet for pharmacological treatment of child and adolescent major depression

Initial evaluation	Obtain child psychiatric and medical history and family psychiatric history. Get baseline electrocardiogram (ECG), complete blood count, and liver function tests now to save time when starting tricyclic antidepressants (TCAs).
Does child or adolescent still meet criteria for major depressive disorder (MDD) at the second visit (or after a week in the hospital)?	If the child or adolescent's depression responds (for whatever reason) after initiating TCAs, the clinician generally continues the medication for 4 months or more. There is a large nonspecific therapeutic effect of talking with someone, discussing symptoms, and knowing that help is available. Many children and adolescents will be dramatically better 1 week after the initial evaluation despite having very severe and long-duration symptoms at presentation. Therefore, initiation of pharmacological intervention should be delayed until at least the second visit.
Consider psychotherapy alone or in combination with antidepressant treatment.	In the absence of experimental data, "clinical intuition" and preference of the child and family must guide the clinician in deciding whether to try psychotherapy alone prior to a trial of antidepressant medication. If medications are used, the clinician must provide considerable psychoeducation and support for the child and family while waiting for the medication to work. As is the case with all child and adolescent psychiatric disorders, contact with the school is usually vital.
Obtain baseline ECG. Make certain a recent physical examination has been done.	The juvenile cardiac system is more sensitive to cardiotoxic effects of TCAs; therefore, ECGs must be obtained more frequently in this population than in adults. A baseline ECG is necessary for comparison purposes and also to rule out Wolff-Parkinson-White syndrome or other congenital conduction abnormalities.

Table 10–1   (continued)

Begin child or adolescent on approximately 1.0 mg/kg/day of imipramine (IMI), desipramine (DMI), or amitriptyline (AMI), or 0.5 mg/kg/day of nortriptyline (NT). Use a tid divided dose for children and a bid or qd dose for adolescents.	In children, these medications have a very short half-life, so a tid divided dosage is important to minimize the peak TCA levels (ECG changes correlate with peak levels) and to prevent anticholinergic withdrawal symptoms between doses. Adolescents can tolerate a less-frequent dosage schedule, which may improve compliance. *In all cases, the parent or guardian must be responsible for medication, not the child or adolescent. These compounds are dangerous or lethal in accidental or deliberate overdose.*
Obtain ECG rhythm strips, heart rate, and blood pressure at each dosage increase.	Limit PR interval to less than 0.21 seconds, QRS interval to less than 30% widening over baseline, heart rate to less than 120 beats/minute, and blood pressure to less than 135 systolic and 85 diastolic.
Increase dose of IMI, DMI, or AMI (in divided doses) every 3–7 days as limited by side effects and ECG. Maximum recommended dosage of these compounds is 5.0 mg/kg/day. Maximum dosage of NT is likely to be less than 2.0 mg/kg/day, but compound must be titrated by plasma level.	Plasma levels should be obtained at a standardized 10–12 hours after the last dose of medication. Plasma level guidelines from adult studies and from the few studies in children and adolescents suggest that for IMI or AMI, the total level of parent compound plus demethylated metabolite (DMI or NT) should be approximately 225 ng/ml. For NT, the total should be in the range of 75–150 ng/ml.

Table 10–1   (continued)

Child or adolescent responds.	Continue medication for minimum of 4 months. At discontinuation, taper medication over 7–10 days. Watch for recurrence of depression at discontinuation. Continue psychoeducation and other support for child and family.
Child or adolescent has minimal or partial response.	Continue medication for at least 6 weeks before deciding that it is not effective. Document adequate plasma response level (child may be a very rapid or a very slow metabolizer of the compound).
Consider: 1) lithium augmentation of TCAs, 2) fluoxetine, or 3) monoamine oxidase inhibitors (MAOIs).	There are no controlled studies of any of these treatments in children or adolescents, but at least some open studies have suggested that each *may* have a part to play in the treatment-refractory MDD in this age group. The use of MAOIs is particularly problematic and the clinician must read in-depth about their use, including their *potentially fatal interactions*, before attempting their use. *Switching between different MAOIs or from an MAOI to a TCA requires a 2-week washout period. Switching from fluoxetine to an MAOI requires a 6-week washout period.*
Consider alternative psychotherapeutic approaches.	Is a cognitive-behavioral approach or an approach based on interpersonal therapy, both of which have demonstrated efficacy in adult major depression, appropriate for this child or adolescent? Are different family, school, or social interventions indicated?

SUMMARY

In summary, scientific studies of pharmacological treatment of adolescent major depression are in their infancy. In prepubertal major depression, multiple plasma level–response studies suggest that there is a relationship between plasma levels in the "therapeutic range" and good clinical outcome. However, double-blind comparisons of medication and placebo do not demonstrate the superiority of medication in most studies, probably because of the high placebo response rate in this population.

In adolescents there are not yet any controlled studies of either pharmacological or psychological treatment of major depressive disorder that demonstrate the superiority of active treatment over placebo. Therefore, the clinician is forced to rely on open treatment data for adolescents, extrapolation from studies in adults, and the few studies available in children.

At present, tricyclic and other antidepressant treatments have a part to play in the treatment of depressed children and adolescents. However, it is clear that today's recommendation may or may not be applicable in several years' time, depending on the outcome of currently ongoing and planned studies. The clinician needs to keep up with this rapidly changing area.

REFERENCES

Dilsaver SC, Greden JF: Antidepressant withdrawal phenomena. Biol Psychiatry 19:237–256, 1984

Geller B: A double-blind placebo-controlled study of nortriptyline in adolescents with major depression. Abstract presented at the annual meeting of the NCDEU (New Clinical Drug Evaluation Unit), Key Biscayne, FL, May 1989

Geller B, Perel JM, Knitter EF, et al: Nortriptyline in major depressive disorder in children: response, steady-state plasma levels, predictive kinetics, and pharmacokinetics. Psychopharmacol Bull 19:62–65, 1983

Geller B, Cooper TB, Farooki ZQ, et al: Dose and plasma levels of nortriptyline and chlorpromazine in nondelusionally depressed adolescents. Am J Psychiatry 142:336–338, 1985

Geller B, Cooper TB, McCombs HG, et al: Double-blind, placebo-controlled study of nortriptyline in depressed children using a "fixed plasma level" design. Psychopharmacol Bull 25:101–108, 1989

Goetz RR, Puig-Antich J, Ryan N, et al: Electroencephalographic sleep of adolescents with major depression and normal controls. Arch Gen Psychiatry 44:61–68, 1987

Goldman-Rakic P, Brown RM: Postnatal development of monoamine content and synthesis on the cerebral cortex of rhesus monkeys. Developmental Brain Research 4:339–349, 1982

Kovacs M, Feinberg TL, Crouse-Novak MA, et al: Depressive disorders in childhood, I: a longitudinal prospective study of characteristics and recovery. Arch Gen Psychiatry 41:229–237, 1984a

Kovacs M, Feinberg TL, Crouse-Novak MA, et al: Depressive disorders in childhood, II: a longitudinal study of the risk for a subsequent major depression. Arch Gen Psychiatry 41:643–649, 1984b

Kramer AD, Feiguine RJ: Clinical effects of amitriptyline in adolescent depression: a pilot study. J Am Acad Child Psychiatry 20:636–644, 1981

Merikangas KR, Leckman JF, Prusoff BA, et al: Familial transmission of depression and alcoholism. Arch Gen Psychiatry 42:367–372, 1985

Petti TA, Conners CK: Changes in behavioral ratings of depressed children treated with imipramine. J Am Acad Child Psychiatry 22:355–360, 1983

Potter WZ, Calil HM, Sutfin TA, et al: Active metabolites of imipramine and desipramine in man. Clin Pharmacol Ther 31:393–401, 1982

Preskorn SH, Weller EB, Weller RA: Depression in children: relationship between plasma imipramine levels and response. J Clin Psychiatry 43:450–453, 1982

Preskorn SH, Weller EB, Weller RA, et al: Plasma levels of imipramine and adverse effects in children. Am J Psychiatry 140:1332–1335, 1983

Preskorn SH, Weller EB, Hughes CW, et al: Depression in prepubertal children: dexamethasone nonsuppression predicts differential response to imipramine vs. placebo. Psychopharmacol Bull 23:128–133, 1987

Puig-Antich J, Goetz R, Hanlon C, et al: Sleep architecture and REM sleep measures in prepubertal major depressive patients: studies during recovery from the depressive episode in a drug-free state. Arch Gen Psychiatry 40:187–192, 1983

Puig-Antich J, Goetz R, Davies M, et al: Growth hormone secretion in prepubertal children with major depression, II: sleep-related plasma concentrations during a depressive episode. Arch Gen Psychiatry 41:463–466, 1984a

Puig-Antich J, Novacenko H, Davies M, et al: Growth hormone secretion in prepubertal children with major depression, I: final report on response to insulin-induced hypoglycemia during a depressive episode. Arch Gen Psychiatry 41:455–460, 1984b

Puig-Antich J, Novacenko H, Davies M, et al: Growth hormone secretion in prepubertal children with major depression, III: response to insulin-induced hypoglycemia after recovery from a depressive episode and in a drug-free state. Arch Gen Psychiatry 41:471–475, 1984c

Puig-Antich J, Goetz R, Davies M, et al: Growth hormone secretion in prepubertal children with major depression, IV: sleep-related plasma concentrations in a drug-free, fully recovered clinical state. Arch Gen Psychiatry 41:479–485, 1984d

Puig-Antich J, Perel JM, Lupatkin W, et al: Imipramine in prepubertal major depressive disorders. Arch Gen Psychiatry 44:81–89, 1987

Puig-Antich J, Goetz D, Davies M, et al: A controlled family history study of prepubertal major depressive disorder. Arch Gen Psychiatry 46:406–418, 1989

Rapoport JL, Buchsbaum M, Weingartner H, et al: Dextroamphetamine: behavioral and cognitive effects on normal prepubertal boys. Science 199:560–563, 1978

Rizack MA: The Medical Letter Handbook of Adverse Drug Interactions. New Rochelle, NY, The Medical Letter, 1989

Ryan ND, Puig-Antich J, Cooper TB, et al: Imipramine in adolescent major depression: plasma levels and clinical response. Acta Psychiatr Scand 73:275–288, 1986

Ryan ND, Puig-Antich J, Ambrosini P, et al: The clinical picture of major depression in children and adolescents. Arch Gen Psychiatry 44:854–861, 1987a

Ryan ND, Puig-Antich J, Cooper TB, et al: Relative safety of single versus divided dose imipramine in adolescent major depression. J Am Acad Child Adolesc Psychiatry 26:400–406, 1987b

Ryan ND, Puig-Antich J, Rabinovich H, et al: Growth hormone response to desmethylimipramine in depressed and suicidal adolescents. J Affective Disord 15:323–337, 1988a

Ryan ND, Puig-Antich J, Rabinovich H, et al: MAOIs in adolescent major depression unresponsive to tricyclic antidepressants. J Am Acad Child Adolesc Psychiatry 27:755–758, 1988b

Ryan ND, Meyer V, Dachille S, et al: Lithium antidepressant augmentation in TCA-refractory depression in adolescents. J Am Acad Child Adolesc Psychiatry 27:371–376, 1988c

Sjoqvist F, Bertilsson L: Clinical pharmacology of antidepressant drugs: pharmacogenetics. Adv Biochem Psychopharmacol 39:359–372, 1984

Strober M: Effects of imipramine, lithium, and fluoxetine in the treatment of adolescent major depression. Abstract presented at the annual meeting of the NCDEU (New Clinical Drug Evaluation Unit), Key Biscayne, FL, May 1989

Weissman MM, Gammon DG, John K, et al: Children of depressed parents: increased psychopathology and early onset of major depression. Arch Gen Psychiatry 44:847–853, 1987

CHAPTER 11

Inpatient Treatment of Depression

Katherine A. Raymer, M.D.

In recent years significant progress has been made in understanding depressive disorders in children and adolescents. However, inpatient treatment has received little attention. Hospital admission often reflects a severe degree of psychopathology and/or the failure of outpatient treatment.

This chapter outlines the essential features of inpatient psychiatric treatment of depressed children and adolescents. Indications for treatment and the general characteristics of an inpatient psychiatric unit are discussed. Treatment issues are examined from the time of admission until discharge. Continuing treatment and follow-up after discharge are emphasized.

INDICATIONS FOR INPATIENT TREATMENT

Specific guidelines for determining the need for hospitalization for depressed children and adolescents have not been developed. However, general guidelines have been put forth by several authors. Irwin (1982a) recommended inpatient treatment for children and adolescents with bizarre and irrational behavior not amenable to outpatient treatment, and with dangerous behavior toward themselves and others.

Parmelee (1986) lists four indications for the psychiatric hospitalization of the adolescent and young adult: the presence of imminent danger to self or others, a prolonged period of disturbing and disruptive behavior in which outpatient intervention has been unsuccessful or refused, lack of progress or persistent resistance to change in outpatient treatment, and the request or requirement by the court for inpatient psychiatric evaluation.

Dalton et al. (1987) noted that the psychiatric hospitalization of preschool children was underinvestigated. They examined contributing factors in 18 cases. Two basic groups emerged: one of autistic children and another of children who had the following four contributing factors: mothers suffering from major psychiatric disorders; fathers not living in the home; alternative placements (such as foster homes) unable to contain the behavior of the

233

child; and a diagnosis of conduct disorder, sometimes associated with depressive disorders.

Frequently, the patient manifests various psychiatric symptoms, including some depressive symptoms that may or may not fulfill any diagnostic criteria. If the symptoms are severe and significantly interfere with daily life, the child or adolescent should be admitted for a comprehensive diagnostic assessment.

When the child or adolescent has a diagnosis of depressive disorder, admission is indicated for suicidality, feelings of hopelessness leading to risk-taking behavior, vegetative symptoms endangering the physical health of the child or adolescent, and the suspicion of physical or sexual abuse. Psychosis complicating any of these symptoms adds urgency to the need for admission. Depressed children and adolescents with a comorbid diagnosis such as alcohol and drug abuse and conduct disorder are at a high risk for suicide (Shafii et al. 1988), and immediate hospitalization is indicated. (See Chapter 1.)

THE INPATIENT UNIT

The various aspects of an inpatient unit, such as physical structure, staff, and programs, will be discussed. According to the American Psychiatric Association's *Standards for Psychiatric Facilities Serving Children and Adolescents* (Prugh 1971, pp. 72–75), "The physical plant . . . must provide a safe and clean environment, which is suitable for the diagnostic, therapeutic and preventive programs that are planned to meet the therapeutic and developmental needs of the children." Adequate and appropriate heating, ventilation, lighting, fire protection, bathing, and toilet facilities are essential. Sleeping areas should provide comfort, dignity, and privacy consistent with the welfare of the patients and the goals of the treatment program. Active and quiet areas, space for each child's possessions, facilities for physical examinations and emergency treatment, centrally placed stations for nursing and child-care personnel, and private space for family interviews and visits are necessary parts of the physical plant. Harper and Geraty (1989) point out that child psychiatry programs require more square feet than adult psychiatry programs and suggest a minimum of 300 square feet of off-ward support space for interview rooms and educational and recreational activities.

Staffing, according to Prugh (1971), should include a qualified medical staff or faculty, preferably a physician who is board certified or experienced in child psychiatry, a nursing service under the direction of a qualified psychiatric nurse, a psychological service under the direction of a fully qualified psychologist, a social work service under the direction of a fully qualified social worker, and a qualified activity therapist. If the unit itself provides an educational program in whole or part, then an educational director and staff that meet the accreditation requirements for special education are needed. The availability of a qualified pediatrician or a physician with training and experience in working with children and of a qualified neurologist with experience in child neurology is also needed. Child-care workers, described as nontraditional professionals whose training and qualifications have not yet been formally standardized, are an essential component of many psychiatric facilities. These individuals function in multiple capacities, such as companions and providers of structure, limits, and rewards.

Harper and Geraty (1989) have observed that child psychiatric inpatient programs require more staff than adult programs and suggest including expressive therapists, speech and language therapists, and physical therapists. Geraty (1989) advises that staff be selected on the basis of training, experience, enthusiasm, love for children and/or families, philosophical consistency with the ideas of the unit, and compatibility with other staff.

Many types of child and adolescent inpatient psychiatric programs have been developed, but few have been described in the literature. Irwin (1982a) described various models, ranging from the inclusion of children on adult psychiatric wards to the more common psychiatric units for children. He identifies the "traditional" model within the latter group as having individual psychotherapy as its core, with the utilization of the child-guidance method of collaborative treatment. Woolston (1989) has reported one of the newer approaches to inpatient treatment of children, the transactional risk model, which is based on changing child-environmental transactions so that positive development occurs. He contrasts this approach to the approach that assumes linear expression of a psychiatric disorder based on a single etiology, in which the focus of hospitalization would be to "cure" the particular problem in the child or family. Zinn (1979) described the various types of programs for inpatient treatment of the adolescent, which differ in terms of conceptual approach, length of stay, the physical site of treatment, a specific age group, "closed" and "open" units, and whether adolescents are mixed with adults.

Kahn and Boyer (1980) reviewed 10 years of adolescent inpatient treatment and also surveyed treatment at adolescent psychiatric facilities across the nation. They found that 12–15% of adolescents hospitalized at either public or private psychiatric units in general hospitals or in psychiatric hospitals had the diagnoses of "affective disorders." Regarding the therapeutic milieu in these inpatient programs, 62.2% had a psychodynamic approach involving individual interaction with patients. Also, 37.7% of the inpatient units used a point system based on behavior therapy principles. In addition, close to 60% of the inpatient units had a levels program in which status and privilege were awarded for adaptive behavior. Studies comparing the outcome of the presenting problem with the type of inpatient treatment program are not available for children and adolescents.

THIRD-PARTY PAYMENTS

Hospital psychiatric treatment in the 1980s changed significantly because of the constraints of third-party payments. Private insurance companies and state-supported medical assistance programs have progressively decreased the number of maximum inpatient days for which they will provide payment and have employed their own physicians to directly or indirectly review treatment for the justification of continuing stay. The clinician has thus been presented with limits on inpatient days for treatment, which have often affected the type and goal of treatment.

Effective treatment in psychiatry is based on accurate diagnosis and formulation. Within child and adolescent psychiatry, diagnosis and formulation require more time for individual and family assessment than they do within adult psychiatry. Due to the significant role of the family in the expression and maintenance of psychopathology, the treatment of children and adolescents is complex, involving the patient not only as an individual but also as a member of the family system.

Because of a limited hospital stay, the clinician often is only able to begin a course of treatment and is not able to fully assess the effectiveness of this treatment over time. The continuation of well-planned treatment is relegated to outpatient follow-up.

TREATMENT

Initially, the decision for hospitalization is made by a member of the medical staff of the hospital, usually on the basis of an initial interview conducted by one or more members of the staff. This initial interview may occur in an emergency setting or by previous arrangement in an outpatient setting. Beyond the initial interview, the admission process is the first contact of the child and family with the physical structure, staff, and program of the inpatient unit.

THE ADMISSION PROCESS

Usually conducted by the nursing staff, possibly with brief contact by the social worker and psychiatrist, the admission process involves the explanation of rules for unit behavior and relevant unit policies (Johnsen 1982; Parmalee 1986). Per written orders of the medical staff, procedures specific for the particular child or adolescent are also explained at this time, such as the use of precautions for a suicidal patient. Facilitating the effective treatment of depression, and indeed any physical or mental illness, is the degree of realistic hope that the patient, the family, and the staff have.

Johnsen (1982) describes the sense of abandonment that the child or adolescent feels upon hospitalization, as well as the feelings of guilt and failure that may arise within parents. The empathic, supporting, and optimistic yet realistic attitude of the admitting and inpatient staff can help significantly in decreasing the patients' and their families' worries and concerns about coming to the hospital.

INITIAL CLINICAL ASSESSMENT AND PLANS

Medical Assessment

Once the child or adolescent has been admitted to the hospital, a period of intensive assessment begins, during which professionals from the disciplines of medicine, nursing, psychology, social work, education, expressive therapy, and occupational/recreation therapy are involved. Generally, the first of these assessments is the medical assessment, encompassing the medical history, physical examination, and investigations (laboratory, radiological, and other) performed or prescribed by a physician assigned to the unit. This physician might be one trained in child psychiatry or pediatrics or one who has experience working with children.

A comprehensive medical history should first be obtained. In evaluation of a patient with possible or probable depression, certain areas of the history warrant special attention. Regarding the medical assessment of children with behavior problems, Strayhorn (1987) emphasizes that the following issues should raise a suspicion of physical illness: a general history of physical complaints, loss of previous intellectual ability or memory, gross impairment in functioning, and inability to explain symptoms on other grounds. The temporal relationship between the ingestion of recreational, prescribed, or over-the-counter drugs to psychiatric symptoms should alert the physician to a possible toxic etiology. Symptoms pertinent to metabolic problems, such as anemia (i.e., skin pallor and an iron-poor diet) or hypothyroidism (i.e., dry skin, coarse hair, and cold intolerance) are also important. A grossly abnormal diet may point to nutritional deficiencies that have behavioral manifestations, such as early protein malnutrition or possibly folic acid deficiency. The physician should inquire about the history of fever or exposure to other persons with infectious illness.

A thorough physical and neurological examination should also be performed as part of the medical assessment. Special attention should be given to the structure and function of particular organs that could be affected by previous illnesses. For example, body temperature (as related to infectious illness), the quality of deep tendon reflexes and thyroid gland size (as related to hypo- or hyperthyroidism), and heart rate and papillary size (as pertains to the ingestion of certain illicit substances) are all essential parts of the physical examination of a patient who may be depressed. Irwin (1982b) feels that nonspecific neurological findings such as uncoordination, "soft" signs, or generalized electroencephalogram (EEG) findings do not necessarily warrant neurological consultation. However, neurological consultation is indicated for either positive localized findings or acute changes in behavior, personality, or cognition that might indicate a space-occupying lesion, infection, trauma, or other central nervous system insult.

Investigations

Laboratory studies that should be prescribed for a child or adolescent with suspected depression include a complete blood count with differential, SMA-18 (general chemistry profile), urinalysis, serum T_4 (total serum thyroxine), serum T_3 (serum triiodothyronine), free thyroid index (a calculation that often helps increase the sensitivity of the T_4 value in detecting hypo- or hyperthyroidism), and thyroid-stimulating hormone (TSH, important in the diagnosis of primary hypothyroidism). Other blood studies that may be necessary, depending on the presenting history, physical examination, and sex and developmental stage of the youngster, include toxin screens of the blood and urine, a serologic test for syphilis, β-human chorionic gonadotropin to exclude pregnancy, and a tuberculin skin test (Irwin 1982b). If the patient has been treated with medication known to affect mood and behavior, then blood levels of the drug should be measured if possible.

The dexamethasone suppression test (DST) is of special interest in the evaluation of a child or adolescent with suspected depression. (See Chapter 3.) As reviewed by Trad (1987), the DST provides information about the pattern of cortisol secretion in a given individual, which is normally suppressed for 24 hours following the administration of dexamethasone. Compared with adults who have other psychiatric disorders, endogenously depressed adults are less likely to show this normal suppression of cortisol secretion. Less is known about the sensitivity and specificity of the DST in children and adolescents, although several studies performed within inpatient populations have suggested some discriminatory value.

Weller et al. (1984) found that 70% of hospitalized prepubertal children meeting the DSM-III criteria (American Psychiatric Association 1980) for major depressive disorder had nonsuppressed cortisol levels on the DST. Hsu et al. (1983) found that 64% of a similar group of adolescents had nonsuppressed levels. Foreman and Goodyer (1988) reported on the measurement of salivary cortisol secretion after oral dexamethasone in a group of depressed inpatients ages 7–16 years, also finding significantly higher levels in this group compared with controls. Although it is not in regular clinical use at this time, the DST may be considered for a given individual as part of a comprehensive evaluation. Other possible biological markers for depressive disorders in children and adolescents, such as the TSH response to thyroid-releasing hormone stimulation and the secretory patterns of the growth hormone, await further study of their validity and reliability before recommendation as a tool for clinical assessment.

While not routinely indicated for the evaluation of primary medical illness, an electrocardiogram at admission is often indicated for the evaluation of ongoing tolerance to psychotropic medication and may well be needed as a baseline study for the later institution of psychotropic medication. (See Chapter 10.) A chest X ray need not be performed unless the history points to the possibility of disease in that area. Similarly, an EEG, computer axial tomography scan, or magnetic resonance imaging scan of the head is reserved for situations in which organicity is suspected.

Nursing Assessment

The first phase of nursing assessment of the depressed child or adolescent usually begins at the time of admission, and, as described by Grossman and Mayton (1988), the second phase continues for about 7–10 days thereafter. The second phase of assessment involves observation and direct interaction with the patient during the daily hospital routine. The nurse is able to develop an individual nursing treatment plan and to contribute to the multidisciplinary plan by verifying the type, amount, and extent of the behaviors present. Family assessments are also an essential part of the nursing process and, along with observation of the patient in the milieu, may result in validation or modification of the original formulation throughout the length of stay.

Nursing diagnoses pertinent to the depressed child or adolescent could highlight vegetative symptoms ("sleep pattern disturbance"), suicidality ("potential for self-directed violence"), hopelessness, or low self-esteem. Short-term nursing goals might be for the patient to learn to identify feelings or to use non-self-destructive methods of coping with feelings. Interventions proposed from the initial nursing assessment could include the implementation of suicide precautions and the reinforcement of appropriate coping measures (Pasquali et al. 1989).

Psychological Assessment

Bolton (1986) describes the tasks that are more or less specific to the clinical psychologist in the multidisciplinary team of the adolescent unit. These can be similarly applied to groups of prepubertal children. The specific tasks are concerned mainly with the investigation of cognitive functioning, which most commonly involves the assessment of intelligence using the Wechsler scales (Wechsler Intelligence Scale for Children—Revised [WISC-R], Wechsler Adult Intelligence Scale—Revised [WAIS-R]). One might find relatively lower scores on performance subtests of the WISC-R or WAIS-R, or one could find decrements in scores over time in a child or adolescent who was depressed. Other components of the psychological assessment could include screens for brain damage or dysfunction; formal tests of educational attainment in reading, spelling, and arithmetic; tests of personality traits; and assessment for the appropriate treatment modality (Bolton 1986). Clues about the presence of a depressive disorder might emerge from projective testing, such as from the identification of themes of loss on the Thematic Apperception Test.

The qualification and quantification of depressive disorder can be further assessed by such methods as structured and semistructured interviews (Kiddie Schedule for Affective Disorders and Schizophrenia [K-SADS], Diagnostic Interview Schedule for Children [DISC], and others), clinician rating scales (Children's Depression Rating Scale—Revised [CDRS-R] and others), self-report measures (Children's Depression Inventory [CDI], Children's Depression Scale [CDS], and others), parent rating measures, peer rating scales, teacher measures, and behavioral assessment (Kolko 1987; Matson 1989). (See Chapter 6.) Recent work has utilized the DISC (Weinstein et al. 1989) and the CDS (Kazdin 1987) in inpatient populations of children and adolescents, finding poor agreement with diagnoses by clinicians for the DISC but finding the suggestion of validity for the CDS.

Psychosocial Assessment

The psychosocial assessment usually is performed by a clinical social worker, with additions by the supervising psychiatrist, the nursing staff, and the primary psychotherapist. This evaluation includes current and past family structures and relationships, biographical information, significant relationships of the primary caregiver(s), significant relationships of the child, characteristics of the various environments with which the child interacts, and the identification of internal and external stresses and strengths of the family. Pertinent to the depressed child or adolescent would be histories of abuse or neglect, maternal deprivation, parental divorce, lack of social supports, low socioeconomic status, and the presence of parental psychopathology, particularly mood disorders.

Educational Assessment

Educational evaluation on an inpatient unit has been described by Schulman (1982), beginning with the request for a comprehensive report from the child's home school. The Wide-Range Achievement Test (WRAT) is then given to assist the teacher with planning the specific educational program.

More detailed and formal testing (such as the Illinois Test of Psycholinguistic Ability) is obtained for nearly half of those admitted to discern a learning disability or the particular strengths and weaknesses of the patient. Beyond the function of providing a meaningful classroom experience, the unit teachers are in the strategic position of observing the child or adolescent in a major "life space" (Redl 1966). Valuable information about depressive symptomatology, including interest and motivation, memory and concentration, self-concept, and peer relationships, is gleaned from such observation and is used by the team in the eventual formulation of a diagnosis.

Art Therapy Assessment

Ulman et al. (1978) note that artistic expression is much more accessible to people between the ages of 4 years and the onset of puberty than at any other time of life. Linesch (1988) points out the adolescent propensity for creativity, which arises from the feelings of self-absorption and isolation involved in separating from the family. The various types of diagnostic drawing procedures are reviewed by Rubin (1978), and one structured approach (the technique of Stimulus Drawings) has been studied for its use in screening children and adolescents for depression (Silver 1988). With the Draw-A-Story test, the author found that both depressed and learning-disabled subjects had fantasies that were significantly more negative.

Literature regarding the characteristics of art expression in depressed children and adolescents is reviewed by Wadeson (1980), who also reports on her systematic study of adults. Findings from pictures produced during times of increased depression included less color, more empty space, less investment of effort or less completeness, more depressive affect or less affect, and a trend toward being more constricted and less meaningful. Wadeson also describes the expression of suicidal feelings in art, including the prevalence of a spiral-shaped figure or a spiral symbol. Conger (1988) identifies death-related imagery (such as headstones), along with themes of hopelessness, helplessness, isolation, anger, and a sense of failure or guilt as possible indications of suicidal risk.

Occupational Therapy and Therapeutic Recreation Assessment

The occupational therapist and therapeutic recreation specialist have assessment as their initial task; ultimately, they will share their findings and develop a plan of treatment with other team members. Literature particular to the depressed child or adolescent is not currently available in either discipline. Indeed, Florey (1989) writes about the dearth of occupational therapy articles focusing on the emotional problems of children. Occupational therapy has been defined as "services to address the functional needs of a child related to the performance of self-help skills, adaptive behavior and play, and sensory, motor, and postural development" (Dunn 1989, p. 717). Peterson and Gunn (1984) note that the purpose of therapeutic recreation, as stated by the National Therapeutic Recreation Society, is the facilitation of the development, maintenance, and expression of an appropriate leisure lifestyle for an individual with physical, mental, emotional, or social limitations. Maximizing the function of a child or adolescent in either occupational therapy or therapeutic recreation has implications for improving a depressed state.

Melia and Weikert (1987) describe the activity therapy assessments on a short-term adolescent psychiatric unit, which evaluate areas of physical functioning, cognitive/task skills, emotional/behavioral skills, interpersonal/social skills, leisure/avocational skills, independent living skills, and vocational skills. Sholle-Martin (1987) reviews the model of human occupation (as put forth by Kielhofner, Burke, and associates) and describes assessment tools that have been effective with child and adolescent psychiatric populations, as well as an assessment battery applicable to the model of human occupation. This assessment battery has been used successfully on a short-term psychiatric and research diagnostic unit. Dunn (1984) notes that the development of assessment procedures for therapeutic recreation programming is in an early stage, but reviews the characteristics of and differences among several of these in use within the field. She describes three phases of therapeutic recreation assessment, which include screening or program placement, pinpointing an area in need of improvement, and monitoring the progress of the patient while he or she is in various programs.

THE TREATMENT PLAN

Because they are now accountable to those not directly involved in treatment, psychiatrists treating children and adolescents in the hospital must justify and document their services. One method of justification required by many reviewing and accrediting organizations is the treatment plan. Treatment plans are additions to the narrative medical record that list in a concise and organized fashion the problems, treatment goals, and methods of attaining these specific goals for each patient. Several approaches for devising a treatment plan have been suggested, such as goal-directed treatment planning (Nurcombe 1989) and focal inpatient treatment planning (Harper and Geraty 1989). The approach for a given unit varies with administrative and clinical philosophy.

The minimal criterion for discharge of a depressed child or adolescent must be that the patient is of no immediate danger to the self or others. This should be stated as a goal on the treatment plan. In behavioral terms, this goal might further be elaborated on by listing the alternative coping behaviors that a child or adolescent will learn to use instead of self-harming acts.

Such behaviors might logically include those that have in the past assisted in coping with suicidal thoughts, such as discussing suicidal feelings with a parent or therapist. The method of treatment for suicidal patients could include individual, family, group, and milieu therapy. Beyond the goal of eliminating suicidal risk, other major goals of treatment based on the reasons for admission could include diagnostic and treatment reformulation in a patient who has not responded to outpatient treatment for depression and development of a therapeutic alliance with a patient who manifests moderate to severe symptoms of depression but who has refused outpatient treatment.

Additionally, the treatment plan in an outpatient setting should address problems, goals, and methods of treatment in the areas of physical health, the family or living environment, peer relationships, the educational and/or occupational setting, and leisure activities. The patient's strength and effective coping abilities should be noted in each area. Periodic updates and revisions of the treatment plan are essential for helping to reorient and refocus members of the treatment team, and they are also needed for utilization review and accrediting agencies.

Milieu Therapy

The time that the patient spends with other patients and the staff outside of the formally structured activities of the treatment program is highly valuable. In the milieu, therapeutic interventions can be applied and reinforced as the patient contends with the routine activities of daily living and with peer and caretaking relationships. Within the framework of treating depression, the milieu staff can, for example, work with a patient behaviorally on obtaining more positive reinforcement from the environment. This work might involve the selective rewarding of behaviors that increase social supports, such as more time spent out of a patient's room or even the initiation of play or interaction with peers. If major psychodynamic themes have been identified as part of the formulation, then the milieu staff can assist the child with expressing and reworking conflict. (See Chapter 7.)

Individual Psychotherapy

During the course of inpatient treatment, individual psychotherapy is the cornerstone of the various interventions. If individual therapy has been used in the outpatient treatment of the depressed child or adolescent, then further clarification and modification of personal issues can be undertaken in the hospital. A therapist not previously acquainted with the patient may be able to provide a new perspective from the vantage point of hospital observation. In individual therapy, depressive themes may become more clear, thereby allowing more appropriate inclusion of other therapies such as family therapy, group therapy, cognitive-behavioral therapy, and/or pharmacotherapy. (See Chapters 7, 8, 9, and 10.)

Specific theoretical orientations have particular applications in the individual therapy of depression in children and adolescents. These include behavioral therapies (for a review, see Hirschfeld and Shea 1989), cognitive-behavioral therapy (Beck et al. 1979; see Chapter 9), and psychodynamic approaches (see Chapter 7).

Group Psychotherapy

Because of developmental proclivity toward peer relationships, most children and adolescents, including those with depressive disorders, are suited for group psychotherapy. Involvement in group therapy decreases social isolation and facilitates peer interactions in other situations on the inpatient unit. In the course of development, peer relationships gain more influence. Because of this, peer feedback has increasingly powerful effects on the thoughts, feelings, and behaviors of children and adolescents. Depressed children or adolescents in group therapy can learn directly and indirectly about themselves, their families, and the issues that affect the course of their depression. (See Chapter 8.)

Pharmacotherapy

If antidepressant medication is indicated in depressed children and adolescents who are hospitalized, the inpatient setting provides the opportunity for close observation of the patient's response. Also, it is easier to make more rapid adjustments in dose or medication type. Probably the most widely used antidepressants for children and adolescents are the tricyclics (e.g., imipramine). On an inpatient unit, the dose can be titrated up relatively quickly while watching for excessive anticholinergic side effects, cardiac rhythm disturbances, side effects referable to other organ systems, and early therapeutic effects. (See Chapter 10.) Daily monitoring of the pulse and blood pressure, periodic checking of the cardiac rhythm strip, and observation for changes in bowel or bladder habits are necessary during this dose adjustment. (See Chapter 10.)

If a patient does not tolerate or responds inadequately to the antidepressant used initially, then hospitalization provides an opportunity for further single or combination medication trials. Combination medication therapy has not been well studied in children and adolescents and thus currently should be reserved for cases of particularly severe depression that have been refractory to more often used pharmacotherapy. Beyond tricyclic antidepressants, the efficacy in childhood and adolescent depression of such agents as the serotonin reuptake–inhibitor fluoxetine and the monoamine oxidase inhibitors is not clear, and these agents should be reserved for special circumstances after careful consideration of the alternatives. (See Chapter 10.)

Family Therapy

Theories about the development and expression of depressive illness in young people all provide for the inclusion of family factors in some way. In turn, the presence of a depressive illness and the hospitalization of a depressed child or adolescent resound throughout the family with various effects. The effects depend on such variables as the number of family members and their relationships to each other and to the patient, the particular expression of the depressive illness (i.e., withdrawn behavior versus aggressive behavior) and its meaning to the family, and the availability of supports outside the family to assist in the response to the crisis. When approaching family therapy in the hospital setting, therefore, one must think of means to modify identified family factors that contribute to symptoms in the child and adolescent, as well as ways to assist the family in coping with stress associated with the deterioration of the patient's functioning. Problems within the realm of the family and home living environment may only begin to be addressed during hospitalization due to their complexity and short lengths of stay in the hospital.

An example of a family factor that might be identified in the expression of depressive disorder could be a social or psychological burden placed on a child by virtue of her or his role within the family. This burden could exceed the child's current capacity, leading to failed efforts and consequent depression. The family therapist might wish to work toward redistributing this burden within the family or to the outside, thus removing to some extent the sense of frustration and failure for the child. A case example follows:

> Jimmy, a 12-year-old male living with his recently divorced mother and 8-year-old sister, was referred by his teachers after a classmate reported that he had written a suicide note. Problems with declining grades, lack of concentration in class, and withdrawal from classroom activities and peers had also been observed. After evaluation and admission, family therapy assessment revealed that following the divorce, Jimmy's mother had added a number of household duties to his list of chores. Also, she had unknowingly been spending a good deal of their time together talking about her sadness and loneliness after his father left. In future family sessions, a more efficient and evenly distributed set of responsibilities for each family member was delineated, and the mother was referred to a local support group for divorced people. On 6-month follow-up, Jimmy described his mood as "happy except when my sister bugs me," and his academic performance had returned to its previous level.

Parents' groups are also helpful adjuncts to the inpatient treatment of depressed youngsters, allowing exchange of ideas about the nature of the illness and the experiences and coping strategies of individual parents.

CONCLUSION

Inpatient psychiatric treatment of depressed children and adolescents should be perceived as one of the means of intervention, rather than as an end in itself. It is part of the treatment process. Whether the patient is discharged to a residential center, partial hospitalization program, or outpatient setting, close follow-up is essential to ensure continuity of treatment, to enhance possibilities for recovery, and to decrease the occurrence of future depressive episodes. Carefully designed, controlled studies on treatment outcome are necessary to understanding which factors increase the effectiveness of inpatient treatment for depression in children and adolescents.

REFERENCES

American Psychiatric Association: Diagnostic and Statistical Manual of Mental Disorders, 3rd Edition. Washington, DC, American Psychiatric Association, 1980

Beck AT, Rush AJ, Shaw BF, et al: Cognitive Therapy of Depression. New York, Guilford, 1979

Bolton D: The clinical psychologist in adolescent psychiatry, in The Adolescent Unit. Edited by Steinberg D. New York, John Wiley, 1986, pp 113–120

Conger D: Suicidal youth: the challenge to art therapy. American Journal of Art Therapy 27:34–44, 1988

Dalton R, Forman MA, Daul GC, et al: Psychiatric hospitalization of preschool children: admission factors and discharge implications. J Am Acad Child Adolesc Psychiatry 26(3):308–312, 1987

Dunn JK: Assessment, in Therapeutic Recreation Program Design, 2nd Edition. Edited by Peterson CA, Gunn SL. Englewood Cliffs, NJ, Prentice-Hall, 1984, pp 267–320

Dunn W: Occupational therapy in early intervention: new perspectives create greater possibilities. Am J Occup Ther 43(11):717–721, 1989

Florey LL: Treating the whole child: rhetoric or reality? Am J Occup Ther 43(6):365–369, 1989

Foreman DM, Goodyer IM: Salivary cortisol hypersecretion in juvenile depression. J Child Psychol Psychiatry 29(3):311–320, 1988

Geraty R: Administrative issues in inpatient child and adolescent psychiatry. J Am Acad Child Adolesc Psychiatry 28(1):21–25, 1989

Grossman J, Mayton K: Applying the nursing process with children, in Psychiatric Nursing, 3rd Edition, No 34. Edited by Wilson HS, Kneisl CR. Redwood City, CA, Addison-Wesley, 1988, pp 916–949

Harper G, Geraty R: Hospital and residential treatment, in Psychiatry, Vol 2, No 64. Edited by Michael A, Cavenor J. New York, JB Lippincott, 1989, pp 1–20

Hirschfeld RMA, Shea MT: Mood disorders: psychosocial treatments, in Comprehensive Textbook of Psychiatry, Vol 5. Edited by Kaplan HI, Sadock BJ. Baltimore, MD, Williams & Wilkins, 1989, pp 933–944

Hsu LKG, Molcan K, Cashman MA, et al: The dexamethasone suppression test in adolescent depression. J Am Acad Child Adolesc Psychiatry 22(5):470–473, 1983

Irwin M: Literature review, in Psychiatric Hospitalization of Children. Edited by Schulman JL, Irwin M. Springfield, IL, Charles C Thomas, 1982a, pp 5–42

Irwin M: Workup, in Psychiatric Hospitalization of Children. Edited by Schulman JL, Irwin M. Springfield, IL, Charles C Thomas, 1982b, pp 242–246

Johnsen BC: Admission, in Psychiatric Hospitalization of Children. Edited by Schulman JL, Irwin M. Springfield, IL, Charles C Thomas, 1982, pp 222–241

Kahn DG, Boyer DN: Inpatient hospital treatment of adolescents. Psychiatr Clin North Am 3(3):513–545, 1980

Kazdin AE: Children's Depression Scale: validation with child psychiatric inpatients. J Child Psychol Psychiatry 28(1):29–41, 1987

Kolko DJ: Depression, in Behavior Therapy With Children and Adolescents: A Clinical Approach. Edited by Hersen M, Van Hasselt VB. New York, John Wiley, 1987, pp 137–183

Linesch DG: Adolescent Art Therapy. New York, Brunner/Mazel, 1988, p 5

Matson JL: Treating Depression in Children and Adolescents. New York, Pergamon, 1989, pp 22–59

Melia MA, Weikert K: Evaluation and treatment of adolescents on a short-term unit. Occupational Therapy in Mental Health 7(2):23–37, 1987

Nurcombe B: Goal-directed treatment planning and the principles of brief hospitalization. J Am Acad Child Adolesc Psychiatry 28(1):26–30, 1989

Parmelee DX: The adolescent and the young adult, in Inpatient Psychiatry, 2nd Edition, No 13. Edited by Sederer LI. Baltimore, MD, Williams & Wilkins, 1986, pp 280–295

Pasquali EA, Arnold HM, DeBasio N: Patterns of conflict and stress in childhood and adolescence, in Mental Health Nursing, 3rd Edition, No 17. St. Louis, MO, CV Mosby, 1989, pp 469–508

Peterson CA, Gunn SL: Therapeutic Recreation Program Design, 2nd Edition. Englewood Cliffs, NJ, Prentice-Hall, 1984, pp 3–8

Prugh DG: Standards for Psychiatric Facilities Serving Children and Adolescents. Washington, DC, American Psychiatric Association, 1971

Redl F: When We Deal With Children. New York, Free Press, 1966

Rubin JA: Child Art Therapy. Cincinnati, OH, Van Nostrand Reinhold, 1978, pp 49–50

Schulman JL: Education, in Psychiatric Hospitalization of Children. Edited by Schulman JL, Irwin M. Springfield, IL, Charles C Thomas, 1982, pp 84–97

Shafii M, Steltz-Lenarsky J, Derrick AM, et al: Comorbidity of mental disorders in the post-mortem diagnosis of completed suicide in children and adolescents. J Affective Disord 15:227–233, 1988

Sholle-Martin S: Application of the model of human occupation: assessment in child and adolescent psychiatry. Occupational Therapy in Mental Health 7(2):3–21, 1987

Silver R: Screening children and adolescents for depression through Draw-A-Story. American Journal of Art Therapy 26:119–124, 1988

Strayhorn JM: Medical assessment of children with behavioral problems, in Behavior Therapy With Children and Adolescents: A Clinical Approach. Edited by Hersen M, Van Hasselt VB. New York, John Wiley, 1987, pp 50–74

Trad PV: Infant and Childhood Depression: Developmental Factors. New York, John Wiley, 1987

Ulman E, Kramer E, Kwiatkowska HY: United States. Craftsbury Common, VT, Art Therapy Publications, 1978, p 20

Wadeson H: Art Psychotherapy. New York, John Wiley, 1980, pp 61–67, 82–104

Weinstein SR, Stone K, Noam GG: Comparison of DISC with clinician's DSM-III diagnoses in psychiatric inpatients. J Am Acad Child Adolesc Psychiatry 28(1):53–60, 1989

Weller EB, Weller RA, Fristad MA: The dexamethasone suppression test in hospitalized prepubertal depressed children. Am J Psychiatry 141:290–291, 1984

Woolston JL: Transactional risk model for short and intermediate term psychiatric inpatient treatment of children. J Am Acad Adolesc Psychiatry 28(1):38–41, 1989

Zinn D: Hospital treatment of the adolescent, in Basic Handbook of Child Psychiatry, Vol 3, No 16. Edited by Noshpitz JD. New York, Basic Books, 1979, pp 263–288

PART III

BIPOLAR DISORDERS IN CHILDREN AND ADOLESCENTS

If you keep a green bough in your heart
the singing bird will come.

Chinese proverb

CHAPTER 12

Bipolar Disorders: Natural History, Genetic Studies, and Follow-up

Michael Strober, Ph.D.

Kraepelin, in his 1921 monograph, *Manic-Depressive Insanity and Paranoia,* commented on the rarity of the onset of manic-depressive disorder before age 10 years. Nonetheless, he cited descriptions by Friedman of "mild forms" of mood disorder in young people with the clinical manifestations of stuporous, delirious, and somnambulistic states. Kraepelin (1921) also referred to a case reported by Liebers of mania of 6 months' duration in a 4-year-old boy. At the same time, Kraepelin alerted us to the fundamentally important role of puberty as a precipitating agent, noting that the "greatest frequency of first attack falls, however, in the period of development with its increased emotional excitability between the fifteenth and twentieth year" (p. 167).

The study of juvenile onset of bipolar disorder carries with it a number of important theoretical and clinical implications. One issue is whether or not certain early childhood behavioral phenomena reliably anticipate the later development of the classic bipolar phenotype. The difficulty here is that, aside from the rare cases of unequivocal mania in prepubertal children, there is no convincing body of longitudinal data that allows prediction of later bipolar disorder on the basis of specific psychopathological attributes. A second issue is whether or not there are specific genetic, biological, or psychosocial factors that constitute a basis for early juvenile onset of illness. Although we have known since the time of Kraepelin that the incidence of bipolar disorder rises sharply with the onset of puberty, only 15–30% of patients experience their first attack prior to age 20 years (Goodwin and Jamison 1984). A final issue is whether or not there are straightforward continuities between the pharmacological management of juvenile- and adult-onset forms of bipolar disorder.

In this chapter the natural history, clinical manifestations, precursors,

251

and longitudinal follow-up of bipolar disorders in children and adolescents will be discussed. Genetic studies of bipolar disorders in adults and their possible implications for children and adolescents are reviewed. A discussion of pharmacological treatment of bipolar disorders in this age group concludes this chapter.

NATURAL HISTORY

Kraepelin was of the opinion that the susceptibility to manic depression could be evoked early in life, an opinion also held by Bleuler (1934). Indeed, several early references to unequivocal circular manic-depressive states in children and young adolescents are discussed in a survey of the literature on juvenile bipolar disorders by Strober et al. (1989). So far as adolescence is concerned, phenotypic similarities of manic and depressive syndromes to the adult forms of expression are well supported by clinical studies (Ballenger et al. 1982; Carlson and Strober 1978; Coryell and Norten 1980; Hassanyeh and Davison 1980; Horowitz 1977; Hsu and Starzynski 1986; Landolt 1957; Olsen 1961; Strober et al. 1988, 1990). However, opinion has been divided on whether or not puberty evokes a more atypical or psychotic coloring of illness. For example, several authors (Ballenger et al. 1982; Landolt 1957; Olsen 1961; Rosen et al. 1983) have remarked on the unusually common presence of schizophreniform features in adolescent patients with bipolar disorder, whereas others (Carlson and Strober 1978; Coryell and Norten 1980; Hassanyeh and Davison 1980; Horowitz 1977; Hsu and Starzynski 1986) concluded that adolescents with bipolar disorder have the same intensity and range of symptoms as adults and a similar incidence of "atypical" features.

Bipolar Disorders in Prepubertal Children and Adolescents

By Kraepelin's (1921) account, fewer than 2% of the onsets of manic-depressive disorder occur before the 10th year of life. Judging from the available literature (Anthony and Scott 1960; Barrett 1931; Coll and Bland 1979; Esman et al. 1983; Feinstein and Wolpert 1973; Kasanin 1930; McKnew et al. 1981; Olkon 1945; Poznanski et al. 1984; Sylvester et al. 1984; Varanka et al. 1988; Varsamis and MacDonald 1972; Weinberg and Brumback 1976), the distinctive features of younger prepubertal manic children include irritability, hyperactivity, destructiveness, and emotional unpredictability, whereas grandiosity, paranoia, and pure manic euphoria become increasingly prominent with the onset of puberty. On the other hand, hyperactivity, pressured speech, and distractibility appear to vary little with age. In regard to the depressive pole, maturational effects on symptom phenomenology are striking. In young children, somatic complaints, general malaise, and tearfulness are commonplace, whereas the more classic melancholic features of profound psychomotor retardation, guilt, delusions, anhedonia, and disruption of neurovegetative functioning are conspicuous hallmarks of bipolar disorder in adolescence (Akiskal et al. 1983; Carlson 1983; Strober and Carlson 1982). What we can infer broadly from these reports is that in very young children pure mania is a relatively uncommon psychopathological syndrome; we are more likely to see mixed cycles of highly variable duration in which affective irritability, agitation, hyperactivity, and disruptive behavior are prominent, giving way to alternating cycles of manic excitement and endogenomorphic depression at the onset of puberty. Just how the ontogeny of biological systems interacts with genetic susceptibility and other intrapsychic developmental changes to affect symptom presentation eludes our understanding at present.

Precursors of Bipolar Disorder

A more intriguing speculation, one that has been encouraged by burgeoning interest in the genetics of bipolar disorder, is that certain behavioral deviances may reflect the developmental anlage of bipolar disorder in young, prepubertal children in whom full-fledged affective pathology is absent. Behavioral patterns purported to represent bipolar "variants" in children include ill-temperedness and explosive tantrums, intermittent hyperactivity and aggressive storms, periodic boisterousness, pressured activity, stupor, and paranoia (Annell 1969; Davis 1979; DeLong 1978; Dyson and Barcai 1970; Frommer 1968; Popper and Famularo 1983; Thompson and Schindler 1976). Intriguing as this concept is, these accounts are problematic conceptually and generate many more questions and diagnostic uncertainties than they answer. True, there is every reason to assume that the form and expression of behavioral propensities tied to a bipolar genotype may differ qualitatively across developmental periods; however, we are unable at the present time to reliably or meaningfully discriminate these hypothesized precursors from the broad spectrum of nonaffective psychiatric disorders whose symptomatic features overlap to a significant degree (e.g., conduct disorder in association with attention-deficit hyperactivity disorder, borderline states, etc.). In the absence of robust and specific biological or genetic markers or longitudinal prospective studies that map out developmental linkages in a methodologically rigorous fashion, it simply is premature, and theoretically unfounded, to conceive of these behavior patterns as anticipating the later development of bipolar disorder in any way that could be useful diagnostically or therapeutically.

Longitudinal Follow-up and Prognosis

Data on the long-term follow-up and prognosis of juvenile bipolar disorder are sparse. Concerning the disorder in adults, we know that 1) it is invariably recurrent, the proportion of patients with multiple episodes ranging from 50–90%, depending on which study one cites (see Goodwin and Jamison 1984); 2) the average manic episode has a duration of roughly 3 months; 3) depressions last 4–6 months on average, though individual variabilities in episode duration and cycle length are quite substantial (Angst 1981; Lundquist 1945; Rennie 1942); 4) the interval between attacks shows a tendency to shorten as the illness progresses (see Goodwin and Jamison 1984); and 5) the rate of chronicity is upward of 20% and may even be higher in patients who enter treatment in mixed or polyphasic (continuously cycling) episodes (Keller 1985).

Whether or not morbidity is influenced to a greater or lesser extent when the disorder begins early in life is not known. In an early study of 1,700 patients, Pollack (1931) noted that among patients whose first hospitalization occurred before age 20 years, 22% had three or more prior episodes. In a 5- to 25-year follow-up of 60 bipolar patients first hospitalized between the ages of 15 and 25 years, Landolt (1957) found that 90% had a relapsing course, whereas Carlson et al. (1977) found that some 20–50% of adolescent-onset bipolar patients remained significantly impaired in their psychological functioning through their adult years. Welner et al. (1979) described the course of 12 bipolar adolescents 8–10 years following discharge; 3 were found to have completed suicide and the remainder were chronically ill with generally poor social-occupational adjustment, repeat hospitalizations, and suicide attempts. Associations between suicidality and bipolar illness have also been reported in a recent case-controlled study by Brent et al. (1988). Finally, episodic drinking, drug abuse, and other complicating comorbid features are not unexpected in young bipolar patients, given that the incidence of these behavioral risk factors in the general population rises significantly at the time of adolescence. In short, even though it cannot be said that juvenile onset confers a decidedly worse course and long-term outcome of bipolar illness (Carlson et al. 1977),. the seriously disruptive social, vocational, intrapsychic, and even psychobiological effects of early developing disorder seem undeniable.

GENETIC STUDIES

The familial nature of bipolar disorder is an incontrovertible fact. Of nearly 20 family studies reviewed by Gershon (1988) and those published subsequently (Andreason et al. 1987; Coryell et al. 1984; Endicott et al. 1985; Gershon et al. 1982; Weissman et al. 1984), nearly all show that the morbidity risk of mood disorders in relatives of patients is elevated threefold over that in the general population. These observations are complemented by twin (Bertelsen et al. 1977) and adoption (Mendlewicz and Rainer 1977; Wender et al. 1986) studies in supporting the existence of a genetic susceptibility factor.

Despite the consistency of family aggregation studies, the mode of inheritance of bipolar disorder remains unknown. Segregation analysis of nuclear families and extended pedigrees has been reported, but results are inconsistent; single major-locus models have received strong or marginal support in some studies (O'Rourke et al. 1983; Price et al. 1985; Rice et al. 1987; Risch et al. 1986), but are explicitly rejected in others (Bucher et al. 1981; Goldin et al. 1983; Tsuang et al. 1985). Furthermore, it has not been possible using these quantitative methods to reliably discriminate among alternative models of familial transmission.

Most workers in this area agree that more recent advances in quantitative and molecular genetics herald a period of unprecedented growth in psychiatric research and will be utilized extensively in coming years to further our understanding of etiological factors. However, these methodologies are not without potential limitations that must be taken into account when integrating genetic findings. In the case of segregation analysis, confounding influences include ascertainment bias, phenocopies, and heterogeneity (Cox and Suarez 1985; Gershon and Goldin 1987; Gershon et al. 1987b; Goldin et al. 1984). Moreover, Goldin et al. (1984) have shown, using simulated pedigree data, that segregation analysis may not possess sufficient sensitivity to detect major-locus transmission of a dichotomous trait under conditions of low to intermediate heterozygote penetrance. However, a locus could be inferred by demonstrating linkage to a genetic marker if phenocopies were rare and linkage was tight. By the same token, the power of linkage analysis can be reduced appreciably under conditions of genetic heterogeneity, moderate recombination, secular changes in incidence, and incomplete knowledge of genetic parameters (Cox and Suarez 1985; Gershon and Goldin 1987). Presumably, the yield in genetic studies would be greater if these methods were applied to specific, more homogeneous subgroups of bipolar disorder.

Genetic Heterogeneity

There is an emerging consensus that more than one disease locus figures in the causation and pathogenesis of bipolar disorder. On the question of X-linked inheritance, several reports have supported linkage of bipolar illness to the X chromosome markers color blindness and glucose-6-phosphate dehydrogenase (G6PD) (Baron 1977; Baron et al. 1987; DelZampo et al. 1984; Mendlewicz and Fleiss 1974; Mendlewicz et al. 1979, 1980; Reich et al. 1969), whereas others have not (Gershon et al. 1979; Leckman et al. 1979). It is conceivable that genetic heterogeneity, which was noted in families investigated by Mendlewicz et al. (1979) and Gershon et al. (1980), accounts for some of the discrepant findings. Consistent with this idea, in an expanded review and analysis of the X-linked hypothesis, Risch and Baron (1982) and Risch et al. (1986) suggest that only some bipolar families segregate for a dominant X-linked gene and that this mode of transmission may be differentially associated with early onset of illness. Supporting this idea, Mendlewicz and associates (1989) have reported evidence of linkage between bipolar illness and a factor IX DNA probe in the Xq27 region, thereby giving further impetus to the investigation of polymorphic DNA markers on the X chromosome in select families. However, a more recent study by Berrettini et al. (1990) failed to replicate linkage to these X chromosome markers.

Also generating controversy are studies examining linkage to the histocompatibility complex mapped to chromosome 6. This literature has been reviewed in detail (Suarez and Croughan 1982; Suarez and Reich 1984), with the majority of studies finding no, or highly equivocal, evidence for linkage to these markers. Nonetheless, Cox and Suarez (1985) have argued that the possibility of linkage between bipolar illness and a locus in the human leukocyte antigen (HLA) region in at least some families cannot be excluded with certainty.

Last, Egeland et al. (1987) have presented evidence for linkage between bipolar disorder and DNA polymorphisms of the insulin gene (INS) and the c-Ha-ras-1 oncogene (HRAS1) region on chromosome 11 in a large Older Order Amish pedigree. However, linkage to this region was ruled out in Icelandic pedigrees studied by Hodgkinson et al. (1987), North American pedigrees studied by Detera-Wadleigh et al. (1987), and, in a more recent expanded analysis of the Amish data, by Kelsoe et al. (1989). Given the inbreeding and isolated structure of the Older Order Amish sect, the lack of reproducible findings is not surprising, especially if multiple gene forms of bipolar disorder do exist. Another point worth noting is that juvenile-onset bipolar disorder seems to be unusually common among the Amish. In a methodological study (Egeland et al. 1987) using the Amish data to assess reliability of various age-at-onset indices, the proportion of bipolar cases with onset of illness prior to age 19 years was 65%, whereas in other series reported in the literature, juvenile onset accounts for no more than 10–30% of cases (Baron et al. 1983; Kraepelin 1921; Loranger and Levine 1979; Winokur et al. 1969).

Age at Onset and Familiality

Studies examining the association between age at onset in bipolar illness and degree of familiality clearly underscore the value of this parameter in genetic analyses. Most studies have shown that relatives of early-onset probands have significantly higher morbidity risk for mood disorders compared with relatives of late-onset probands (Baron et al. 1981; Gershon et al. 1982; Goetzl et al. 1974; James 1975; Johnson and Leeman 1977; Mendlewicz et al. 1972; Rice et al. 1987; Stenstedt 1952; Winokur 1975). While secular trends in the incidence of unipolar depression and bipolar disorder (Gershon et al. 1987a; Klerman et al. 1985) must be taken into account when interpreting these associations, Rice et al. (1987) have shown that age at onset in bipolar probands independently and significantly predicts familial risk even after this variable is statistically controlled. Even so, conclusions regarding the broader genetic significance of age at onset have been limited by the use, in most studies, of a single age cutoff (usually ages 30–40 years) to separate probands into early- versus late-onset types.

To determine whether juvenile-onset bipolar illness indexed a genetically more severe expression of the disorder, we examined in blind fashion lifetime rates of psychiatric illness among 115 first-degree relatives of 50 adolescents with bipolar I disorder and 71 first-degree relatives of 31 age-matched schizophrenic controls (Strober et al. 1988). Unipolar depression and bipolar disorder aggregated only in relatives of the bipolar group. Significant loading of mood disorder was also found among second-degree relatives (see Tables 12–1 and 12–2).

Especially noteworthy is the 14.8% lifetime rate of bipolar disorder among first-degree relatives, substantially higher than the values reported in adult family-genetic studies, which range from 3% to 6% (Coryell et al. 1984; Endicott et al. 1985; Gershon et al. 1982; Rice et al. 1987; Weissman et al. 1984).

Table 12–1. Lifetime rates of psychiatric illness in first-degree relatives of bipolar and schizophrenic probands

Diagnosis in relatives	No. of relatives Bipolar probands (n = 115)	Schizophrenic probands (n = 71)	P value
By hierachy			
Schizophrenia	0	2 (2.8)	NS
Schizoaffective, bipolar	0	0	NS
Schizoaffective, depressed	0	0	NS
Major affective disorder	34 (29.6)	3 (4.2)	.0001
Bipolar	17 (14.8)[a]	0	.002
Unipolar	17 (14.8)	3 (4.2)	.05
Cyclothymic personality	0	0	NS
Chronic, intermittent depression	3 (2.6)	2 (2.8)	NS

Note. Numbers in parentheses are percentages.
[a]Includes one case of bipolar II disorder; risks for bipolar I and bipolar II disorder among first-degree relatives are 13.9% and 0.9%, respectively.
Source. Reproduced with permission from Strober M, Morrell W, Burroughs J, et al: A family study of bipolar I disorder in adolescence: early onset of symptoms linked to increased familial loading and lithium resistance. J Affective Disord 15:255–268, 1988. Copyright 1988 Elsevier Science Publishers.

Familial rates were also analyzed in bipolar probands separated by age at first onset of psychiatric abnormalities (see Table 12–3). This comparison revealed that the rate of bipolar illness in parents of the 15 probands with prepubertal onset of illness was 3.5 times that in parents of probands who were psychiatrically well prior to onset of mood disorder in adolescence (30.0% versus 8.6%, respectively; $P < .03$). The childhood diagnoses given to the 15 probands classified as prepubertal onset, based on careful review of data from the psychiatric history provided by parents, included conduct disorder plus attention-deficit hyperactivity disorder ($n = 12$), dysthymia plus obsessive-compulsive disorder ($n = 1$), dysthymia plus major depression ($n = 1$), and dysthymia plus separation anxiety disorder ($n = 1$).

This finding fits with the general idea that there may be some very early onsets of illness in which the prepubertal expression of affective temperamental abnormalities is linked to a more severe bipolar genotype and a correspondingly greater lifetime risk of affective illness in relatives. Similar findings and conclusions have been reported by Dwyer and DeLong (1987).

In sum, it is increasingly evident that the inheritance of bipolar disorder is complex and resists simple genetic analysis. In this regard, no longer is it tenable to assume that affected individuals comprise a genetically unitary population; rather, susceptibility may be transmitted by genes at more than one X chromosome and autosomal locus, one or more of which may uniquely define a juvenile-onset phenotype.

Table 12–2.   Lifetime rates of schizophrenia, unspecified psychosis, and major affective disorder in second-degree relatives

	No. of relatives		
Diagnosis in relatives	Bipolar probands ($n = 408$)	Schizophrenic probands ($n = 250$)	P value
Schizophrenia	2 (0.5)	9 (3.6)	.005
Unspecified functional psychosis	3 (0.7)	5 (2.0)	NS
Major affective disorder	63 (15.4)	10 (4.0)	.0001
Bipolar	23 (5.6)	2 (0.8)	.003
Unipolar	40 (9.8)	8 (3.2)	.002

Note. Numbers in parentheses are percentages. Second-degree relatives include grandparents, aunts, and uncles.

Source. Reproduced with permission from Strober M, Morrell W, Burroughs J, et al: A family study of bipolar I disorder in adolescence: early onset of symptoms linked to increased familial loading and lithium resistance. J Affective Disord 15:255–268, 1988. Copyright 1988 Elsevier Science Publishers.

PHARMACOLOGICAL TREATMENT

At least nine controlled studies attest to the superiority of lithium over placebo in reducing recurrences of episodes in adults with bipolar disorder (Cole et al. 1986; Prien 1983). When study data are pooled, relapse rates of patients receiving lithium over a 1- to 2-year period of prophylactic treatment average 35%, compared to a 90% relapse rate for patients receiving placebo; however, lithium appears to be somewhat more effective in preventing recurrences of mania than in preventing recurrences of depression. These same studies suggest that risk of relapse is greatest during the initial year of preventative treatment and that early relapse tends to predict future recurrences (Abou-Saleh and Coppen 1986; Dunner et al. 1976; Prien et al. 1974). These controlled data are in line with uncontrolled, naturalistic reports of frequent, and sometimes rapid, reoccurrence of illness upon discontinuation

Table 12–3.   Lifetime rates of major affective disorders in relatives of bipolar probands with prepubertal versus adolescent onset of illness

| | No. of diagnoses in relatives of: | | | | | | |
| | Prepubertal-onset probands | | | Adolescent-onset probands | | | |
Relative[a]	Unipolar	Bipolar	Total	Unipolar	Bipolar	Total	P value[b]
Parents							
Mothers (15/35)	3 (20.0)	3 (20.0)	6 (40.0)	7 (20.0)	3 (8.6)[c]	10 (28.6)	NS
Fathers (15/35)	1 (6.7)	6 (40.0)	7 (46.7)	4 (11.4)	3 (8.6)	7 (20.0)	NS
Total (30/70)	4 (13.3)	9 (30.0)	13 (43.3)	11 (15.7)	6 (8.6)[c,d]	17 (24.3)	.10
Siblings							
Sisters (2/15)	1 (50.0)	1 (50.0)	2 (100.0)	0	1 (20.0)	1 (20.0)	[e]
Brothers (2/6)	0	0	0	1 (16.7)	0	1 (16.7)	[e]
Total (4/21)	1 (25.0)	1 (25.0)	2 (50.0)	1 (9.1)	1 (9.1)	2 (18.2)	[e]
All first-degree							
relatives (34/81)	5 (14.7)	10 (29.4)	15 (44.1)	12 (14.8)	7 (8.6)	19 (23.5)	.05
All second-degree							
relatives (126/282)	19 (15.1)	9 (7.1)	28 (22.2)	21 (7.4)	14 (5.0)	35 (12.4)	.02

Note.   Numbers in parentheses are percentages.
[a]Number of relatives of prepubertal-onset probands/number of relatives of adolescent-onset probands. [b]Statistical tests conducted on combined rate of unipolar and bipolar disorder in relatives of prepubertal-onset versus adolescent-onset probands. [c]Includes one case of bipolar II disorder; risks for bipolar I and bipolar II disorder in mothers of adolescent-onset probands are 5.7% and 2.9%, respectively. [d]Risks for bipolar I and bipolar II disorder in parents of adolescent-onset probands are 7.1% and 1.4%, respectively. Among all first-degree relatives, the risks are 7.4% and 1.2%, respectively. [e]Numbers are too small for statistical analysis.
Source.   Reprinted with permission from Strober M, Morrell W, Burroughs J, et al: A family study of bipolar I disorder in adolescence: early onset of symptoms linked to increased familial loading and lithium resistance. J Affective Disord 15:255–268, 1988. Copyright 1988 Elsevier Science Publishers.

of lithium therapy (Baastrup et al. 1970; Cordess 1982; Grof et al. 1970; Mander 1986; Sashidharan and McGuire 1983; Small et al. 1971).

By contrast, the available data on lithium use in children and adolescents are sparse. A variety of case reports hint at potentially beneficial effects, yet the measures used to document efficacy, compliance, and adequacy of serum levels are poorly described and the period of follow-up is usually too brief to allow even a tentative statement about prophylactic value (Campbell et al. 1984; Youngerman and Canino 1978).

Annell (1969) described improvement on lithium in a diagnostically heterogeneous sample of 12 juveniles, 2 of whom exhibited manic-depressive cycles. Successful use of lithium in treating hypomanic states in a small series of children has also been reported by Frommer (1968). Four late-adolescence patients included in a large study by Van der Velde (1970) of adults with manic-depressive disorder were all seen as markedly improved with lithium therapy. Horowitz (1977) described 8 adolescents, 7 of whom manifested classic mania with prominent psychotic features; all patients were reported to have experienced complete remission on lithium alone. Two children with definite mania were among 6 subjects described by Brumback and Weinberg (1977). Each experienced prolonged remission following initiation of treatment with lithium, whereas the remainder, some of whom had prominent depressive and psychotic symptoms, showed minimal improvement or exacerbations of symptoms. Carlson and Strober (1978) reported that 3 of 6 manic adolescents diagnosed by Research Diagnostic Criteria (Robbins et al. 1982) showed a markedly positive response to lithium, while the remaining 3 demonstrated only partial improvement. At follow-up, which averaged 18 months, lithium appeared to have prophylactic value in the 3 adolescents who had the best initial response, whereas recurrences were seen in the other 3 patients. Another report of 10 adolescent patients with mania concluded that lithium was effective in 6 of the 7 treated patients, as judged by the significantly shorter duration of episodes in this group compared with the episodes in the 3 patients not treated with lithium (Hassanyeh and Davison 1980). And in one of the few studies of prepubertal children to apply DSM-III diagnostic criteria for mania (American Psychiatric Association 1980), Varanka et al. (1988) found that each of 10 prepubertal children, who also demonstrated prominent psychotic features, improved significantly when treated with lithium alone, beginning an average of 11 days after the start of treatment.

Lithium has also been reported to be strikingly effective in some children and young adolescents with cyclic behavioral disorders suggesting bipolar illness (Davis 1979; DeLong 1978; DeLong and Aldershoff 1987) and in psychiatrically ill children of lithium-responsive bipolar parents (DeLong and Aldershoff 1987; Dyson and Barcai 1970; McKnew et al. 1981). However, these are anecdotal accounts, the validity of which has yet to be established with certainty.

Fewer studies have used randomized, double-blind, placebo-controlled methods to assess lithium's effectiveness in children. In one (Gram and Rafaelson 1972), a diagnostically mixed group of 18 patients was studied, including 2 patients with probable bipolar disorder; both of these children showed significantly greater improvement during the 6 months that they received lithium compared with the 6 months that they received placebo. Similarly, DeLong and Nieman (1983) found significantly greater overall improvement in 11 manic children during a 3-week period of lithium treatment than during a 3-week period of placebo treatment.

Lithium Treatment and Relapse

To extend these findings, I (Strober et al. 1990) recently completed a naturalistic study of lithium maintenance therapy in 37 adolescents whose bipolar I disorder had been stabilized with lithium during inpatient hospitalization. Patients were then followed prospectively for 18 months to compare failure rates among those who were compliant with the recommended maintenance treatment and those who discontinued therapy with the drug. Thirteen patients were noncompliant, whereas 13 patients continued treatment without interruption. The relapse rate among the noncompliant group was 92.3% (12 of 13 relapsed) compared to 37.5% (9 of 24) among the lithium-compliant patients. Relapse was most common in the first 12 months of follow-up and was associated with additional relapses thereafter. Relapsing and nonrelapsing patients were not found to differ in age, sex, number of episodes prior to index hospitalization, or family history of bipolar illness. To our knowledge, this is the first attempt to assess prospectively the early course of maintenance lithium therapy in adolescents with bipolar disorder using strict diagnostic criteria. Because of the uncontrolled nature of the study, it is not known for certain whether these relapses were the cause or effect of lithium discontinuation, or if noncompliant patients were biased in unknown ways toward greater chronicity or lithium refractoriness. For example, Himmelhoch and Garfinkel (1986) have noted an unusually high proportion of adolescents among lithium-resistant bipolar patients that they have studied. Likewise, our group (Strober et al. 1988) has reported that a prepubertal history of aggression-hyperactivity among adolescent manic patients increases the likelihood of resistance to lithium during treatment of the acute episode. Nonetheless, these findings suggest that preventative therapy with lithium may be an essential part of the overall management of bipolar disorder in adolescents.

In short, we know little at present about the generality of lithium effects in children and adolescents with bipolar disorder, or about the utility and differential efficacy of alternative antimanic compounds. These remain issues of obvious theoretical and practical importance to researchers and clinicians alike.

CONCLUSION

Although Kraepelin refers to a case of mania of 6 months' duration in a 4-year-old boy, the recognition and diagnosis of bipolar disorders in preschool and school-age children are still a matter of controversy. However, we are now in a much better position to recognize, diagnose, and treat bipolar disorders in adolescents.

Precursors of bipolar disorders in children are irritability, hyperactivity, destructiveness, and emotional unpredictability. In adolescence, manic euphoria, grandiosity, and paranoia become more prominent. Distractibility, pressured speech, and hyperactivity are present in both children and adolescents. The presence of bipolar disorders, hypomania, and depressive disorders in the family should alert the clinician to the possibility of bipolar disorder in children or adolescents. Accurate diagnosis is important for appropriate pharmacological treatment, follow-up, and education of the patient and the family in treating this cyclic but chronic mental disorder.

REFERENCES

Abou-Saleh MT, Coppen A: Who responds to prophylactic lithium? J Affective Disord 10:115–125, 1986

Akiskal HS, Walker P, Puzantian VR, et al: Bipolar outcome in the course of depressive illness: phenomenologic, familial, and pharmacologic predictors. J Affective Disord 5:115–128, 1983

American Psychiatric Association: Diagnostic and Statistical Manual of Mental Disorders, 3rd Edition. Washington, DC, American Psychiatric Association, 1980

Andreasen NC, Rice J, Endicott J, et al: Familial rates of affective disorder. Arch Gen Psychiatry 44:461–469, 1987

Angst J: Course of affective disorders, in Handbook of Biological Psychiatry. Edited by van Praag H. New York, Marcel Dekker, 1981, pp 225–242

Annell A: Lithium in the treatment of children and adolescents. Acta Psychiatr Scand Suppl 207:19–30, 1969

Anthony J, Scott P: Manic-depressive psychosis in childhood. J Child Psychol Psychiatry 1:53–72, 1960

Baastrup PC, Poulson JC, Schou M, et al: Prophylactic lithium: double-blind discontinuation in manic-depressive disorders. Lancet 2:326–330, 1970

Ballenger JC, Reus VI, Post RM: The "atypical" clinical picture of adolescent mania. Am J Psychiatry 139:602–606, 1982

Baron M: Linkage between an X-chromosome marker (deutan color-blindness) and bipolar affective illness. Arch Gen Psychiatry 34:721–725, 1977

Baron M, Mendlewicz J, Klotz J: Age-of-onset and genetic transmission in affective disorders. Acta Psychiatr Scand 64:373–380, 1981

Baron M, Risch N, Mendlewicz J: Age at onset in bipolar-related major affective illness: clinical and genetic implications. J Psychiatr Res 17:5–18, 1983

Baron M, Risch N, Hamburger R, et al: Genetic linkage between X-chromosome markers and bipolar affective illness. Nature 326:289–292, 1987

Barrett AM: Manic-depressive psychosis in childhood. International Clinics 3:205–211, 1931

Berrettini WH, Goldin LR, Gelernter J, et al: Chromosome markers and manic–depressive illness: rejection of linkage to Xq 28 in nine bipolar pedigrees. Arch Gen Psychiatry 47:366–376, 1990

Bertelsen A, Harvald B, Hauge M: A Danish twin study of manic-depressive disorders. Br J Psychiatry 130:330–351, 1977

Bleuler E: Textbook of Psychiatry. New York, Macmillan, 1934

Brent DA, Perper JA, Goldstein CE, et al: Risk factors for adolescent suicide. Arch Gen Psychiatry 45:581–588, 1988

Brumback RA, Weinberg WA: Mania in childhood, II: therapeutic trial of lithium carbonate and further description of manic-depressive illness in children. Am J Dis Child 131:1122–1126, 1977

Bucher KD, Elston R, Green R, et al: The transmission of manic-depressive illness, II: segregation analysis of three sets of family data. J Psychiatr Res 16:65–78, 1981

Campbell M, Perry R, Green WH: Use of lithium in children and adolescents. Psychosomatics 25:95–106, 1984

Carlson GA: Bipolar affective disorders in childhood and adolescence, in Affective Disorders in Childhood and Adolescence: An Update. Edited by Cantwell DP, Carlson GA. New York, Spectrum, 1983, pp 61–83

Carlson GA, Strober M: Manic-depressive illness in early adolescence: a study of clinical and diagnostic characteristics in six cases. J Am Acad Child Psychiatry 17:138–153, 1978

Carlson GA, Davenport YB, Jamison K: A comparison of outcome in adolescent and late onset bipolar manic-depressive illness. Am J Psychiatry 134:919–922, 1977

Cole JO, Chiarello RJ, Merzel APC: Psychopharmacology update: long-term pharmacotherapy of affective disorders. McLean Hospital Journal 11:106–138, 1986

Coll PG, Bland R: Manic depressive illness in adolescence and childhood. Can J Psychiatry 24:255–263, 1979

Cordess C: "Rebound" mania after lithium withdrawal? (letter). Br J Psychiatry 141:431, 1982

Coryell W, Norten SG: Mania during adolescence. J Nerv Ment Dis 168:611–613, 1980

Coryell W, Endicott J, Reich T, et al: A family study of bipolar II disorder. Br J Psychiatry 145:49–54, 1984

Cox NJ, Suarez BK: Linkage analysis for psychiatric disorders, II: methodological considerations. Psychiatr Dev 4:369–382, 1985

Davis RE: Manic-depressive variant syndrome of childhood: a preliminary report. Am J Psychiatry 136:702–705, 1979

DeLong GR: Lithium carbonate treatment of select behavior disorders suggesting manic-depressive illness. J Pediatr 93:689–694, 1978

DeLong GR, Aldershoff AL: Long-term experience with lithium treatment in childhood: correlation with clinical diagnosis. J Am Acad Child Psychiatry 26:398–394, 1987

DeLong GR, Nieman GW: Lithium induced changes in children with symptoms suggesting manic-depressive illness. Psychopharmacol Bull 19:258–265, 1983

DelZampo M, Bochetta A, Goldin L, et al: Linkage between X-chromosome markers and manic-depressive illness. Acta Psychiatr Scand 70:282–287, 1984

Detera-Wadleigh SC, Berrettini WH, Goldin LR, et al: Close linkage of c-Harvey-ras-1 and the insulin gene to affective disorder is ruled out in three North American pedigrees. Nature 325:806–808, 1987

Dunner DL, Fleiss JL, Fieve RR: Lithium carbonate prophylaxis failure. Br J Psychiatry 129:40–44, 1976

Dwyer JT, DeLong GR: A family history study of twenty probands with childhood manic-depressive illness. J Am Acad Child Psychiatry 26:176–180, 1987

Dyson L, Barcai A: Treatment of lithium-responding patients. Curr Ther Res 12:286–290, 1970

Egeland JA, Gerhard DS, Pauls DL, et al: Bipolar affective disorders linked to DNA markers on chromosome 11. Nature 325:783–787, 1987

Endicott J, Nee J, Andreasen N, et al: Bipolar II: combine or keep separate? J Affective Disord 8:17–28, 1985

Esman AH, Hertzig M, Aarons S: Juvenile manic depressive illness: a longitudinal perspective. J Am Acad Child Psychiatry 22:302–304, 1983

Feinstein SC, Wolpert EA: Juvenile manic-depressive illness. J Am Acad Child Psychiatry 12:123–136, 1973

Frommer EA: Depressive illness in childhood, in Recent Developments in Affective Disorders. Edited by Coppen A, Walk A. Kent, England, Headybros, 1968

Gershon E: Genetics, in Manic-Depressive Illness. Edited by Goodwin FK, Jamison KR. London, Oxford University Press, 1988, pp 373–401

Gershon ES, Goldin LR: The outlook for linkage research in psychiatric disorders. J Psychiatr Res 21:541–550, 1987

Gershon ES, Targum SD, Matthysse S, et al: Color blindness not closely linked to bipolar illness. Arch Gen Psychiatry 36:1423–1434, 1979

Gershon ES, Mendlewicz J, Gastpar M, et al: A collaborative study of genetic linkage of bipolar manic-depressive illness and red/green color blindness. Acta Psychiatr Scand 61:319–338, 1980

Gershon ES, Hamovit J, Guroff J, et al: A family study of schizoaffective, bipolar I, bipolar II, unipolar, and normal controls. Arch Gen Psychiatry 39:1157–1167, 1982

Gershon ES, Hamovit JH, Guroff JJ, et al: Birth-cohort changes in manic and depressive disorders in relatives of bipolar and schizoaffective patients. Arch Gen Psychiatry 44:314–319, 1987a

Gershon ES, Merril CR, Goldin LR, et al: The role of molecular genetics in psychiatry. Biol Psychiatry 22:1388–1405, 1987b

Goetzl U, Green R, Whybrow P, et al: X-linkage revisited—a further family history study of manic-depressive illness. Arch Gen Psychiatry 31:665–672, 1974

Goldin LR, Gershon ES, Targum SD, et al: Segregation and linkage analysis in families of patients with bipolar, unipolar, and schizoaffective mood disorders. Am J Hum Genet 35:274–287, 1983

Goldin LR, Cox NJ, Pauls DL, et al: The detection of major loci by segregation and linkage analysis: a simulation study. Genet Epidemiol 1:285–296, 1984

Goodwin FK, Jamison KR: The natural course of manic-depressive illness, in The Neurobiology of Mood Disorders. Edited by Post RM, Ballenger JC. Baltimore, MD, Williams & Wilkins, 1984, pp 20–37

Gram LF, Rafaelson OJ: Lithium treatment of psychotic children and adolescents. Acta Psychiatr Scand 48:253–260, 1972

Grof P, Cakuls P, Dostal T: Lithium drop-outs: a follow-up study of patients who discontinued prophylactic treatment. Acta Psychiatr Scand 5:162–169, 1970

Hassanyeh F, Davison K: Bipolar affective psychosis with onset before age 16: report of 10 cases. Br J Psychiatry 137:530–539, 1980

Himmelhoch JM, Garfinkel ME: Sources of lithium resistance in mixed mania. Psychopharmacol Bull 22:613–620, 1986

Hodgkinson S, Sherrington R, Gurling H, et al: Molecular genetic evidence for heterogeneity in manic depression. Nature 325:805–806, 1987

Horowitz MM: Lithium and the treatment of adolescent manic-depressive illness. Diseases of the Nervous System 38:480–483, 1977

Hsu LKG, Starzynski JM: Mania in adolescence. J Clin Psychiatry 47:596–599, 1986

James NM: Early- and late-onset bipolar affective disorder. Arch Gen Psychiatry 34:715–717, 1975

Johnson GFS, Leeman MM: Analysis of familial factors in bipolar affective illness. Arch Gen Psychiatry 34:1074–1083, 1977

Kasanin J: The affective psychoses in children. Am J Psychiatry 10:897–926, 1930

Keller MB: Chronic and recurrent affective disorder: incidence, course, and influencing factors, in Chronic Treatments in Neuropsychiatry. Edited by Kemali D, Racagni G. New York, Raven, 1985, pp 111–120

Kelsoe JR, Ginns EI, Egeland JA, et al: Re-evaluation of the linkage relationship between chromosome 11p loci and the gene for bipolar affective disorder in the Older Order Amish. Nature 342:238–243, 1989

Klerman GL, Lavori PW, Rice J, et al: Birth-cohort trends in rates of major depressive disorder among relatives of patients with affective disorder. Arch Gen Psychiatry 42:689–693, 1985

Kraepelin E: Manic-Depressive Insanity and Paranoia. Translated by Barclay RM and edited by Robertson GM. Edinburgh, E & S Livingstone, 1921

Landolt AB: Follow-up studies on circular manic-depressive reactions occurring in the young. Bull NY Acad Med 33:65–73, 1957

Leckman JF, Gershon ES, McGinnis MH, et al: New data do not suggest linkage between the Xq blood group and bipolar illness. Arch Gen Psychiatry 36:1435–1441, 1979

Loranger AW, Levine PM: Age at onset of bipolar illness. Arch Gen Psychiatry 35:1345–1348, 1979

Lundquist G: Prognosis and course in manic-depressive psychoses: a follow-up study of 319 first admissions. Acta Psychiatrica Neurologica 35 (suppl 1):1–96, 1945

Mander AJ: Is lithium justified after one manic episode? Acta Psychiatr Scand 73:60–67, 1986

McKnew DH, Cytryn L, Buchsbaum MS, et al: Lithium in children of lithium-responding parents. Psychiatr Res 4:171–180, 1981

Mendlewicz J, Fleiss J: Linkage studies with X-chromosome markers in bipolar (manic-depressive) and unipolar (depressive) illness. Biol Psychiatry 9:261–264, 1974

Mendlewicz J, Rainer J: Adoption study supporting genetic transmission in manic-depressive illness. Nature 268:327–329, 1977

Mendlewicz J, Fieve RR, Rainer JD: Manic-depressive illness: a comparative study of patients with and without family history. Br J Psychiatry 120:523–530, 1972

Mendlewicz J, Linkowski P, Guroff JJ, et al: Color blindness linkage to bipolar manic-depressive illness: new evidence. Arch Gen Psychiatry 36:1442–1449, 1979

Mendlewicz J, Linkowski P, Wilmotte J: Linkage between 6-phosphate dehydrogenase deficiency and manic-depression psychosis. Br J Psychiatry 134:337–342, 1980

Mendlewicz J, Simon P, Sevy S, et al: Polymorphic DNA marker on X-chromosome and manic depression. Lancet 1:1230–1232, 1989

Olkon DM: Essentials of Neuro-Psychiatry. Philadelphia, PA, Lea & Febiger, 1945

Olsen T: Follow-up study of manic-depressive patients whose first attack occurred before the age of 19. Acta Psychiatr Scand Suppl 162:45–51, 1961

O'Rourke DH, McGuffin P, Reich J: Genetic analysis of manic depressive illness. Am J Phys Anthropol 62:51–59, 1983

Pollack HM: Recurrence of attacks in manic-depressive psychoses. Am J Psychiatry 11:568–573, 1931

Popper C, Famularo R: Child and adolescent psychopharmacology, in Developmental Behavioral Pediatrics. Edited by Levine MD, Carey WB, Gross RT. Philadelphia, PA, WB Saunders, 1983, pp 280–298

Poznanski EO, Israel MC, Grossman J: Hypomania in a four year old. J Am Acad Child Psychiatry 23:105–110, 1984

Price AR, Kidd KK, Pauls DL, et al: Multiple threshold models for the affective disorders: the Yale-NIMH collaborative study. J Psychiatr Res 19:553–546, 1985

Prien RF: Long-term prophylactic pharmacologic treatment of bipolar illness, in

Psychiatry Update: The American Psychiatric Association Annual Review, Vol 2. Edited by Grinspoon L. Washington, DC, American Psychiatric Press, 1983, pp 303–318

Prien RF, Caffey FM, Klett CJ: Factors associated with treatment success in lithium carbonate prophylaxis. Arch Gen Psychiatry 31:189–192, 1974

Reich T, Clayton PJ, Winokur G: Family history studies, V: the genetics of mania. Am J Psychiatry 125:1358–1369, 1969

Rennie TAC: Prognosis in manic-depressive psychosis. Am J Psychiatry 98:801–814, 1942

Rice J, Reich T, Andreasen NC, et al: The familial transmission of bipolar illness. Arch Gen Psychiatry 44:441–450, 1987

Risch N, Baron M: X-linkage and genetic heterogeneity in bipolar-related disorder: reanalysis of linkage data. Ann Hum Genet 46:153–166, 1982

Risch N, Baron M, Mendlewicz J: Assessing the role of X-linked inheritance in bipolar-related major affective disorder. J Psychiatr Res 20:275–288, 1986

Robbins DR, Alessi NE, Cook SC, et al: The use of the Research Diagnostic Criteria (RDC) for depression in adolescent psychiatric inpatients. J Am Acad Child Psychiatry 21(3):251–255, 1982

Rosen LN, Rosenthal NE, van Dusen PH, et al: Age at onset and number of psychotic symptoms in bipolar I and schizoaffective disorder. Am J Psychiatry 140:1523–1525, 1983

Sashidharan SP, McGuire RJ: Recurrence of affective illness after withdrawal of long-term lithium treatment. Acta Psychiatr Scand 68:126–133, 1983

Small JB, Small IF, Moore DF: Experimental withdrawal of lithium in recovered manic-depressive patients: a report of five cases. Am J Psychiatry 127:1555–1559, 1971

Stenstedt A: A study in manic-depressive psychosis. Acta Psychiatrica Neurologica Scandinavica Supplementum 79:1–111, 1952

Strober M, Carlson G: Bipolar illness in adolescents: clinical, genetic and pharmacologic predictors in a three- to four-year prospective follow-up. Arch Gen Psychiatry 39:549–555, 1982

Strober M, Morrell W, Burroughs J, et al: A family study of bipolar I disorder in adolescence: early onset of symptoms linked to increased familial loading and lithium resistance. J Affective Disord 15:255–268, 1988

Strober M, Hanna G, McCracken J: Bipolar disorder, in Handbook of Child Psychiatric Diagnosis. Edited by Last C, Hersen M. New York, John Wiley, 1989, pp 299–316

Strober M, Morrell W, Lampert C: Relapse following discontinuation of lithium maintenance therapy in adolescents with bipolar I illness: a naturalistic study. Am J Psychiatry 147:457–461, 1990

Suarez BK, Croughan J: Is the major histocompatibility complex linked to genes that increase susceptibility to affective disorders? A critical appraisal. Br J Psychiatry 7:19–27, 1982

Suarez BK, Reich T: HLA and affective disorder. Arch Gen Psychiatry 41:22–27, 1984

Sylvester CE, Burke PM, McCauley EA, et al: Manic psychosis in childhood. J Nerv Ment Dis 172:12–15, 1984

Thompson RJ, Schindler FH: Embryonic mania. Child Psychiatry Hum Dev 6:149–154, 1976

Tsuang MT, Bucher KD, Fleming JA, et al: Transmission of affective disorders: an application of segregation analysis to blind family data. J Psychiatr Res 19:23–29, 1985

Van der Velde C: Effectiveness of lithium carbonate in the treatment of manic-depressive illness. Am J Psychiatry 127:121–127, 1970

Varanka TM, Weller RA, Weller EB, et al: Lithium treatment of manic episodes with psychotic features in prepubertal children. Am J Psychiatry 145:1557–1559, 1988

Varsamis J, MacDonald SM: Manic depressive disorder in childhood. Can J Psychiatry 17:279–281, 1972

Weinberg WA, Brumback RA: Mania in childhood. Am J Dis Child 130:380–385, 1976

Weissman MM, Gershon ES, Kidd KK, et al: Psychiatric disorders in the relatives of probands with affective disorders: the Yale University-National Institute of Mental Health Collaborative Study. Arch Gen Psychiatry 41:13–21, 1984

Welner A, Welner Z, Fishman R: Psychiatric adolescent inpatients: a 10-year follow-up. Arch Gen Psychiatry 36:698–700, 1979

Wender PH, Kety SS, Rosenthal D, et al: Psychiatric disorders in biological and adoptive families of adopted individuals with affective disorders. Arch Gen Psychiatry 43:923–928, 1986

Winokur G: The Iowa 500: heterogeneity and course in manic-depressive (bipolar) illness. Compr Psychiatry 16:125–131, 1975

Winokur H, Clayton PJ, Reich T: Manic Depressive Illness. St. Louis, MO, CV Mosby, 1969

Youngerman J, Canino IA: Lithium carbonate use in children and adolescents. Arch Gen Psychiatry 35:216–224, 1978

CHAPTER 13

Bipolar Disorders:
Clinical Manifestations, Differential
Diagnosis, and Treatment

Caroly S. Pataki, M.D.
Gabrielle A. Carlson, M.D.

Bipolar disorders in children and adolescents include the same core components present in the adult form, i.e., episodic clinical manifestations meeting diagnostic criteria for mania, hypomania, and major depression. In this young age group, one or more episodes of major depression may precede an initial episode of mania by months or in some cases by years (Angst et al. 1973; Dunner et al. 1976; Perris 1968).

The essential phenomenology of major depression appears to be the same at all ages, although specific symptoms vary in frequency and intensity in various age groups. The frequency of somatic complaints, auditory hallucinations, and depressed appearance is highest in prepubertal depressed children and tends to decrease with age, whereas other symptoms such as diurnal mood variation, delusions, psychomotor retardation, and anhedonia become more frequent as age increases. Other symptoms, including suicidal ideation, insomnia, and poor concentration, seem to occur with equal frequency in every age group (Carlson and Kashani 1988; Carlson and Strober 1983; Kashani and Carlson 1987; Ryan et al. 1987). (See Chapter 13.)

Mania, which distinguishes bipolar disorder from depressive disorders, is characterized by elevated or irritable mood, increased physical activity, decreased need for sleep, grandiose thinking, and excessive involvement in pleasurable activities, all of which produce marked impairment in functioning. Since discrete manic episodes seem to occur rarely in prepubertal children, it is unclear whether the chronic syndromes comprised of severe hyperactivity, temper outbursts, and instability of mood, in conjunction with family histories of bipolar illness, that are seen in prepubertal children are in fact related to bipolar disorder.

Few data, so far, support the notion of a premorbid behavioral profile in children and adolescents that is predictive of future development of bipolar disorder. In adolescents and young adults who present with a major depression, however, a constellation of features has been identified that is associated with future bipolar disorder. An acute onset of a depression characterized by hypersomnia, psychomotor retardation, mood-congruent psychotic features, and a genetic "loading" for mood disorder appears to predict an eventual bipolar course (Akiskal et al. 1983; Strober and Carlson 1982).

Although specific observable markers of bipolar disorder have not yet been delineated in individuals without affective episodes, studies of high-risk groups are elucidating differences in behavior and adjustment in these individuals as early as the toddler years. For instance, toddlers of a bipolar parent appear to exhibit higher levels of aggression, impaired social behavior, and disturbed attachment to mothers when compared with toddlers of nonpsychiatric control mothers (Gaensbauer et al. 1984; Zahn-Waxler et al. 1984). In spite of some methodological problems that make the above findings tentative, these studies suggest that deviant behaviors may be discernible early on in high-risk groups. Presently, we cannot predict which high-risk individuals will develop bipolar disorder.

CLINICAL MANIFESTATIONS OF BIPOLAR DISORDERS IN CHILDREN AND ADOLESCENTS

Bipolar disorder by definition must include clinical manifestations of a manic or a hypomanic episode. Up to approximately one-third of adults with major depression are likely to develop a manic episode after one or more episodes of depression (Clayton 1981). Higher rates of manic episodes seem to develop in individuals with recurrent depressions (Akiskal et al. 1978). Thus, the clinical picture and corresponding diagnosis of major depression may be present prior to the clinical picture of bipolar disorder. The risks of an eventual manic episode in depressed individuals must be kept in mind.

Depression

The onset of major depression may be acute or insidious, but is most obvious in a child without preexisting psychopathology. Preschool depressed children who are not able to verbalize their depressed feelings often appear sad or listless. Depressed school-age children are less enthusiastic and often show a decreased interest in usual activities, but pervasive anhedonia is generally not prevalent until age increases (Carlson and Kashani 1988). Depressed adolescents, on the other hand, may exhibit severe hopelessness, hypersomnia, and a more generalized withdrawal from activities and social interactions (Ryan et al. 1987). (See Chapter 1.)

Irritability. Irritability is a phenomenon that can be present during a major depressive episode or in mania. To determine whether irritability in a child is a component of an affective episode, it is important to delineate the chronology of this behavior with respect to other affective symptoms. When it occurs along with poor frustration tolerance, inability to finish tasks, and poor attention span, irritability may be a feature associated with attention-deficit hyperactivity disorder or a feature of the disruptive behavior disorders. When irritability is present in the context of a new pattern of behavior, however, it may be an important affective symptom. Interestingly, defiance and aggressive outbursts, and potentially the full syndrome of conduct disorder, have been found to occur in some cases *following* the onset of a depressive episode, particularly in males (Kovacs et al. 1988; Puig-Antich 1982).

Anxiety. Anxiety is frequently a part of the clinical picture of major depression among children. It ranges from an occasional symptom to a concurrent anxiety disorder. About half of the children with school phobia seem to have a co-occurring major depression and separation anxiety disorder (Bernstein and Garfinkel 1986; Hershberg et al. 1982). Kovacs et al. (1989) found coexisting anxiety disorders (most frequently separation anxiety disorder) in 41% of 104 children with depressive disorders. In the 30 children who had major depression and anxiety, the anxiety disorders predated the depression in two-thirds of the cases. It is notable that "school phobia" is not uncommonly reported in the past histories of bipolar patients, prior to the onset of mood disorder (Hassanyeh and Davison 1980).

Vegetative symptoms. Vegetative symptoms occur in depressed individuals of all ages, although they seem to be more prominent as age increases. Initial insomnia is frequently reported in prepubertal depressed children and young adolescents, while terminal insomnia and diurnal mood variation are more common in older adolescents and adults (Baker et al. 1971; Carlson and Strober 1979; Mitchell et al. 1988). Somatic complaints, on the other hand, such as stomachaches and headaches, are most frequently reported by younger depressed children, as compared with depressed adolescents and adults (Carlson and Kashani 1988).

Suicidal ideation. Suicidal ideation is a common symptom in every age group of patients with depressive disorders. Completed suicide, however, rarely occurs in prepubertal children but continues to show an increasing prevalence throughout adolescence (Shaffer 1985; Shaffer and Fisher 1981). Adolescents tend to choose more lethal methods of attempting suicide than their younger depressed counterparts, thereby increasing the risk of completion (Carlson et al. 1987; Ryan et al. 1987). Thus, the risk of suicide is an important one to recognize in adolescents with bipolar disorder.

Psychotic symptoms.   Certain psychotic symptoms in the context of a major depressive episode are not uncommon in prepubertal children. Auditory hallucinations are reported in approximately one-third of prepubertal children with major depression, yet in most cases the hallucinations are not experienced as disruptive to daily activities (Chambers et al. 1982). Auditory hallucinations are reported less frequently among adolescents with major depression than among younger children. Other psychotic symptoms such as delusions are reported in over 10% of adolescents with major depression, which exceeds the rate for adults (Strober et al. 1981).

Psychotic symptoms during episodes of depression and mania are associated with an early onset of bipolar disorder (Ballenger et al. 1982; Rosen et al. 1983; Varanka et al. 1988). Furthermore, a profile in adolescence of depression with psychotic features, along with hypersomnia and a genetic "loading" for mood disorder, appears to be predictive of future development of bipolar disorder (Strober and Carlson 1982). Some evidence suggests that the younger the individual is at the onset of a mood disorder, the more likely it is that psychotic features will be present. It is not clear whether the psychosis represents a more severe form of the illness or points out the propensity of younger individuals to display psychotic symptoms during an affective episode.

Mania

Mania is less common than depression in children, and unless its onset is acute, it may be more difficult to diagnose. In its most extreme form, mania is characterized by frenetic activity, florid psychotic features, grandiose delusions, expansive mood, racing thoughts, lack of insight, and grossly poor judgment. When its onset is acute and the symptoms are extreme, mania is relatively easy to diagnose. The major difficulty is that although classic mania has been well documented in adolescents (Joyce 1984; Loranger and Levine 1978; Winokur et al. 1969), given the high frequency of psychotic symptoms occurring in younger bipolar patients, misdiagnoses of schizophrenia in this population are not uncommon (Carlson and Strober 1978). In less severe forms, however, mania shares some features with a number of other behavioral syndromes, which in children include attention-deficit hyperactivity disorder, oppositional defiant disorder, conduct disorder, cyclothymia, and hypomania, and in adolescents and adults include various personality disorders.

Mania in preadolescents.   There have been only a limited number of published case reports of mania in the preadolescent population (Carlson 1984; Poznanski et al. 1984; Varanka et al. 1988; Weinberg and Brumback 1976), although it is possible that cases are being overlooked (Weller et al. 1986b). Among case reports in the youngest children, up to 8 years of age, irritability, mood lability, coexisting psychopathology (often attention-deficit disorders), and an absence of discrete episodes of true grandiose thinking were characteristic (Carlson 1984). In older children, 9–12 years of age, more well-defined episodes were reported that include euphoric mood and grandiose thinking. In all of the cases of prepubertal mania, hyperactivity, high levels of distractibility, and pressured speech were present, whereas vegetative symptoms were reported only in some cases (Carlson 1984).

Mania versus hyperactivity. As with depressive episodes, mania is most easily diagnosed when it presents acutely and when it represents a clear departure from a baseline state. The difficulty occurs in attempting to determine whether a prepubertal child with chronic psychopathology such as a combination of attention-deficit hyperactivity disorder and aggressive conduct disturbance is actually experiencing a manic episode. Symptoms shared by the above combination of disruptive behavior disorder syndromes and mania include a high activity level, poor frustration tolerance, impulsivity, intrusive behavior, and, in some cases, aggressive outbursts and a decreased need for sleep. The relationship between the chronic behavior disorders of childhood and the diagnostically distinct entity of mania that generally presents in adolescence or young adulthood is controversial. A clinical syndrome seen in childhood characterized by hyperactivity, affective storms, disturbed interpersonal relationships, and a family history of bipolar disorder in the absence of psychotic symptoms was described by Davis (1979) as a manic-depressive variant. Secondary features reported in this entity included sleep disturbance, an abnormal electroencephalogram (EEG), "minimal brain dysfunction," enuresis, and "neuropathology." In such clinical cases, a positive response to lithium treatment strengthened the hypothesis that this syndrome is related to bipolar disorder. Similar behavioral syndromes have been reported in the course of studying the children of bipolar parents (Dyson and Barcai 1970). DeLong (1978) reported on a sample of children who responded to lithium and exhibited the following symptoms: explosive anger, hostility, poor attention, and distractibility.

There is no doubt that a complex relationship exists between the disruptive behavior disorders in childhood and bipolar disorder. An important distinguishing feature between these behavior disorders and bipolar disorder is the frequent occurrence of psychotic features in young individuals with mania and an absence of psychosis in the other disorders (Varanka et al. 1988).

Family studies of children with disruptive behavior disorders (Biederman et al. 1987; Lahey et al. 1988) and follow-up studies (Gittelman et al. 1985) do not support the notion of the disruptive disorders of childhood generally representing juvenile forms of mania. On the other hand, there have been a number of reports of adolescents and adults with bipolar disorder who report past histories consistent with hyperactivity, conduct disturbance, and a variety of other psychiatric symptoms in the prepubertal period (Akiskal et al. 1985; Carlson 1983; Strober et al. 1988). The evidence so far suggests that the disruptive behavior disorders in childhood have an association with future development of bipolar disorder, particularly in individuals with a family history of mood disorder. Adolescent bipolar individuals with childhood histories of attention-deficit hyperactivity disorder and/or conduct disorder may represent a subgroup with more severe disorder than adolescent bipolar individuals without prior psychopathology (Strober et al. 1988).

DIFFERENTIAL DIAGNOSIS

When a bipolar disorder begins with a relatively mild episode in adolescence, it is often attributed to "adolescent turmoil." Despite the anecdotal association of adolescence with transitional occurrences of emotional lability, moodiness, and periods of depression, it is now generally accepted that behavioral disturbance severe enough to cause impairment in social, occupational, or academic functioning is evidence of a psychiatric disorder rather than a universal developmental phase (Graham and Rutter 1985).

It is much more difficult to differentiate mood disorder from developmental variation when functional impairment is not a criterion for the diagnosis. Cyclothymia, for example, is currently defined by periods of depressive symptoms alternating with hypomanic episodes that include features of mania in the absence of functional impairment. Thus, it may be difficult to demarcate the onset of this disorder in an individual who has always been "moody." On the other hand, in cases where there is social and occupational impairment, it may be difficult to draw the line between cyclothymia and bipolar disorder. A progression from cyclothymia to bipolar disorder is reported in adolescent relatives of bipolar individuals (Akiskal et al. 1985). See Table 13–1 for a description of the current DSM-III-R criteria (American Psychiatric Association 1987) for the bipolar disorders and for cyclothymia.

Bipolar Disorder Versus Schizophrenia

One of the most important considerations in the differential diagnosis of bipolar disorder is schizophrenia. Like mania, schizophrenia often occurs in adolescence or young adulthood and presents with psychotic symptoms. The active phases of schizophrenia and acute mania may be indistinguishable. It is important, therefore, to pay attention to the chronology of symptoms. Moreover, it is critical not to disregard affective symptomatology simply because psychotic features are present. In some reported cases, for example, mood disorder in adolescents was misdiagnosed as schizophrenia due to a misinterpretation of the affective symptoms (Carlson and Strober

1978). That is, depressed appearance, psychomotor retardation, and flat affect were not considered important diagnostic symptoms in the presence of thought-blocking, nonaffective hallucinations, and non-mood-specific delusions. It is now recognized that the younger the patient is at the onset of bipolar disorder, the more likely psychotic symptoms, even "schizophreniform symptoms," are to occur (Ballenger et al. 1982; Carlson and Strober

Table 13–1.   DSM-III-R classification of bipolar disorders and cyclothymia

BIPOLAR I DISORDER

Bipolar disorder, manic
- Manic episode (includes all criteria for hypomania plus disturbance sufficient to cause functional impairment in occupational or social activities)
- May be mild, moderate, or severe
- May have mood-congruent or mood-incongruent psychotic features
- If there has been a previous episode of mania, the current episode need not meet full criteria

Bipolar disorder, depressed
- Has had one or more past manic episodes
- Current major depressive episode
- If there has been a previous major depressive episode, the current episode need not meet full criteria

Bipolar disorder, mixed
- Current episode involves full symptomatic picture of both manic and major depressive episodes (except for the 2-week duration criteria for depressive symptoms)

Bipolar disorder not otherwise specified
- Disorders with manic or hypomanic features that do not meet the criteria for any specific bipolar disorder
- Includes "bipolar II"—at least one hypomanic episode and at least one major depressive episode, but never either a manic episode or cyclothymia

CYCLOTHYMIA
- At least 1 year of numerous hypomanic episodes and numerous periods with depressed mood that do not meet full criteria for major depression
- Never a period of more than 2 months in the year in which symptoms are not present
- No clear evidence of a manic or major depression during the year

1978; Joyce 1984; Rosen et al. 1983). In spite of the high frequency of the above symptoms in adolescent bipolar patients, psychosis in bipolar illness is not limited to the young and cannot be explained on the basis of age alone (Carlson and Strober 1978).

Finally, there are several psychiatric disorders, including anorexia nervosa (Hsu et al. 1984) and school phobia (Hassanyeh and Davison 1980), that are reported to occur in individuals who later develop bipolar disorder. In addition, there have been reports of polydrug abuse in relatives of bipolar individuals (Akiskal et al. 1985). The specific nature of the relationship of the above disorders to bipolar illness remains unclarified.

EPIDEMIOLOGY

The reported prevalence of bipolar disorder has fluctuated with changes in the diagnostic criteria being used. During the years when DSM-III (American Psychiatric Association 1980) was current, from 1980 to 1987, mania was defined by sustained symptoms of 1 week's duration without any operational criteria for severity. In the current DSM-III-R, a manic episode no longer has a duration criterion, but is now defined as a disturbance that includes social or occupational impairment and that presumably must last long enough to result in this impairment. Hypomania is currently defined as an entity that resembles mania with the exception of the criterion of impairment.

The impact of using various criteria is seen in a recent epidemiological survey of 14- to 16-year-olds, in whom the prevalence of bipolar disorder according to DSM-III criteria was found to 0.7% (Kashani et al. 1987). Only one subject met the full criteria for mania. When DSM-III-R criteria were used, 7.3% of the adolescents would have qualified for either a manic or hypomanic episode because they met the duration criteria. According to DSM-III-R, without specific impairment or duration criteria, 13.3% of the adolescents would at least have met criteria for hypomania because they endorsed four or more symptoms of mania during a structured interview.

The lifetime prevalence of mania, according to DSM-III criteria, based on a survey of three community sites ranged from 0.6% to 1.1% (Robins et al. 1984). In this epidemiological study, prevalence was broken down into various age groups; in the youngster group (ages 18–24 years), lifetime prevalence of mania was found to be 1.3%. Lifetime prevalence of major depression in this age group is 5.4%. Thus, the prevalence of mania in the 14- to 16-year-old population (0.7%) appears to be close to the lifetime prevalence of mania in young adults. The prevalence of mania and thus of bipolar disorder continues to increase over the age of 25 years.

FAMILIAL TRANSMISSION

It is well known that mood disorders tend to run in families, yet the exact modes of transmission and the genetic relationship of the various clinical presentations are still under investigation. Studies of concordance of bipolar illness in twins have clearly shown a significantly higher concordance in monozygotic twins (65%) compared with dizygotic twins (14%) (Nurnberger and Gershon 1982). In studies of adopted probands with bipolar illness, 31% of their biological parents were found to have bipolar or bipolar spectrum illness compared to 2% of the adoptive parents of the probands (Mendlewicz and Rainer 1977).

Another approach to uncovering the mode of transmission of the affective syndromes is to examine the prevalences of the various clinical presentations in relatives of probands diagnosed with each of the entities in question. The issue of whether unipolar depression (major depressive disorder and/or dysthymia), bipolar I disorder (mania or mania and depression), and bipolar II disorder (hypomania and depression) are correctly designated as distinct entities, as opposed to manifestations of differing severity on one continuous spectrum of mood disorders, is considered in the family studies summarized in Table 13–2.

Bipolar disorder is much more commonly found in relatives of probands with bipolar I disorder than in relatives of probands with bipolar II disorder or unipolar depression (3.9% versus 1.1% and 0.6%, respectively). Furthermore, bipolar II disorder is significantly more common in relatives of probands with that diagnosis than in relatives of probands with either bipolar I disorder or unipolar depressive disorder (8.2% versus 4.2% and 2.9%, respectively). Relatives of probands in each of the three groups, however, seem to show approximately the same prevalence of unipolar depression. In general, these data lend support to the notion that bipolar I disorder, bipolar II disorder, and unipolar depression are genetically distinct entities (Andreasen et al. 1987).

Table 13–2. Frequency of bipolar and unipolar illness in interviewed relatives of affectively ill probands

	Percentage of relatives with diagnosis		
Diagnosis	Bipolar I probands (*n* = 569)	Bipolar II probands (*n* = 267)	Unipolar probands (*n* = 1,171)
Bipolar I	3.9	1.1	0.6
Bipolar II	4.2	8.2	2.9
Unipolar	22.8	26.2	28.4

Source. Adapted from Andreasen et al. 1987.

In another study, Rice et al. (1987) found that the risk for bipolar disorder ranged from 1.5% to 10.2% for relatives of bipolar probands, compared to a range of 0.3% to 4.41% for relatives of unipolar probands. However, Gershon et al. (1982) pointed out that there is no definitive basis for concluding that a separate genetic etiology exists for each mood disorder and suggested a "multifactorial model fit" for mood disorders. This hypothesis is based on the fact that mood disorders appear to be highly prevalent within a limited number of families; within those families there seems to be a graded liability for presentation of mood disorders such that unipolar depression is manifested when liability is less and bipolar disorder is manifested when liability is greater.

After examining familial aggregation of probands with bipolar II disorder, Endicott et al. (1985) concluded that this disorder is distinct from bipolar I disorder and from unipolar depression, although it is a clinically heterogeneous entity insofar as co-occurring psychopathology and treatment response are concerned. The above conclusion was based in part on the following findings: 1) a larger proportion of bipolar II patients have a prior history of other mental disorders; 2) bipolar II patients more frequently manifest chronic somatic symptoms such as migraine headaches; and 3) the relatives of bipolar II probands exhibit a higher prevalence of bipolar II disorders than bipolar I disorders, although there is some evidence that a subgroup of bipolar II probands do switch to bipolar I disorder.

Strober et al. (1988) reported heterogeneity in adolescent bipolar I patients. In their study, the rate of bipolar I disorder in relatives of adolescent bipolar probands was 14.8% (see Chapter 12). In contrast, Andreasen et al. (1987) reported a much lower rate of 5.8% for all relatives of bipolar adult probands. It appears that early onset of illness may be indicative of more severe illness. Furthermore, first-degree relatives of probands with prepubertal psychiatric disorders were found to have a fourfold higher prevalence of bipolar I disorder than relatives of probands without prepubertal psychopathology (29.4% versus 7.4%). This is shown in Table 13–3.

An additional distinction in the prepubertal-onset group was poorer response to lithium treatment. Psychopathology in prepubertal children includes attention-deficit disorder with hyperactivity plus conduct disorder in approximately 80% of these probands and dysthymia and an anxiety disorder in most of the rest of the group.

In spite of strong evidence for the heritability of bipolar disorder from family, twin, and adoption studies (Bertelsen et al. 1977; Gershon et al. 1982; Mendlewicz and Rainer 1977), the precise mode of transmission is still under investigation. The lack of straightforward Mendelian patterns of inheritance of bipolar disorder (that is, single locus, autosomal dominant or recessive, or X-linked) has made it more difficult to determine the transmission route

Table 13–3. Lifetime rates of major mood disorders in relatives of bipolar probands with prepubertal versus adolescent onset of psychiatric illness

| | Percentage of first-degree relatives with diagnosis | |
| | Prepubertal-onset probands | Adolescent-onset probands |
Diagnosis	($n = 34$)	($n = 81$)
Bipolar I	29.4	7.4
Unipolar	14.7	14.8

Source. Adapted from Strober et al. 1988.

(Merikangas et al. 1989). Linkage studies have identified several genetic markers that appear to be associated with bipolar illness in certain pedigrees. For example, a number of investigators have found evidence in some pedigrees of a link between genetic markers for color blindness or glucose-6-phosphatase deficiency on the X chromosome and the presence of bipolar illness (Baron et al. 1987; Mendlewicz and Rainer 1974; Reich et al. 1969). In other pedigrees, however, linkage to the above genetic markers was not demonstrated, leading to the conclusion that there may be multiple modes of transmission of bipolar illness (Berrettini et al. 1990).

Other initial evidence of a linkage between bipolar illness and markers on the short arm of chromosome 11 in an Amish pedigree (Egeland et al. 1987) has recently been reanalyzed, incorporating new individuals into the pedigree and with some changes in clinical status, leading to a reduced likelihood that a major gene for bipolar illness is linked to markers on chromosome 11 (Kelsoe et al. 1989). Studies in other pedigrees have failed to confirm linkages of specific genetic markers to bipolar illness (Detera-Wadleigh et al. 1987; Hodgkinson et al. 1987). Thus far, there is some evidence to support the notion of genetic heterogeneity in the transmission of bipolar illness, yet the specific modes still need further clarification.

The finding that the lifetime prevalence of mood disorders in relatives of bipolar individuals has increased with new generations over the last seven decades is described as a "cohort effect" (Gershon et al. 1987). Although the mechanism of this phenomenon is not known, it implies that some influence of the environment leads to an increased expression of this disorder over time.

Overall, there is ample evidence that genetically determined factors contribute to the development of the bipolar disorders, but the specific modes of genetic transmission and the relationships among unipolar, bipolar I, and bipolar II disorders still remain controversial. In adolescents, determining which individuals have increased genetic vulnerability and identification of additional factors responsible for early expression of the disorder require further investigation.

TREATMENT

The most direct approach to treatment in bipolar disorder is used when the index episode is mania. However, since depression often precedes manic episodes in many bipolar individuals, initial treatment is frequently aimed at ameliorating depression (Angst et al. 1973; Dunner et al. 1976; Perris 1968).

A complication of tricyclic and other antidepressant treatments of depression in bipolar individuals is the potential precipitation of a manic episode. Additional risks of antidepressant use in bipolar patients include the possibility of promoting the development of a rapidly cycling bipolar syndrome (Wehr et al. 1988). Thus, it is important to evaluate the risk of bipolar disorder in any individual presenting with depression. As mentioned earlier, when depression is characterized by psychomotor retardation, hypersomnia, and psychosis in conjunction with a family history of bipolar illness, there is a significant risk for the development of bipolar disorder (Akiskal et al. 1983; Strober and Carlson 1982). In such cases, it may be prudent to treat the patient with lithium or a combination of lithium plus antidepressants instead of antidepressants alone.

Lithium Therapy

Lithium has been used in children and adolescents to treat a variety of behavioral disturbances, as well as in small samples of patients with discrete episodes of mania. In a review by Youngerman and Canino (1978), only 20 of 78 children successfully treated with lithium had symptoms that closely resembled current diagnostic criteria for bipolar disorder. Fifty-eight responders had some related symptoms but were unlike bipolar patients or were not clinically described. DeLong and Aldershof (1987) reported on a 10-year follow-up of lithium treatment in children with a variety of behavioral profiles. Children diagnosed according to DSM-III met criteria for disorders including bipolar disorder, major depression, attention-deficit disorder, conduct disorder, and several combinations of these disorders. In addition to DSM-III disorders, several other categories were included, such as emotionally unstable character disorder (Campbell et al. 1978), offspring of a lithium-responsive parent, and affective, aggressive, explosive, and developmental disorders. The utility of lithium was demonstrated in the bipolar group as well as in numerous other groups in which explosive and aggressive behaviors were prominent, even in the absence of a cycling course. It remains to be determined whether the heterogeneous group of children who are positive responders to lithium are best viewed as having atypical bipolar disorders.

In addition to initiating a trial of lithium in children with typical bipolar presentations, current consensus would support a trial of lithium in children with refractory behavior disorders who have positive family histories of bipolar disorder, in children with psychotic presentations and affective components, and in adolescents who present with major depression and who are in high-risk groups for bipolar illness. In these cases, however, when behavioral symptoms are chronic, or the episodes are atypical, determination of positive response is less clear-cut.

Preparation for lithium therapy. Prior to starting lithium treatment, a complete blood count (CBC) should be done, along with laboratory screening tests documenting renal and thyroid function and a panel of general electrolyte and blood chemistries. These should include a serum blood urea nitrogen determination, as well as measurements of thyroid-stimulating hormone and T_4 (thyroid hormone). A routine urinalysis to rule out proteinuria or other microscopic abnormalities is required; a 24-hour urine collection for creatinine clearance is helpful. An electrocardiogram should also be done documenting normal cardiac function.

Lithium dosage and side effects. The dosage of lithium necessary to produce therapeutic plasma levels appears to be related to body weight. Lithium therapy may be safely started at approximately 30 mg/kg/day (Weller et al. 1986a). This dosage may be increased by 300 mg every 3 days if the serum level is not within the therapeutic range. Lithium is often started at a dose of 300 mg per day in prepubertal children, and the dose is increased by 300 mg until a therapeutic level is reached. To ascertain a steady-state level in the blood, maintain the dose for 5 days so that the final blood level will be attained. The therapeutic serum level (0.6–1.2 mEq/L) is the same for all ages. Children tend to have a high renal clearance of lithium and, in some cases, may require higher doses than adults to achieve the same blood level. Lithium is usually given in divided doses to minimize side effects. Common side effects include polyuria, polydipsia, diarrhea, and weight gain. Nausea, vomiting, sedation, slurred speech, ataxia, and change in sensorium are common signs of toxicity. Continued follow-up of renal status, thyroid status, and blood chemistry is recommended.

The decision to start lithium therapy is based both on the severity and frequency of the episodes and on the impairment they cause. If the episodes of depression and mania are tempered but still present after lithium therapy has been initiated, lithium is probably required on a prophylactic basis. In cases where episodes are no longer discernible, a drug holiday should be planned to coincide with a time when relapse, if it occurs, would be least catastrophic.

A recent naturalistic follow-up study of lithium-responsive bipolar adolescents found a relapse rate of 38% in those who continued to receive lithium prophylactically for a full 18 months, compared to a relapse rate of 92%

in those who discontinued the medication prior to the end of the 18-month period (Strober et al. 1990). Of those adolescents who relapsed while on medication within the first 9 months, only 21% relapsed thereafter. Thus, response to lithium over the first 6–12 months may predict longer-term response. (See Chapter 12.)

Lithium and neuroleptics.   In cases of acute mania with florid psychotic symptoms, initial treatment with neuroleptics is sometimes advisable to control unmanageable behavior while lithium is being introduced. The dosage of neuroleptics should be kept as low as possible to minimize potential neurotoxicity that may arise from the combination, as well as to guard against severe extrapyramidal symptoms, to which bipolar patients may be unusually sensitive (Goodwin and Roy-Byrne 1987; Nasrallah et al. 1988).

In situations where therapy with tricyclic antidepressants has been initiated prior to lithium therapy and mood cycles are not responsive to the combination, lithium should be tried by itself, since it is possible that it is more efficacious alone (Wehr and Goodwin 1979).

Medical complications that potentially contraindicate the use of lithium include renal impairment, endocrine abnormalities, and cardiac problems such as conduction defects. Additionally, in individuals with seizure disorders and bipolar illness, in whom both lithium and neuroleptics may increase the risk of a seizure, other pharmacological interventions such as carbamazepine therapy are indicated.

In some adults with bipolar disorder with no evidence of psychosis, lithium is used with the benzodiazepines, particularly clonazepam, instead of with neuroleptics. Also, in some adults with bipolar disorder, lithium is combined with other medications such as propranolol, carbamazepine, or valproic acid. Data on children and adolescents with bipolar disorder are not available in order to make a recommendation for or against these combinations.

Carbamazepine

Carbamazepine, a well-established anticonvulsant used in adults and children, has been noted in a number of published reports to improve attention, social behavior, and mood in epileptic patients (Ballenger and Post 1980). It has been used in several open trials in children who exhibit an array of psychiatric symptoms, including "episodic dyscontrol" syndromes and psychotic disorders (for a review, see Evans et al. 1987). A controlled study of bipolar adults treated with carbamazepine (Ballenger and Post 1980) found that it had antimanic effects that were observed within the first week of treatment and antidepressant effects that occurred after 2 weeks of treatment. Individuals who responded to carbamazepine had blood levels ranging between 7 and 12 µg/ml. The initial dosage was 200 mg bid, and the final dosage ranged from 600 to 1,200 mg/day.

There are not yet any systematic studies delineating the efficacy of carbamazepine for the treatment of affective disorders in children. There have been some case reports documenting the efficacy of carbamazepine in bipolar adolescents who are unresponsive to lithium (Hsu 1986). In general, the dosages used in children with psychiatric disorders are similar to those recommended in children for seizure control, that is, a starting dose of 100 mg bid. Incremental increases of 100 mg daily can be made using a tid or qid regimen until the best response is obtained. The daily dose should not exceed 1,000 mg/day (*Physicians' Desk Reference* 1990). The rare but most serious side effects of carbamazepine are hematopoietic disturbances such as agranulocytosis and aplastic anemia. It is currently recommended that red and white blood cell counts be monitored on a weekly basis for the first 3 months of treatment and monthly thereafter (*Physicians' Desk Reference* 1990). Less serious side effects include nausea, drowsiness, and blurred vision (Evans et al. 1987). Additional behavioral side effects have also occasionally been noted, including irritability, hyperactivity, and aggressivity (Evans et al. 1987).

There has also been a case report of successful electroconvulsive therapy treatment of acute severe mania in a 12-year-old girl who was unable to be managed pharmacologically in the initial phases of her mania due to intolerance of psychotropic medications (Carr et al. 1983).

Psychosocial Intervention

Given the complex set of symptoms in bipolar disorder, the most serious of which is the risk of suicide, it is important to address the spectrum of psychosocial difficulties in bipolar patients with a combination of individual psychotherapy where indicated, family education and therapy, and interpersonal skills interventions when possible. (See Chapters 7, 8, and 9.)

CHILDREN OF PATIENTS WITH BIPOLAR DISORDERS

Children of parents with bipolar disorders are more likely to manifest affective symptoms than children of nonpsychiatrically ill parents because of genetic vulnerability as well as longitudinal exposure to the affective disturbance. Studies comparing psychopathology in children of bipolar parents with that in children of normal parents have found a significantly higher rate of a variety of psychiatric disorders (although not specifically mood disorders) in the children of bipolar parents (Decina et al. 1983; Gershon et al. 1985; Grigoroiu-Serbanescu et al. 1989). Commonly diagnosed disorders in the proband children compared with the children of normal parents are conduct disorders (17% versus 5%), attention-deficit disorder (14% versus 8%), and separation anxiety disorder (24% versus 14%). No significant difference was found in the rate of major depression (10% in probands and 14% in controls) or in the rate of minor affective disorder (28% versus 24%) (Gershon et al. 1985).

In another study, the psychopathology in the children of bipolar parents was characterized by a dimension called "instability" that consisted of emotional instability, poor frustration tolerance, shallowness in schoolwork, poor peer relationships, and symptoms of anxiety (Grigoroiu-Serbanescu et al. 1989). Thus, although it is clear that children in this high-risk group are demonstrating poor adjustment, the relationship between these traits and the development of future bipolar disorder remains as yet poorly defined.

CLINICAL COURSE

The issue of whether adolescent-onset bipolar illness implies a natural history and outcome that differ from those of adult-onset bipolar illness remains investigational. In the adult literature, outcome in bipolar illness was found to be variable with respect to the functional impairment that persisted over time. In an outcome review in several hundred bipolar patients from numerous studies, from 15% to 53% of individuals were found to be chronically disabled (Coryell and Winokur 1982; Goodwin and Jamison 1984). In adult bipolar patients, an index pure manic episode for which treatment is sought seems to resolve in up to 50% of patients within 5 weeks; an index pure depressive episode is expected to resolve in 50% of patients in 9 weeks; and an index episode characterized by mixed depressive and manic symptoms may take up to 14 weeks to resolve in 50% of patients (Keller et al. 1986).

Features of Slower-Recovery Episodes

Clinical features associated with slower recovery include psychotic symptoms, endogenous features, severity of depression, psychomotor retardation, and alcoholism (M.B. Keller, unpublished data, cited in Keller 1987). Further investigation is needed to clarify the pattern by which episodes of depression and mania occur; however, it appears that episodes may increase in frequency over a period of time, after which a more stable cycle develops in which episodes are likely to occur once or twice per year (Clayton 1981; Coryell and Winokur 1982). It appears that patients with mixed cycles are at highest risk for chronic illness: 32% were likely to remain ill after 1 year, compared to chronic illness in only 7% of the patients who had manic symptoms alone (Keller et al. 1986).

Longitudinal Studies

Longitudinal studies of adolescent-onset bipolar disorder have been less numerous than those of adult-onset bipolar disorder. Thus far, the following observations have been made. In one study comparing outcome in adolescent- and adult-onset bipolar patients, 28 adolescent-onset bipolar patients were followed over a mean time of 19 years (Carlson et al. 1977). Of these, 60% were considered to have a good social outcome, 20% were significantly impaired but functional, and 20% were considered chronically ill. There was one suicide within the follow-up period. Eighteen had an index episode of depression, 10 had an index episode of mania, and 2 were considered to be rapid cyclers. There were no differences found between the clinical presentations of the adolescents and the adults; the outcomes of the adolescent-onset patients were generally similar to those of the adult-onset patients. Early-onset bipolar disorder patients were noted to be earning less money than adult-onset bipolar patients, and more of them were unmarried. In a report on 35 juvenile bipolar patients followed over a period of 20 years, 83% were noted to have original diagnoses of schizoaffective disorder and, compared with individuals who had onsets after age 20 years, the early-onset group manifested significantly more psychotic symptoms (McGlashan 1988). Early-onset patients did not require hospitalization more frequently than patients with later onsets; there was no difference in treatment or in the rate of suicide.

Childhood and early adolescent onset of bipolar illness, however, is associated with an increased risk for this illness in relatives (Dwyer and DeLong 1987; Strober et al. 1988). Moreover, adolescent bipolar patients with past histories of childhood psychopathology (it is unclear whether this is affective symptomatology) have a poorer response to lithium. The longitudinal data that do exist suggest that in treatable and uncomplicated bipolar disorder, an early age at onset probably does not worsen the prognosis of the disorder (Carlson et al. 1977; McGlashan 1988).

The following case points out the challenge of diagnosis and management of an adolescent with acute bipolar disorder.

CASE HISTORY

Bob is a 15-year-old adolescent who is the oldest male in a family of five siblings. As a young boy, Bob was characterized by his mother as being the most outspoken, provocative, and mischievous of her children. He was often rebellious toward his parents and received harsh punishments from his father. He and his brother were known in the neighborhood for their frequent pranks and practical jokes. In school, however, Bob was described as a somewhat shy and socially awkward boy who had difficulty making friends and generally kept to himself. Academically, he had no specific learning disabilities and had maintained a B average. Bob had always attended parochial school, where he encountered strict rules, but he had managed to stay out of trouble. Aside from a history of chronic nocturnal enuresis, the family was not concerned about Bob's adjustment.

Family History

Bob's home life was chronically chaotic due to severe marital conflict between his parents, which often turned into physical altercations and at times involved some of the children. There was also a great deal of physical fighting between Bob and his siblings that sometimes escalated to dangerous proportions. Bob's father, a successful businessman, was described as volatile, authoritarian, and critical. He was especially punitive toward Bob, for whom he had unusually high expectations. Bob's mother was known as the family "chatterbox" in her own family when she was growing up, and she also described herself as a "daredevil." Bob's mother was noted to be a rather entertaining conversationalist who spoke in a rapid, pressured manner and who exhibited a perpetually cheery and mildly euphoric mood that was infectious, even in the face of great adversity. She reported that she had a chronically high energy level and that she had never deviated from this state. The family history was positive for a maternal aunt who had a recurrent psychotic illness of late onset that was episodic and required multiple hospitalizations. The diagnosis was unknown. There was a history of alcoholism in the maternal grandfather and depression in one of the maternal aunts. On the paternal side, the father was described as explosive and moody. His family was known for their high achievers and quick tempers. Of Bob's siblings, one sister had learning disabilities and aggressive outbursts. Two of his brothers were also enuretic. Bob had little past medical history other than an allergy to bee stings and a sensitivity to promethazine hydrochloride, which he had used for nausea and to which he had developed a dystonic reaction.

Early Symptoms

When Bob was 13 years old, he went through a period in which he was particularly argumentative, irritable, and hostile. He instigated fights with his siblings, and he appeared to be antagonistic and unhappy with himself and his family. He was taken to a psychotherapist, who saw him irregularly over a period of 3 months. According to the therapist, Bob resented being the one identified as the family member with "problems" and he rarely opened up to the therapist. On those occasions when he did, he would become tearful when describing the troubled family relationships. Bob was felt by his therapist to be depressed and to have poor self-esteem. There was no history of a change in appetite, no sleep disturbance noted, and no suicidal ideation.

Bob's mental status did not change drastically during the 3 months of therapy. Bob's mother reported that there was a gradual improvement in Bob's mood and level of hostility by the end of the therapeutic intervention. Episodes of slamming doors, throwing objects, and instigating fights with his siblings diminished over the next several months.

Imipramine-Induced Psychosis

Bob was doing relatively well in the tenth grade when he was started on a low dose of imipramine to treat the enuresis that was still plaguing him. He continued to receive 25 mg per day for approximately 3 weeks, but he then decided to double the dose since it didn't seem to be working. Several nights later, Bob's parents noticed that he suddenly was insomniac and hyperkinetic and spent the entire night writing voluminous notes to each member of his family detailing how much he loved them. By the next morning, Bob was beginning to rant. He disclosed that he was receiving personal messages from the television, that he had the power to control his siblings from afar, and that the devil was attempting to communicate through him. He was preoccupied with sex and extremely agitated, masturbating in front of his siblings and urinating and defecating in the living room. His mother called the pediatrician, who concurred with the mother's suggestion to try a promethazine hydrochloride suppository that she had at home to diminish his agitation. Bob continued in the same fashion during the course of the night and was brought to the emergency room the next morning in a disoriented and agitated state, experiencing auditory and visual hallucinations.

Hospitalization

While in the emergency room, Bob had a severe dystonic reaction, which responded to diphenhydramine hydrochloride. When his dystonia subsided, a small dose of haloperidol was administered. On admission, he required physical restraints and was virtually incoherent. Over the next 24 hours, his level of arousal and coherence waxed and waned. When alert, he verbalized continuously in a loud, pressured, and grandiose manner. He did not sleep at all during this period and could barely stop raving long enough to swallow food, which had to be spoon-fed to him.

Due to the waxing and waning of his level of arousal and orientation, a delirium of unknown etiology was at first considered. An organic workup, including a CBC, electrolytes, and liver, renal, and endocrine studies, was done and found to be negative. A lumbar puncture, a computed tomography scan, and an EEG were done and were all negative. There were no signs of current or recent infectious process. To rule out a central anticholinergic delirium, a physostigmine challenge was done and was negative. In view of the negative medical workup and the strikingly grandiose psychotic symptomatology, a diagnosis of delirious mania was made. Neuroleptics and anti-parkinsonian medications were continued, but shortly thereafter these medications were discontinued due to recurrent severe extrapyramidal side effects. Over the next week, Bob slept only several hours. He was able to recognize his doctors at times, although he seemed to believe that all of the female staff were his wives and he was still intermittently confused about where he was. Bob was in perpetual motion, intermittently agitated, and still psychotic and delusional. Bob expressed bizarre grandiose ideas such as, "I am God," and admitted to feeling that his thoughts were racing. On some days he would start out the day more subdued and, over the course of the day, would become silly and regressed, giggle uncontrollably, and end up grossly incoherent. He spent most of the next week verbalizing in a grandiose stream of consciousness and, for the most part, was unable to differentiate reality from his expansive delusions.

Treatment With Lithium and Carbamazepine

Lithium was started and titrated up to a dose of 1,800 mg per day and a blood level of 1.1 mEq/L. After several weeks of therapeutic levels of lithium treatment, Bob's activity level had diminished somewhat and he was experiencing periods in which he muttered incoherently with clang associations and hypersexual delusions. He occasionally verbalized that the staff were lying to him and often spit out his food, believing that it might be poisoned. Carbamazepine at a dose of 1,000 mg per day was added to his lithium regimen, with a resulting blood carbamazepine level of 6 mcg/dl. Over the next few weeks, Bob's mental status gradually improved.

Three weeks after the combination of medications was established, Bob began to have longer periods of sitting quietly and he was calm enough to begin attending school in the hospital. He was oriented, able to groom himself, and generally cooperative. In fact, he appeared to be sluggish and his parents confirmed that his activity level was lower than it had been prior to his illness. He avoided eye contact and appeared to be mildly depressed, although he denied feeling sad or having suicidal ideation. His affect was flat and his responses were characterized by long latency periods, but his speech was nonpressured and his thoughts were coherent. There was no evidence of persistent delusions or hallucinations. He answered questions directly and made little spontaneous conversation. He seemed to be both anxious and embarrassed that he could not remember what had happened to him over the past 2 months.

Psychiatric Follow-up

Over the next few weeks while Bob continued to recuperate in this mildly depressed state without much change in his mental status, the family was educated about his illness. They were counseled regarding the importance of regular psychiatric follow-up and the need for a less stressful home environment for Bob during his recuperation period. The family agreed to make an effort to be less critical and more supportive of Bob, and his school was cooperative in offering him special help to make up for missed work. Bob was discharged on the combination of lithium and carbamazepine because he continued to do well. After discharge, Bob came sporadically to scheduled appointments and the household appeared to be persistently chaotic. His periodic blood lithium levels showed significant fluctuation, and Bob admitted that he was not taking his medications on a regular basis. In spite of this, Bob continued to function relatively well, although he was having some increased difficulty concentrating on his schoolwork. His depressed appearance diminished over the following 2 months, and he seemed to be more spontaneous in his interactions, especially with his siblings. Despite discussions with the family regarding the advisability of maintaining the medications until a reasonable time was planned to discontinue them, such as the end of the school year, 4 months after discharge Bob took himself off both medications. At the end of a 6-month period Bob was still doing well, without further episodes of depression or mania.

CONCLUSION

Bipolar disorder, when it presents in its classic form in adolescence, appears to have the same characteristics, treatment response, and natural history as it does in adults. Adolescents with bipolar disorders appear to have an increased genetic loading for the illness. Those who have an onset of psychiatric symptoms before pubescence may represent a distinct subgroup with an even greater risk of mood disorders in family members, as well as a poorer response to lithium treatment (Strober et al. 1988). Disruptive behavioral syndromes in prepubertal children may mask manic or hypomanic tendencies. Some of these children may develop bipolar disorders in adolescence. However, at the present time, we are not able to predict which of these children will develop bipolar disorders.

REFERENCES

Akiskal HS, Bitar AH, Puzantian VR, et al: The nosological status of neurotic depression—a prospective three- to four-year examination in light of the primary-secondary and unipolar-bipolar dichotomies. Arch Gen Psychiatry 35:756–766, 1978
Akiskal HS, Parks W, Puzantian VR, et al: Bipolar outcome in the course of depressive illness. J Affective Disord 5:115–128, 1983
Akiskal HS, Downs J, Jordan P, et al: Affective disorders in referred children and

younger siblings of manic-depressives: mode of onset and prospective course. Arch Gen Psychiatry 42:996–1003, 1985

American Psychiatric Association: Diagnostic and Statistical Manual of Mental Disorders, 3rd Edition. Washington, DC, American Psychiatric Association, 1980

American Psychiatric Association: Diagnostic and Statistical Manual of Mental Disorders, 3rd Edition, Revised. Washington, DC, American Psychiatric Association, 1987

Andreasen NC, Rice J, Endicott J, et al: Familial rates of affective disorder: a report from the National Institute of Mental Health Collaborative Study. Arch Gen Psychiatry 44:461–469, 1987

Angst J, Baastrup P, Grof P, et al: The course of monopolar depression and bipolar psychosis. Psychiatria Neurologia Neurochirurgia 76:489–500, 1973

Baker M, Dorzab J, Winokur G, et al: Depressive disease: classification and clinical characteristics. Compr Psychiatry 12:354–365, 1971

Ballenger JC, Post RM: Carbamazepine (Tegretol) in manic-depressive illness: a new treatment. Am J Psychiatry 137:782–790, 1980

Ballenger JC, Reus VI, Post RM: The "atypical" presentation of adolescent mania. Am J Psychiatry 139:602–606, 1982

Baron M, Risch N, Hamburger R, et al: Genetic linkage between X-chromosome markers and bipolar affective illness. Nature 326:289–292, 1987

Bernstein GA, Garfinkel BD: School phobia: the overlap of affective and anxiety disorders. J Am Acad Child Psychiatry 25:235–241, 1986

Berrettini WH, Goldin LR, Gelernter J, et al: X-chromosome markers and manic depressive illness: rejection of linkage to Xq28 in nine bipolar pedigrees. Arch Gen Psychiatry 47:366–373, 1990

Bertelsen A, Harvald B, Hauge MA: A Danish twin study of manic depressive disorders. Br J Psychiatry 130:330–351, 1977

Biederman J, Munir K, Knee D: Conduct and oppositional disorder in clinically referred children with attention deficit disorder: a controlled family study. J Am Acad Child Adolesc Psychiatry 26:724–727, 1987

Campbell M, Schulman D, Rapoport J: The current status of lithium therapy in child and adolescent psychiatry. J Am Acad Child Psychiatry 14:95–105, 1978

Carlson GA: Bipolar affective disorders in childhood and adolescence, in Affective Disorders in Childhood and Adolescence. Edited by Cantwell DP, Carlson GA. New York, SP Medical & Scientific Books, 1983, pp 61–84

Carlson GA: Classification issues of bipolar disorders in childhood. Psychiatr Dev 4:273–285, 1984

Carlson GA, Kashani JH: Phenomenology of major depressive from childhood through adulthood: analysis of three studies. Am J Psychiatry 145:1222–1225, 1988

Carlson GA, Strober M: Manic-depressive illness in early adolescence: a study of clinical and diagnostic characteristics in six cases. J Am Acad Child Psychiatry 17:138–153, 1978

Carlson GA, Strober M: Affective disorders in adolescence. Psychiatr Clin North Am 2:511–526, 1979

Carlson GA, Strober M: Affective disorders in adolescence, in Affective Disorders in Childhood and Adolescence: An Update. Edited by Cantwell D, Carlson GA. New York, Spectrum Publications, 1983, pp 85–96

Carlson GA, Davenport YB, Jamison K: A comparison of outcome in adolescent and late-onset bipolar manic-depressive illness. Am J Psychiatry 134:919–922, 1977

Carlson GA, Asarnow JR, Orbach I: Developmental aspects of suicidal behavior. J Am Acad Child Adolesc Psychiatry 26:186–193, 1987

Carr V, Dorrington C, Schrader G, et al: The use of ECT for mania in childhood bipolar disorder. Br J Psychiatry 143:411–415, 1983

Chambers WJ, Puig-Antich J, Tabrizi MA, et al: Psychotic symptoms in prepubertal major depressive disorder. Arch Gen Psychiatry 39:921–927, 1982

Clayton PJ: The epidemiology of bipolar affective disorder. Compr Psychiatry 22:31–43, 1981

Coryell W, Winokur G: Course and outcome, in Handbook of Affective Disorders. Edited by Paykel ES. New York, Guilford, 1982, pp 93–106

Davis RE: Manic-depressive variant syndrome of childhood: a preliminary report. Am J Psychiatry 136:702–706, 1979

Decina P, Kestenbaum CJ, Farber S, et al: Clinical and psychological assessment of children of bipolar probands. Am J Psychiatry 140:548–553, 1983

DeLong GR: Lithium carbonate treatment of select behavior disorders in children suggesting manic-depressive illness. J Pediatr 93:689–694, 1978

DeLong GR, Aldershof AL: Long term experience with lithium treatment in childhood: correlation with diagnosis. J Am Acad Child Psychiatry 26:389–394, 1987

Detera-Wadleigh SD, Berrettini WH, Goldin LR, et al: Close linkage of c-Harvey-ras-1 and the insulin gene to affective disorder is ruled out in three North American pedigrees. Nature 325:806–808, 1987

Dunner DL, Fleiss JL, Fieve RL: The course and development of mania in patients with recurrent depression. Am J Psychiatry 133:905–908, 1976

Dwyer JT, DeLong GR: A family history of twenty probands with childhood manic-depressive illness. J Am Acad Child Adolesc Psychiatry 26:176–180, 1987

Dyson WL, Barcai A: Treatment of children of lithium-responding parents. Curr Ther Res 12:286–290, 1970

Egeland JA, Gerhard DS, Pauls DL, et al: Bipolar affective disorders linked to DNA markers on chromosome 11. Nature 325:783–787, 1987

Endicott J, Nee J, Andreasen N, et al: Bipolar II: combine or keep separate? J Affective Disord 8:17–28, 1985

Evans RW, Clay TH, Gualtieri CT: Carbamazepine in pediatric psychiatry. J Am Acad Child Adolesc Psychiatry 26:2–8, 1987

Gaensbauer TJ, Harmon RJ, Cytryn L, et al: Social and affective development in infants with a manic-depressive parent. Am J Psychiatry 141:223–229, 1984

Gershon ES, Hamovit J, Guroff JJ, et al: A family study of schizoaffective, bipolar

I, bipolar II, unipolar, and normal control probands. Arch Gen Psychiatry 39:1157–1167, 1982

Gershon ES, McKnew D, Cytryn L, et al: Diagnoses in school-age children of bipolar affective disorder patients and normal controls. J Affective Disord 8:283–291, 1985

Gershon ES, Hamovit JH, Guroff JJ, et al: Birth cohort changes in manic and depressive disorders in relatives of bipolar and schizoaffective patients. Arch Gen Psychiatry 44:314–319, 1987

Gittelman R, Mannuzza S, Shenker R, et al: Hyperactive children almost grown up. Arch Gen Psychiatry 42:937–947, 1985

Goodwin FK, Jamison KR: The natural course of manic-depressive illness, in Neurobiology of the Mood Disorders. Edited by Post RM, Ballenger JC. Baltimore, MD, Williams & Wilkins, 1984, pp 20–37

Goodwin FK, Roy–Byrne P: Treatment of bipolar disorders, in Psychiatry Update: American Psychiatric Association Annual Review, Vol 6. Edited by Hales RE, Frances AJ. Washington, DC, American Psychiatric Press, 1987, pp 81–108

Graham P, Rutter M: Adolescent disorders, in Child and Adolescent Psychiatry. Edited by Rutter M, Hersen L. London, Blackwell Scientific Publications, 1985, pp 351–367

Grigoroiu-Serbanescu M, Christodorewcu D, Jipescu I, et al: Psychopathology in children aged 10–17 of bipolar parents: psychopathology rate and correlates of the severity of the psychopathology. J Affective Disord 16:167–179, 1989

Hassanyeh F, Davison K: Bipolar affective psychosis with onset before age 16: report of 10 cases. Br J Psychiatry 137:530–539, 1980

Hershberg SG, Carlson GA, Cantwell DP, et al: Anxiety and depression disorders in psychiatrically disturbed children. J Clin Psychiatry 43:358–361, 1982

Hodgkinson S, Sherrington R, Gurling H, et al: Molecular genetic evidence for heterogeneity in manic depression. Nature 325:805–806, 1987

Hsu LKG: Lithium resistant adolescent mania. J Am Acad Child Adolesc Psychiatry 25:280–283, 1986

Hsu LKG, Holder D, Hindmarsh D, et al: Bipolar illness preceded by anorexia nervosa in identical twins. J Clin Psychiatry 45:262–266, 1984

Joyce PR: Age of onset in bipolar affective disorder and misdiagnosis as schizophrenia. Psychol Med 14:145–149, 1984

Kashani JH, Carlson GA: Seriously depressed preschoolers. Am J Psychiatry 144:348–350, 1987

Kashani JH, Beck NC, Heoper EW, et al: Psychiatric disorders in a community sample of adolescents. Am J Psychiatry 144:584–589, 1987

Keller MB: Differential diagnosis, natural course and epidemiology of bipolar disorders, in Psychiatry Update: American Psychiatric Association Annual Review, Vol 6. Edited by Hales RE, Frances AJ. Washington, DC, American Psychiatric Press, 1987, pp 10–31

Keller MB, Lavori PW, Coryell W, et al: Differential outcome of episodes of illness in bipolar patients: pure manic, mixed/cycling and pure depressive. JAMA 256:3138–3142, 1986

Kelsoe JR, Ginns EF, Egeland JA, et al: Re-evaluation of the linkage relationship between 11p loci and the gene for bipolar affective disorder in the Old Order Amish. Nature 342:238–243, 1989

Kovacs M, Paulauskas S, Gatsonis C, et al: Depressive disorders in childhood, III: a longitudinal study of comorbidity with and risk for conduct disorders. J Affective Disord 15:205–217, 1988

Kovacs M, Gatsonis C, Paulauskas SL, et al: Depressive disorders in childhood, IV: a longitudinal study of comorbidity with and risk for anxiety disorders. Arch Gen Psychiatry 46:776–782, 1989

Lahey BB, Piacentini JC, McBurnett K, et al: Psychopathology and antisocial behavior in the parents of children with conduct disorder and hyperactivity. J Am Acad Child Psychiatry 27:163–170, 1988

Loranger AW, Levine PM: Age of onset of bipolar affective illness. Arch Gen Psychiatry 35:1345–1348, 1978

McGlashan TH: Adolescent versus adult onset of mania. Am J Psychiatry 145:221–224, 1988

Mendlewicz J, Rainer JD: Morbidity risk and genetic transmissions in manic depressive illness. Am J Hum Genet 25:692–701, 1974

Mendlewicz J, Rainer JD: Adoption study supporting genetic transmission in manic-depressive illness. Nature 265:327–329, 1977

Merikangas KR, Spence A, Kupfer DJ: Linkage studies of bipolar disorder: methodologic and analytic issues: report of MacArthur Foundation workshop on linkage and clinical features in affective disorders. Arch Gen Psychiatry 46:1137–1141, 1989

Mitchell J, McCauley E, Burke PM, et al: Phenomenology of depression in children and adolescents. J Am Acad Child Adolesc Psychiatry 27:12–20, 1988

Nasrallah HA, Churchill CM, Hamden-Allan G: Higher frequency of neuroleptic-induced dystonia in mania than in schizophrenia. Am J Psychiatry 145:1455–1456, 1988

Nurnberger JI, Gershon E: Genetics, in Handbook of Affective Disorders. Edited by Paykel ES. Edinburgh, Churchill-Livingston, 1982, pp 126–145

Perris C: The course of depressive psychoses. Acta Psychiatr Scand 238–248, 1968

Physicians' Desk Reference, 44th Edition. Oradell, NJ, Medical Economics Company, 1990

Poznanski EO, Israel MC, Grossman J: Hypomania in a four-year-old. J Am Acad Child Psychiatry 23:105–110, 1984

Puig-Antich J: Major depression and conduct disorder in prepuberty. J Am Acad Child Psychiatry 21:118–128, 1982

Reich T, Clayton PJ, Winokur G: Family history studies, V: the genetics of mania. Am J Psychiatry 125:1358–1369, 1969

Rice J, Reich T, Andreasen NC, et al: The familial transmission of bipolar illness. Arch Gen Psychiatry 44:441–447, 1987

Robins LN, Helzer JE, Weissman MM, et al: Lifetime prevalence of specific psychiatric disorders in three sites. Arch Gen Psychiatry 41:949–958, 1984

Rosen LN, Rosenthal NE, Van Dusen PH, et al: Age at onset and number of psychotic symptoms in bipolar I and schizoaffective disorder. Am J Psychiatry 140:1523–1524, 1983

Ryan ND, Puig-Antich J, Ambrosini P, et al: The clinical picture of major depression in children and adolescents. Arch Gen Psychiatry 44:854–861, 1987

Shaffer D: Depression, mania, and suicidal acts, in Depression in Young People: Developmental and Clinical Perspectives. Edited by Rutter M, Hersov L. New York, Guilford, 1985, pp 383–396

Shaffer D, Fisher P: The epidemiology of suicide in children and young adolescents. J Am Acad Child Psychiatry 20:545–565, 1981

Strober M, Carlson GA: Bipolar illness in adolescents with major depression: clinical, genetic and psychopharmacologic predictors in a three- to four-year prospective follow-up investigation. Arch Gen Psychiatry 39:549–555, 1982

Strober M, Green J, Carlson GA: Phenomenology and subtypes of major depressive disorder in adolescents. J Affective Disord 3:281–290, 1981

Strober M, Morrell W, Burroughs J, et al: A family study of bipolar I disorder in adolescence: early onset of symptoms linked to increased familial loading and lithium resistance. J Affective Disord 15:255–268, 1988

Strober M, Morrell W, Lampert C, et al: Relapse following discontinuation of lithium maintenance therapy in adolescents with bipolar I illness: a naturalistic study. Am J Psychiatry 147:457–461, 1990

Varanka TM, Weller EB, Fristad MA: Lithium treatment of manic episodes with psychotic features in prepubertal children. Am J Psychiatry 145:1557–1559, 1988

Wehr TA, Goodwin FK: Rapid cycling in manic-depressives induced by tricyclic antidepressants. Arch Gen Psychiatry 36:555–559, 1979

Wehr TA, Sack DA, Rosenthal NE, et al: Rapidly cycling affective disorder: contributing factors and treatment responses in 51 patients. Am J Psychiatry 145:179–184, 1988

Weinberg WA, Brumback RA: Mania in childhood: case studies and literature review. Am J Dis Child 130:380–385, 1976

Weller EB, Weller RA, Fristad MA: Lithium dosage guide for prepubertal children: a preliminary report. J Am Acad Child Psychiatry 25:92–95, 1986a

Weller RA, Weller EB, Tucker SG, et al: Mania in prepubertal children: has it been underdiagnosed? J Affective Disord 11:151–154, 1986b

Winokur G, Clayton PJ, Reich T: Manic Depressive Illness. St. Louis, MO, CV Mosby, 1969

Youngerman J, Canino I: Lithium carbonate use in children and adolescents: a survey of the literature. Arch Gen Psychiatry 35:216–224, 1978

Zahn-Waxler C, McKnew DH, Cummings M, et al: Problem behaviors and peer interactions of young children with a manic-depressive parent. Am J Psychiatry 141:236–240, 1984

Index

Psychoanalysis. *See* Psychotherapy
Psychoanalytic model of
    depressive disorder, 52
Psychological autopsy, 168–169
Psychopharmacological research,
    152
Psychotherapy
    countertransference, 161
    duration, 172–174
    dynamic
        and adolescents, 168–172
        in children, ages 3–6 years,
            163–165
        defense mechanisms in, 159
        group therapy, 185–186
        and infant's therapy, 161–163
        principles of, 158
        in school-age children,
            165–168
        therapeutic process, 159–160
    historical perspective, 157–158
    infant-parent mode, 162
    in inpatient treatment, 243–244
    outpatient, 173–174
    resistance, 160–161
    transference, 160
    use of videotape, 167–168
Puberty onset and depression, 32

R
Realistic Thoughts Worksheet,
    205–210
Regression, in depressed children,
    13
Research Diagnostic Criteria, 68,
    141, 260
Research needs cited
    biological correlates and
        suicidal behavior, 124
    developmental chronobiology,
        109
    developmental psycho-

pathology and depressive
    disorders, 12–13
dexamethasone suppression
    test, prognostic value, 73–74
epidemiological survey, 57
group psychotherapy and
    outcome, 194
HPA axis dysfunction, 72
infants and DSM-III(-R) criteria,
    44
integrating assessment data, 151
mania-depression cycles, 284
neurobiological studies, 82
personality factors in depressive
    disorders, 54, 57
pharmacological treatments, 57
prevalence of cyclothymia in
    children/adolescents, 45
psychosocial treatments, 57
standardized criteria, 56–57
thyroid-stimulating hormone
    measurement, 78
Risk factors of depressive disorders
    age, 46, 256–258
    biological factors, 47–52
    gender-related, 46–47
    genetic, 51
    psychological, 52–54
    race-related, 47
    social, 54–55
    sociodemographic, 46–47
    socioeconomic status, 47

S
San Diego Suicide Study, 117
Schedule for Affective Disorders
    and Schizophrenia—
    Children's Version, 139–142,
    149
Schedule for Affective Disorders
    and Schizophrenia, 120
Schizophrenia, in diagnosing
    bipolar disorders, 274–276